ABNORMATIVITIES: QUEER/GENDER/EMBODIMENT
Scott Herring, Series Editor

PREVENTION

GENDER, SEXUALITY, HIV, AND THE MEDIA IN CÔTE D'IVOIRE

CHRISTINE CYNN

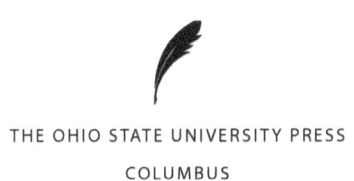

THE OHIO STATE UNIVERSITY PRESS
COLUMBUS

Copyright © 2018 by The Ohio State University.
All rights reserved.

Library of Congress Cataloging-in-Publication Control Number: 2018020066

Cover image: Aboudia. Untitled, 2013. Acrylic and mixed media on canvas, 198 x 124 cm (00557). Image courtesy Jack Bell Gallery, London.

Cover design by Susan Zucker
Text design by Juliet Williams
Type set in Adobe Minion Pro

CONTENTS

List of Illustrations		vi
Acknowledgments		ix
INTRODUCTION		1
CHAPTER 1	AIDS as an "Imaginary Syndrome": Humor as Negotiation of Racism, Austerity, and the Single-Party State	18
CHAPTER 2	Popular Satiric State Television Programs and HIV Prevention	50
CHAPTER 3	Regulating Female Reproductive Potential: Abortion and Family as HIV Prevention	95
CHAPTER 4	The Melodrama and the Social Marketing of HIV Prevention	138
CHAPTER 5	"Stay away from unhealthy places": Sex Work, Condoms, and the NGO	169
AFTERWORD		203
Bibliography		209
Index		229

ILLUSTRATIONS

FIGURE 1.1	Sketch of "Moussa"	28
FIGURE 1.2	AIDS is there... IT KILLS	46
FIGURE 1.3	Ivorian athlete Gabriel Tiacoh	47
FIGURE 1.4	Emaciated bodies as index of the truth of AIDS	48
FIGURE 1.5	Television spot: "AIDS is not a joke. It exists."	49
FIGURE 2.1	Badoté's body marked by sores	70
FIGURE 2.2	Sores on Badoté's face	71
FIGURE 2.3	Kaloua as boss	72
FIGURE 2.4	Woman handing her partner the condom she demands that they use	76
FIGURE 2.5	Kaloua to Delta: "Do you see the tears that flow?"	79
FIGURE 2.6	Kaloua's tears convert to laughter as Delta weeps offscreen	80
FIGURE 2.7	Wintin Wintin to woman: "Do you know that I love you?"	87
FIGURE 2.8	Patas monkey looks on skeptically	88
FIGURE 2.9	Wintin Wintin relaxing with his condom [chaussettes, or socks] on	89

FIGURE 2.10	Wintin Wintin insisting that he did not come	90
FIGURE 2.11	Woman to Wintin Wintin: "Isn't this your sperm in my hand?"	91
FIGURE 3.1	Jeanne and Sister Catherine	102
FIGURE 3.2	Supervisor with Kouako	104
FIGURE 3.3	Prudence Condoms campaign	115
FIGURE 3.4	"Life" advising the group about anal mucous membranes	120
FIGURE 3.5	Agent of progress Kafongo	125
FIGURE 3.6	A mysterious fortuneteller	126
FIGURE 3.7	Slow dissolve of Mado screaming in labor	127
FIGURE 3.8	Fatou believing that she is barred from producing children	130
FIGURE 3.9	Reverse shot of the children playing in the schoolyard	131
FIGURE 4.1	Adams as he attempts to put a condom on a prosthetic penis	154
FIGURE 4.2	Adams's mother warning her daughter-in-law	155
FIGURE 4.3	Juliette urging Nathalie to calm down	161
FIGURE 4.4	Nathalie's mother overhearing Alex trying to end his engagement	162
FIGURE 4.5	Nathalie and Alex arguing about testing for HIV	163
FIGURE 4.6	Nathalie and her mother	164
FIGURE 5.1	Condoms being used to sell drinks of water	176
FIGURE 5.2	Second wife learning that "in your blood . . . there is the AIDS virus"	186
FIGURE 5.3	Doctor reminding women, "Trust is good, but Prudence is best"	194
FIGURE 5.4	Amah as entrepreneur engaged in "real work"	197
FIGURE 5.5	Amah and Boni celebrating	200
FIGURE 5.6	Fortuna instructing a support group about HIV/AIDS	201

ACKNOWLEDGMENTS

ALTHOUGH RESEARCH and writing can be solitary enterprises, many people have participated directly and indirectly in this book's production, and I am happy to publicly acknowledge them.

I would never have finished graduate school and become an academic without the support of Lisa Estreich, Kim F. Hall, and Hiram Pérez. I am inspired by Hiram's and Kim's brilliant scholarship and continue to rely on their advice as I navigate through the university. Lisa helped me locate sources, edited drafts, dug a path in the snow, and mailed me letters, for which I thank her. At certain critical moments, Sarita See offered clear-eyed counsel that I appreciate even more in retrospect.

A Fulbright research and teaching award from the Council for International Exchange of Scholars in Abidjan, Côte d'Ivoire, made it possible for me to begin this project. In Abidjan, Konan Amani was—and continues to be—an invaluable colleague and friend. Aghi Bahi, Koffi Olivier Koffi, and Angèle Gnako were generous with their time and expertise. I thank Brahima Koné and Mamadou Zongo for translating song lyrics for this book (though all responsibility for errors are mine), as well as Jeff Barnes and Alexis Don Zigré for patiently responding to my many questions. Kamagaté Allassana was an indefatigable fellow traveler. I am glad that Ama is still in my life, along with Aïcha, Matou, Kadi (Christine!), and Malik. They are busily engaged in building futures that I eagerly await to see unfold.

The Andrew W. Mellon Foundation provided a postdoctoral fellowship in the Women's, Gender and Sexualities Department at Barnard College, and I thank Abosede George, Rebecca Jordan-Young, Tally Kampen, Irena Klepfisz, Amanda Swarr, Neferti Tadiar, and especially Janet Jakobsen for providing such a congenial space for me to engage in research. The Director of Africana Studies at Barnard, Kim F. Hall, invited me to split the fellowship, and the years I spent working with her, and teaching for and traveling with the program, continue to inform and inspire my scholarship. In New York City, a queer reading group that included Lisa Estreich, Maja Horn, Hiram Pérez, and Chi-ming Yang provided generative feedback on early drafts of chapters.

At Andover, Steph Curci, Jeff Domina, Tasha Hawthorne, Tom Kane, LaShonda Long, Temba Maqubela, Megan Paulson, and Flavia Vidal were welcoming friends and colleagues, and I am grateful for the support that enabled me to continue to research and write. At Virginia Commonwealth University, a Humanities Research Center Residential Fellowship made it possible for me to spend a semester engaging with Leigh Ann Craig, Kathryn Shively, and Sachi Shimomura in rich interdisciplinary collaborations and conversations that have shaped this book. The Humanities Research Center and the Global Education Office provided funding to conduct essential research in Paris. The Humanities Research Center also awarded travel grants that enabled me to attend conferences where I presented portions of this book in Montreal and Utrecht, and I am very grateful to the center and to its director, Richard Godbeer. A reading group that included Myrl Beam, Jesse Goldstein, Samaneh Oladi Ghadikolaei, Brandi T. Summers, and Cristina Stanciu read significant portions of this manuscript and encouraged me to clarify some of my claims. I am as grateful for their sharp readings as for their good-humored camaraderie and snacks. As I have made my way through VCU, Karen Rader has been a wonderful friend and mentor. I deeply appreciate her support and that of Kathy Ingram, Chair of the Department of Gender, Sexuality and Women's Studies, as well as the friendship of Liz Canfield and Jenny Rhee. Students have been indispensable in putting this book together, and I appreciate the careful work of Danielle Deshazor, Memunatu Koroma, Frankie Ann Mastrangelo, Leah Thomas, and especially Alexius Houchens.

Jennifer Brier and Vinh-Kim Nguyen were kind enough to read early drafts of what became a book proposal and, eventually, this book. Karen M. Booth, Ashley Currier, and Adeline Masquelier were tremendously encouraging readers, and I thank them for their valuable comments and suggestions. Kristen Elias Rowley at The Ohio State University Press has been a vital supporter and a judicious editor who helped to make the publication process much less stressful than I had feared. Many thanks to her and to Scott Herring, the editor of the Abnormativities Series, in which I am proud to participate. The lively cover art is by Aboudia, and I am grateful to the artist and Jack Bell Gallery for permitting me to reproduce it. A community in Richmond, which has included Elaine Bragg, Gigi and Stephen Curtin, Alyson Davis, Tania Fernandez, Sonali Gulati, Rosana McGann and Phyllis Aqui-Anwar, Nikhil and Urvi Neelakantan, and Beth Seward, have helped on the home front. Friends from long ago have seen me through multiple iterations of my work and life: Susan Caskie, Mare Diaz, Jen Holleran, Kit Leaning, Rob Shin, and Jen Sinton. Liam A. Donohoe has been a stalwart supporter during all these years.

Finally, I thank Hyoun-Shin, Kenneth, Di, Michael, Jen, Pat, Mike, Tonya, Karen, Rob, Milo, Nico, Isaac, Isla, and especially Ibrahim, who has grown up alongside this book and who has so persistently and persuasively reminded me when I must set it aside and why I must finish it.

The questions that eventually led to this book were first posed to me by women living with HIV whom I met in Abidjan. Almost all of them have since passed away, and their absences haunt this book.

INTRODUCTION

> More philosophically, it may be supposed that the present as experience of a time is precisely that moment when different forms of absence become entangled [s'enchevêtrent]: absence of those presences that are no longer here and that one remembers (memory [la mémoire]), and absence of those others who are not here yet and are anticipated (utopia).
> —ACHILLE MBEMBE, *ON THE POSTCOLONY*[1]

> Boys will be serious with girls who make them wait.
> —*SUPER GIRL*, 2009 HIV PREVENTION SHORT, CÔTE D'IVOIRE

IN SUB-SAHARAN Africa, according to the United Nations (UN), about 25.5 million people were living with HIV/AIDS in 2016—69% of the global total. Of an estimated one million AIDS-related deaths globally in 2016, the majority—730,000—were in sub-Saharan Africa.[2] While the epidemic has been identified as most severe in Southern Africa, where an estimated one in five adults lives with HIV/AIDS, prevalence in Central and West Africa has also been significant, peaking at about 10% among adults in Côte d'Ivoire, the highest in a region where only an estimated 42% of people living with HIV were aware of their HIV status.[3] In 2016, UNAIDS estimated that 460,000 were living with HIV/AIDS in Côte d'Ivoire, with approximately 20,000 new HIV infections and 25,000 AIDS-related deaths that year.[4]

---

1. Mbembe, *On the Postcolony,* 16 (translation modified); Mbembe, *De la postcolonie,* 37.
2. UNAIDS, *Data: 2017,* 14.
3. According to UNAIDS, in 2016, estimated adult prevalence (ages fifteen to forty-nine) in South Africa was 18.9%. UNAIDS, *Country Fact Sheets, 2016*; PEPFAR, "Côte d'Ivoire Country Operational Plan," 4; UNAIDS, *Data: 2017,* 48. According to World Bank data, in 2016, Côte d'Ivoire had a total estimated population of almost 23.7 million. World Bank, *Data, Côte d'Ivoire,* http://data.worldbank.org/country/cote-divoire.
4. UNAIDS, *Data: 2017,* 58.

As these statistics indicate, the 2010 UN goals of zero new infections and zero AIDS-related deaths have not been achieved, and the need to limit the spread of HIV/AIDS, especially in sub-Saharan Africa, remains as imperative as ever.[5] After delayed governmental responses in most countries, including the United States, the media—and visual media in particular—have been consistently deployed as an essential tool for prevention. This media seeks to persuade the public to try to imagine and then effect alternative ways of conducting themselves, of forming communities and families, and of forging identities. By definition, it displays a resolute futurity; it focuses on instigating action in anticipation of and in order to avert something—HIV infection—before it comes. But in the etymology of the word *prevention*, a trace of the converse persists in a now obscure definition of the term: "The coming, action, or occurrence of one person or thing before another, or before the due time; previous occurrence."[6]

This book explores HIV prevention media in the now obsolete, latter sense of what has previously happened, to analyze how the past informs and inflects present-day articulations of the anticipated future, the utopia of the first epigraph of this introduction. As Paula Treichler observed almost two decades ago, "The [HIV/AIDS] epidemic has become a symbolic arena for other struggles, many seemingly far from health care."[7] HIV prevention media in Côte d'Ivoire serves as a particularly productive site to begin to understand some of these struggles and their significations. By representing what it defines as proper gendered sexual behavior as the condition of possibility for envisioned futures, this media is deeply embedded in the past and reiterates the conflations of modernity, progress, and health, structuring prior colonial and postcolonial interventions. At the same time, HIV prevention media in Côte d'Ivoire engages with local, as well as global, dynamics and processes and responds actively to contemporary political and economic crises—especially conflicts around state retrenchment and around citizenship and national belonging—also rooted in the past. HIV prevention media—and the media itself—are products of what Achille Mbembe has so suggestively described as the postcolony's "*time of entanglement* [italics in original]."[8]

---

5. UNAIDS, *2011–2015 Strategy*, 7. These goals have since been scaled down. In 2015, new goals targeted are that by 2020, 90% of people living with HIV know their status; 90% of those diagnosed with HIV infection are receiving sustained antiretroviral treatment; and 90% of those on antiretroviral treatment have attained viral suppression. UNAIDS, *90-90-90*, 1.

6. *Oxford English Dictionary Online*, s.v. "prevention, n."

7. Treichler, *How to Have Theory in an Epidemic*, 233.

8. Mbembe, *On the Postcolony*, 16. The term *entanglement* [l'enchevêtrement] does not appear in the French here: "*le temps en cours, celui de l'existence et de l'expérience.*" Mbembe, *De la postcolonie*, italics in original, 36. Nor is the noun in the sentence translated into English:

The status of the HIV/AIDS epidemic as exceptional, as unprecedented crisis propelling unprecedented responses, has obscured the extent to which HIV prevention media builds on prior interventions, for example, into family formations, and supports multiple overlapping and divergent agendas and interests.[9] The lack of attention to these histories and agendas has facilitated the dominance of individual behavior change in HIV prevention efforts, as epitomized by the 2009 *Super Girl* HIV prevention campaign television short exhorting girls and young women in Côte d'Ivoire to abstain from sex: "Boys will be serious with girls who make them wait!" This media's emphasis on individual responsibilization identifies heteronormative gendering and sexual relations as the solution to HIV/AIDS. By advocating particular gendered sexualities and families as necessary for health and life, HIV prevention media acts as a particularly powerful global discourse disseminating heteronormative norms and ideals.

At the same time, such prevention strategies elide the material conditions and inequities—the structural violence—that underpin and heighten the epidemic and provide further justification for donor-mandated austerity measures, including those reducing health-care expenditures, despite increasing needs resulting from HIV/AIDS.[10] Marking a return to free-market economic approaches and a shift away from Keynesian policies and the so-called welfare state, neoliberalism operates, as Wendy Brown describes, as a "confusing signifier" for "deregulation, marketization, and privatization of all public goods, a forthright attack on the public sector, and the beginnings of casting every human endeavor and activity in entrepreneurial terms."[11] HIV prevention media prescribes what Lisa Duggan identifies as neoliberalism's "key terms"—privatization and personal responsibility—as the most effective method to deal with HIV/AIDS, as well as with economic and political crises, the conditions of precarity that exacerbate the spread of HIV/AIDS, and that HIV/AIDS in turn exacerbates.[12]

"As an age, the postcolony encloses multiple *durées* made up of discontinuities, reversals, inertias, and swings that overlay one another, interpenetrate one another, and envelope one another: an *entanglement* [qui se superposent, s'enchevêtrent et s'enveloppent les unes et les autres]." Mbembe, *On the Postcolony*, 14, italics in original; Mbembe, *De la postcolonie*, 34. However, the term does appear as a central concept elsewhere in the French edition. Mbembe, *De la postcolonie*, 20, 95. I retain the English term here in part to mark another process marked by entanglements—that of translation.

9. Robinson, *Intimate Interventions*, 37–69.

10. Farmer, "An Anthropology of Structural Violence," 307. See also Farmer, "On Suffering and Structural Violence," 24–25.

11. Brown, "Neoliberalized Knowledge," 118.

12. Duggan, *The Twilight of Equality?* 12.

However, foreign funders did not simply dictate AIDS policies and attendant prevention efforts consolidating heteronormative gendering touted as "empowerment." HIV prevention messages were disseminated on Ivorian state media as part of a long genealogy of educational programming explicitly framed as enabling postcolonial national development. They shored up the waning authority of a single-party state confronting deepening economic crises and converged with the potent rhetoric of ethnonationalist conflicts associating proper family and proper reproduction with political legitimacy. As this book contends, close readings of HIV prevention media shed light on how efforts by both global AIDS policies and the state media to define and produce proper gendered heterosexualities and families are deeply entangled in both colonial and postcolonial histories.

BIOPOLITICS AND STATE SOVEREIGNTY

Growing recognition of the epidemic's impact in Côte d'Ivoire coincided with the economic crises following the oil embargos of the 1970s and sharp declines in the prices of coffee and cocoa, the country's primary export crops. After the 1993 death of the country's first president, Félix Houphouët-Boigny, political and economic instability intensified, culminating in two civil wars and the division of the country from 2002 to 2011. *Prevention* centers on a selection of HIV prevention media in Côte d'Ivoire during the critical two-decade period from the first two reported AIDS cases from 1985 to 2005, shortly after implementation of the U.S. President's Emergency Plan for AIDS Relief (PEPFAR), which remains a major funder of HIV prevention and treatment in focus countries, including Côte d'Ivoire. Extending and revising earlier colonial and postcolonial campaigns, HIV prevention messages sought—and continue to seek—to encourage the creation of nuclear families and to inculcate self-discipline to limit the spread of the HIV epidemic.

A first wave of visual and written media promoting HIV prevention from 1985 to 1993—newspaper and journal articles, films, videos, and television shows—served as sites of uneven negotiation with the demands of state and foreign lenders, not only over effective responses to HIV/AIDS but also over structural adjustment policies and attendant austerity measures, which prevention messages portrayed as implemented by a strong paternalistic state headed by Houphouët-Boigny. By contrast, a latter wave of HIV prevention visual media from the early 1990s and onward has been increasingly consonant with the mandates of its foreign funders, especially the United States. This later media insists on the central role of the corporation and the nongovernmental organization (NGO) for support services. Circulating amidst increasingly violent struggles around citizenship and land tenure, it portrays companionate, heterosexual, monogamous marriage enabling production of the HIV-negative child as the single most hopeful form for the future.[13]

In seeking to transform behavior in the name of individual and public health, and in defining who must be worked on to live and who will be left to die, HIV prevention media constitutes a particularly trenchant technique of what Michel Foucault has defined as biopolitics. In brief but influential comments, Foucault characterized disciplinary techniques as targeting individual bodies and behaviors, and the biopolitical as referring to "the set of mechanisms through which the basic biological features of the human species become the object of a political strategy, of a general strategy of power." One of Foucault's central insights in his late lectures on biopolitics was modernity's mutual inscription of politics and biology, political and biological life, a shift he describes as the moment when the "ancient right to take life or let live was replaced by a power to foster life or disallow it to the point of death."[14] According to Foucault, this shift corresponds with what he describes as the emergence of liberalism, a new mode of European political governance in the nineteenth century that concerns itself with the health not of the individual but of the body politic, the body of the population, whose life is secured through the elimination or the letting die of those deemed an unhealthy threat to the population. Biopower operates at the conjunction of discipline applied on individual bodies and regulatory controls on entire populations, with sexuality a privileged site of application because it "exists at the point where body and population meet," in other words, where discipline and regulation intersect.[15]

Drawing from Foucault's analyses, Giorgio Agamben links biopolitics with the foundation of the modern state. For Agamben, modern sovereignty is inaugurated through the establishment of states of exception, suspensions of the law that become the rule, and through the power to identify who will be permitted to die. He defines *homo sacer* as the person who cannot be sacrificed but can be killed with impunity.[16] As I will discuss in more detail in chapter 3 in the context of abortion as a form of HIV prevention, *homo sacer*

---

13. Sociologist Anna Esacove has traced how U.S. AIDS policy in sub-Saharan Africa prescribes what she terms "love matches," a heterosexual relationship configured as modern, between rational, autonomous individuals. Esacove, *Modernizing Sexuality*, 47–48. See also O'Manique, *Neoliberalism and AIDS Crisis*, 10.
14. Foucault, *The History of Sexuality*, 138.
15. Foucault, *"Society Must Be Defended,"* 145.
16. Agamben, *Homo Sacer*, 71–74.

has served as a productive figure for critiquing some of the new systems of exclusion produced in the wake of the HIV/AIDS epidemic—and HIV prevention media in Côte d'Ivoire does seem to correspond particularly neatly to such analyses. During periods of rising xenophobia linked to struggles around citizenship and land ownership, HIV prevention media sought to establish how, when, and which bodies should engage in certain sexual acts, reproduce, and be incorporated in properly constituted families and communities. HIV prevention media identified some—particularly homosexuals, sex workers, and intravenous drug users, as well as members of certain groups marked as Muslim, Northern, and foreign—as inassimilable to the community and nation. In defining conditions of reproductive legitimacy, prevention media expanded and reinforced forms of social and political exclusion framing economic and political—and, eventually, military—crises, especially the setting of "stranger/foreigner" against citizen in the mobilization of ethnonationalist claims of belonging known as Ivoirité.[17]

However, as Jean Comaroff points out, while evocative, Agamben's *homo sacer* as allegory for state sovereignty can prove reductive: "It blurs precisely what demands specification to plumb the shifting political significance of AIDS in contemporary Africa, for example."[18] In the case of Côte d'Ivoire, HIV prevention media has a number of named producers—both foreign funders and the state—and the deployment of the media in Côte d'Ivoire to advance pedagogical projects has a history fraught with contradictions. The biopolitics of HIV prevention media do not index a modern state sovereign, so much as multiple, fluctuating, at times conflicting interests and players, including the Ivorian state, as well as multilateral and bilateral foreign funders who finance most HIV prevention campaigns—and the media itself. Challenging binaries of foreign/local, hegemonic/subversive, authentic/inauthentic, and even commercial/educational, HIV prevention visual media can be described more accurately in terms of what Sarah Nuttall has characterized as the ambiguous and asymmetric networks, entanglements, reciprocities, creolizations, and cohabitations that characterize diverse conditions and contexts in contemporary sub-Saharan Africa.[19]

HIV prevention media depicts as successful the transformations that it attempts to instigate. It represents individuals and communities absorbing

---

17. Akindès, "The Roots of Military-Political Crisis"; Babo and Droz, "Conflits fonciers"; Cutolo, "Modernity, Autochthony and the Ivorian Nation"; Dembélé, "La Construction"; Dembélé, "Côte d'Ivoire"; Dozon, "La Côte d'Ivoire"; Marshall-Fratani, "The War of 'Who Is Who'"; McGovern, *Making War in Côte d'Ivoire*.

18. Comaroff, "Beyond Bare Life," 209.

19. Sarah Nuttall provides a salient overview of such scholarship. Nutall, *Entanglement*.

prevention messages, initiating the changes promoted, and, as a result, either avoiding or containing the spread of HIV. The media thereby portrays publics being called into being by HIV prevention campaigns, the kinds of publics that the media seeks to summon into existence—a self-referential mode consistently invoked by media mandated to serve the interests of the single-party state in Côte d'Ivoire.[20] Even popular satiric shows airing on state television, and columns and comics published in the state press that mocked the didacticism of state educational campaigns, nevertheless reinforced the campaigns' messages. HIV/AIDS prevention media makes more starkly visible some of the complex dynamics already at play in Ivorian state media, dynamics that disrupt the foundational categories of much of the scholarship on postcolonial visual arts.

VISUAL MEDIA IN CÔTE D'IVOIRE

Côte d'Ivoire was established as a French colony in 1893. Health policies imposed by the French provided ideological and technical support for colonial rule and contributed to the generation of resentments based on ethnic and regional divisions leading to the outbreak of war in 2002.[21] Health systems in the country developed as part of larger colonial organizational and administrative efforts classifying different ethnic and linguistic groupings and regions into hierarchies according to their ability to participate in colonial enterprises. After World War I, France increasingly viewed Côte d'Ivoire as a major market for its exports and as an important source of raw materials. The French encouraged internal migration from the north but also from the center (deemed Baoulé), as well as west (Bété) migration, and from the Upper Volta (now Burkina Faso), to provide labor, especially to the southeastern and central western agricultural production zones. Maintaining a healthy African labor force became a source of concern, and hygienic and preventive measures were focused on the agricultural zones, an inequitable distribution of resources along regional and ethnic lines that by the 1930s reflected deepening inequities between the north and south, an internal border maintained throughout and after World War II. The abolition of forced labor in 1946 led to a wave of new migration, mostly in the central west, and by the 1950s, French colonists and Ivorian political elites were already confronting tensions between migrant laborers and so-called autocthones. The establishment of

---

20. For a particularly influential account of the production of publics and those subordinated to them, see Warner, *Publics and Counterpublics*, 66.

21. Arnold, *Imperial Medicine*, 19; Dozon, *Les Clefs de la crise ivoirienne*, 116.

new postwar development plans for health infrastructure by 1960 included the building of hospitals and a basic health system, with some preventive and hygiene campaigns directed at endemic diseases. These plans were similarly concentrated in the south and center west.[22]

In contrast to leaders of neighboring countries, the country's first president, Félix Houphouët-Boigny—who was trained as a medical doctor—envisioned modern nationhood as intimately bound to the former colonial power. Following independence from the French in 1960, Houphouët-Boigny essentially continued the French colonial mode of governance relying on control of land use and distribution of income from agricultural exports.[23] Like the French, Houphouët-Boigny encouraged labor migration from the north and from neighboring countries with promises of land, voting rights, and social services provided by a sprawling state bureaucracy. For Houphouët-Boigny, the French language was integral to national unification and to the maintenance of close ties with France, links that he viewed as in turn facilitating national economic development and modernization—synonymous objectives entailing the country's integration into global capitalist markets. The country's first constitution established French as the only official language among over sixty identified by colonial taxonomies, and in the decades following formal independence, France—with Houphouët-Boigny's support—continued to exert significant political, economic, and cultural influence.[24] That influence encompassed Ivorian radio, television, and film, which received major financing and technical support from the French government, as well as from other multilateral and bilateral funders. Much of the media and major educational initiatives, like the Educational Television Program [Le Programme d'éducation télévisuelle (PETV)], relied primarily on external financing and technical support. However, Houphouët-Boigny and the single-party state controlled the media for the first thirty years after independence and enlisted it to promote economic development, define and educate proper subjects of the modern nation, and strengthen and legitimize the rule of Houphouët-Boigny and of the country's sole political party, the Democratic Party of Côte d'Ivoire [Parti democratique de la Côte d'Ivoire–Rassemblement démocratique africain (PDCI)].

The conditions—and contradictions—of the production of HIV prevention media replicate those of prior state educational campaigns, with multi-

---

22. Gaber and Patel, "Tracing Health System Challenges," 701–3; Dozon, *Les Clefs*, 81, 83; Lasker, "Role of Health Services," 283; Chauveau, "Question foncière," 98–99.

23. Chauveau, "Question foncière," 101.

24. Boutin and N'Guessan, "Citoyenneté," 125–26; Chauveau and Dozon, "Au Coeur."

lateral organizations and foreign governments, especially France, and, to an increasing extent, the United States, providing the majority of funding and technical support for the national struggle against HIV/AIDS in the country.[25] Like much of Francophone African cinema, educational HIV/AIDS visual media—especially television—incorporates Ivorian coproducers, as well as Ivorian (and other African) directors, actors, musicians, and crew, but it relies principally on foreign financing.[26] However, while most Francophone African films are written and directed by Africans, they are distributed primarily in European markets. In contrast, HIV prevention media, also written and directed by Africans (closely overseen by foreign technical experts), is intended exclusively for African audiences and generally does not screen outside the subcontinent. HIV prevention visual media broadcasts on state television, and videos and DVD copies are distributed locally and regionally for free or at a low cost.

Although purportedly—and, as I discuss later, debatably—noncommercial, and represented as essential to nation-building, television and film promoting HIV prevention hardly conforms to the kind of liberatory educational cinema envisioned by the Pan African Federation of Filmmakers [Fédération Panafricaine des Cinéastes (FEPACI)]. In their 1973 Algiers Charter, FEPACI sought to reclaim cinema as an instrument of decolonization and a corrective to colonial images of Africa and of Africans that justified France's civilizing mission and that incorporated select colonial subjects into evolutionary narratives of progress. Early HIV prevention visual media in Côte d'Ivoire does not merely buttress the "ideological and economic ascendance of the imperialist powers" any more than it can be characterized as a resistant cinema contesting "cultural domination."[27] Theories of spectatorship, especially of the male, racializing, and imperial gaze familiar from Anglophone film scholarship prove similarly inadequate in accounting for the complex imbrications

---

25. According to the Ivorian government, from 2006 to 2009, international funders provided 89% of funding to the struggle against HIV/AIDS, the Ivorian government, 8%. République de Côte d'Ivoire and Conseil National de Luttle contre le SIDA, *Rapport National 2012*, 27.

26. On the shifting role of the French government in Francophone African film production, see de Turégano, "The New Politics of African Cinema."

27. Diawara, *African Cinema*, 53–54; Bakari, "Algiers Charter," 25–26 [La Charte d'Alger, 65]; Bloom, *French Colonial Documentary*, 123. Film critics such as Alexie Tcheuyap and Kenneth W. Harrow have more recently argued that film scholarship itself too readily embraced FEPACI's dogmatic perspective on African cinema and assumed a univocality that never actually existed. Tcheuyap, *Postnationalist African Cinema*, 12–13; Tcheuyap, "Comedy of Power, Power of Comedy," 25–27; Harrow, *Postcolonial African Cinema*, xi. See also Thackway, *Africa Shoots Back*, 44–45.

of interests involved in the production and dissemination of HIV prevention education and their shifting messages and meanings.[28]

From the mid-1980s to early 1990s, HIV prevention media facilitated state- and lender-mandated cutbacks and mediated conflicts they generated to legitimize the weakening power of Houphouët-Boigny. Much of the media from the late 1990s and onward enforces U.S. perspectives on HIV prevention issues that encompass sex work and abortion but that, like prior media, engages with local debates and comments on intensifying political and economic crises in the country. The media and the strategies it urges viewers to deploy do not just reflect agendas of foreign funders; they also replicate the terms of previous and ongoing interventions to remake families, create laborers, provide social services, and define identities. HIV prevention media; the conditions of its production; and its fluctuating, contradictory messages and objectives cannot be viewed through either/or frameworks of neo-imperialism or of Afrocentrism, as another case of Western hegemony in sub-Saharan Africa or of Africans mobilizing African models in response to crisis.[29]

Thus far, there have been no in-depth analyses in the Francophone African context of HIV prevention visual media. Previous studies, especially in English, have been restricted mainly to Southern Africa, where the HIV/AIDS epidemic is most pronounced, and to the province of public health, where experts have focused more on developing new HIV prevention campaigns than on closely analyzing specific examples of existing media.[30] When particular productions have been studied, they are evaluated almost exclusively for their efficacy in reaching targeted audiences and attaining predetermined goals.[31] For example, Population Services International, the producers of *AIDS*

---

28. Mulvey, "Visual Pleasure and Narrative Cinema"; De Lauretis, *Technologies of Gender*; Kaplan, *Looking for the Other*; Mayne, *Woman at the Keyhole*; Rony, *Third Eye*; Barlet, *African Cinemas*; Everett, *Returning the Gaze*.

29. Genova, *Cinema and Development*, 128–29; Andrade-Watkins, "France's Bureau of Cinema," 213; Ukadike, *Black African Cinema*, 70–71.

30. Noar, "A 10-Year Retrospective." The scholarship on HIV prevention media, performance, and art in South Africa (which necessarily engages with the Thabo Mbeke's government's responses to established scientific understandings of HIV and AIDS and the refusal to roll out antiretroviral treatment) is extensive. See, for example, Allen, "Art Activism"; Barz and Cohen, *The Culture of AIDS*; Beinart and Dawson, *Popular Politics and Resistance*; Fassin, *When Bodies Remember*; Grünkemeier, *Breaking the Silence*; Hoad, "Miss HIV and Us." From the perspective of communications, Louise M. Bourgault offers a comparative analysis of oral narratives—songs, stories, and chants—and dance, television, and theatrical performances educating about HIV/AIDS in Mali and in South Africa and relates them to what she describes as "African" performance. Bourgault, *Playing for Life*.

31. Bertrand et al., "Systematic Review"; Noar et al., "A 10-year Systematic Review"; Zoungrana et al., *La Prevention*; Guenou, *Impact d'une campagne*; Shapiro and Meekers, "Target Audience."

in the City [*Sida dans la cité*]—a series that this book discusses in depth—funded studies of the second version of the program, which showed that episodes were widely viewed and that "the propensity to use condoms increases with the individual's level of exposure to 'SIDA dans la Cité.'"[32] African film and video scholarship has not adequately supplemented such self-promoting, instrumentalist analyses with detailed readings of particular HIV prevention visual media, the specific circumstances in which they are disseminated, and the conventions upon which they rely.

Similarly, although foreign funders have financed almost all HIV prevention campaigns in Côte d'Ivoire, continuing discussions and debates about the educational and political roles of the visual arts in Francophone West Africa and about the dominant role of foreign producers in African film have neglected to address HIV prevention visual media. Despite vocal critiques of neoliberal approaches to HIV/AIDS that have influenced my own writing, including Vinh-Kim Nguyen's *The Republic of Therapy* and Claire Laurier Decoteau's *Ancestors and Antiretrovirals*, and explicitly feminist critiques, such as Colleen O'Manique's *Neoliberalism and AIDS Crisis in Sub-Saharan Africa*, no scholarship has yet considered HIV prevention media as a technique and a by-product of neoliberalism. Nor does pathbreaking research on representations of sexualities focusing mostly on Southern and Eastern Africa address how HIV prevention media seeks to reshape conceptions of proper gendering, sexualities, families, and individual behavior.[33] *Prevention: Gender, Sexuality, HIV, and the Media in Côte d'Ivoire* brings together these different strands of scholarship in order to enrich, as well as to expand, conversations in fields that do not often engage with each other. To the extent that HIV prevention media centers on the promotion of heterosexual monogamy and family, queer and feminist theory's trenchant critiques of racialized and gendered sexual normativities serve as useful analytics. In order to better account for the sexual and gender norms produced by HIV prevention campaigns as they dovetail with both prior and contemporaneous subject-building projects, this book

---

32. Shapiro, Meekers, and Tambashe, "Exposure," 313. (*Sida* is the French acronym for syndrome immunodéficitaire acquis, or syndrome d'immunodéficience acquise.) The capitalization of the French for AIDS, or sida, has changed over time. Initially, the word was generally capitalized: SIDA. Usage eventually shifted to "Sida" and more recently to "sida," although the different conventions overlapped. This book will follow the capitalization used in the original source cited.

33. See, for example, Tamale's *African Sexualties*; Hoad's *African Intimacies*; Epprecht's *Heterosexual Africa?* Rachel Sullivan Robinson details how HIV prevention policies have built on prior interventions into the family, but her book does not draw from the humanities. Robinson, *Intimate Interventions*. See also Esacove, *Modernizing Sexuality*.

supplements their critiques with scholarship on neoliberalism and postcolonial media.

ADDITIONAL COMMENTS ON METHOD

I came to this project through prior engagements in struggles against HIV/AIDS as a community organizer and Reproductive Rights Program Coordinator working with low-income and homeless people living with HIV/AIDS in New York City. My research has since expanded to focus on global prevention efforts, especially after the 2003 enactment of PEPFAR, a multibillion-dollar initiative that mandated emphasis both on abstinence until marriage and on fidelity and monogamy in its global HIV prevention efforts. In order to get a better sense of what was happening on the ground, I spent a year as a Fulbright researcher and professor at the national university in Abidjan, Côte d'Ivoire, one of PEPFAR's initial focus countries. During this trip and four subsequent visits ranging from one to four months, I spent countless hours with women who had tested HIV-positive and subsequently been forced out of their households, often with their children.

Many of the women I met explained their expulsion from their households as the culmination of complicated series of events, and they viewed their situations as exacerbated as much as alleviated by their interactions with the NGO that provided them temporary shelter and other services. Such complexities were not legible in the organization's funder reports—that I helped to edit—of stigmatization and ignorance remedied by education, job training, and family reintegration represented as signs of women's successful empowerment. I allude to these conversations and the gaps they highlight not to offer evidence of formal fieldwork or to assign blame, but to underscore that I approach and attempt to respond to some of the questions raised by my research and by the women in Abidjan in the speculative and interpretive registers enabled by my training in literary and film analysis. Although I scavenge from other disciplines, and this book is necessarily deeply interdisciplinary, I draw extensively from the humanities to critique specific examples of HIV prevention media and the narratives that they promulgate about HIV and its prevention.[34] A central argument of this book is that the humanities can make vital contributions to discussions that have generally been limited to the purview of the sciences, and to a lesser extent, the social sciences.

---

34. On scavenging as queer method, see Currier and Migraine-George, "Queer Studies/African Studies," 282–83.

Feminist anthropologists emphasize the importance of attending to both the multiplicity of meanings generated by the media and viewers who resist dominant messages encoded in television. As Lila Abu-Lughod insists, "One cannot simply analyze the overt messages of plot and character, just as one should not limit oneself to the study of reception."[35] However, television and film messages prove far from self-evident or univocal, as all texts inhabit contested fields of representation, and signification is irreducible to a text's declared instrumental or technical functions. In other words, the meanings generated by visual media do not align seamlessly with the media's stated objectives or with the intentions of producers—whose agendas do not always align with each others'—just as the impact of visual media always exceeds individual viewers' recounting. In attempting to situate HIV prevention media in the contexts of local, national, and global dynamics and debates, I recognize the importance of alternative, unofficial modes of HIV prevention education and of persistent and ongoing efforts to challenge the processes that I detail. Further accounting for these mobilizations would require additional expertise and result in scholarship that would serve as a welcome supplement to mine.

This book's point of departure is the recognition of the chasm between the lived experiences of those exposed to HIV prevention messages and the idealized versions represented on-screen, of characters who assimilate prevention messages and either alter their behavior or, acting as negative examples, suffer dire consequences. That said, I do not attempt to close the gap, for example, by delineating how epidemiological categories, such as "men who have sex with men," or "MSM," have been taken up and modified in unanticipated ways.[36] Rather than offer case histories or ethnographies of resistant subjects of health interventions, this book critiques the production and dissemination of dominant HIV prevention narratives and the terms that they set about HIV and HIV prevention and, by extension, about identities, community, and belonging.

In so doing, *Prevention* retains deliberate and sustained focus on individual productions of HIV prevention media. It relies on close readings to trace how that media recapitulates terms and technologies of prior educational efforts in its intensified scrutiny of gendering, sexualities, and sexual behavior and in its identification of particular kinds of families as forms of protection. My approach to this media has been determined in part by my own training as a literary and film critic, but it also best corresponds to the book's argument about the importance of attending to dominant discourses

---

35. Abu-Lughod, "Egyptian Melodrama," 117.
36. Thomann, "HIV Vulnerability"; Thomann, "Zones of Difference."

of heteronormative sexualities as they were embedded in broader political and economic projects. These dominant discourses and how they are entangled in prior educational campaigns must be better understood in order to draw attention to how health interventions targeting gender and sexualities have dovetailed with neoliberal agendas and local political struggles, as well as to better contend with the terms of such interventions and the futures they promise.

The RTI archives in Abidjan are understaffed and underfunded, and I was not able to obtain clean copies of many of the programs that I was able to locate, as will be visible in some of the stills captured from videos and DVDs incorporated in the individual chapters. Despite the issues with archival research and the importance of radio as a mode of communication in Côte d'Ivoire, I concentrate almost exclusively on the press and on visual materials, a focus determined by the historical importance of television in educational campaigns. Nevertheless, I suggest that many of the conclusions that I draw about HIV prevention visual media could apply to radio programming. On the other hand, although many of the HIV prevention video series produced in Côte d'Ivoire have circulated throughout the region, the specificities of production and dissemination of HIV prevention media and its significations vary according to the particularities of local histories and experiences. I hope that the Ivorian case can offer insights into dynamics operating elsewhere and that this book will lead to broader comparative conversations around the kinds of normativities produced and promoted by HIV prevention campaigns.

As I detail in the first chapter, "AIDS as an 'Imaginary Syndrome': Humor as Negotiation of Racism, Austerity, and the Single-Party State," initially the Ivorian government was slow to officially respond to AIDS, but the satiric *Moussa* column in the state weekly *Ivoire Dimanche* offered consistent commentary about the growing epidemic. As a Guignol, Moussa vulgarized and satirized official edicts but reratified them in a process that Achille Mbembe describes as enabling the state to reinforce and render accessible its rule. Written in the voice of the marginalized male urban migrant, the column used the language of the streets, "Popular French of Abidjan," or *nouchi,* and a crude, sexual humor to challenge racialized and sexualized definitions of Africa and African AIDS. In depictions of HIV/AIDS as a crisis of white modernity, the column conflated sexual and economic austerity as necessary to preserve and protect the nation. *Moussa* thereby rationalized the abdication of state responsibility for social welfare and state cutbacks. It worked to facilitate the implementation of structural adjustment policies and to reinforce neoliberal ideologies of individual responsibility undergirding them and, simultaneously, to shore up Houphouët-Boigny and his control of the single-party state. In its portrayals of HIV, *Moussa* promoted austerity as a specifically Ivorian version of development and of Ivorian identity, with sexual self-control as moral alternative to foreign models of development—and as a solution for HIV.

While the first chapter focuses on early press commentary, chapter 2, "Popular Satiric State Television Programs and HIV Prevention," shifts to analyze popular early satiric state television programs representing HIV prevention campaigns: the 1989 "AIDS" and 1993 "Joke to Kill" episodes of *How's it going?* and the "500 CFA If You Don't Come" skit from *Wintin Wintin and Old Headscarf* (the exact broadcast date of the latter is unknown but is probably early 1990s). As examples of koteba performance, the humorous productions deployed satire and parody in their depictions of HIV prevention. In the 1989 *How's it going?* the male office worker who refuses to comply with warnings is swiftly punished with illness and ostracism. As massive strikes eventually led to the country's first multiparty elections and to the liberalization of the media in 1990, the television episodes broadcast on the state channel necessarily avoided any overt reference to ongoing economic and political upheaval. The "Joke to Kill" episode of *How's it going?* and the "500 CFA If You Don't Come" skit from *Wintin Wintin and Old Headscarf* represent recalcitrant heterosexual male characters subverting and openly defying HIV prevention messages about condom usage. But their resistance is directed entirely against their female sexual partners, as the shows effectively displace any critique of or resistance to state and foreign donor policies into a comic staging of gender conflict in which the unruly male prevailed. Ironically, female characters' awareness of HIV prevention measures and attempts to implement them render them the unwitting targets of the episodes' humor.

In 1992, seroprevalence among pregnant women in Abidjan, the largest city and the economic capital of Côte d'Ivoire and of the region, was estimated at 15%, and multiple television series represented mother-to-child HIV transmission as requiring dramatic intervention. Chapter 3, "Regulating Female Reproductive Potential: Abortion and Family as HIV Prevention," discusses media from 1993 to 2003 that targeted pregnant women and women who tested HIV-positive. Initially, as indicated by Kitia Touré's series of four short films, *Gestures or Life* (1993), women in Côte d'Ivoire who tested HIV-positive were urged never to reproduce, and if pregnant when they tested positive, to terminate their pregnancies. Although unofficially approved by the state, these recommendations violated both state and religious prohibitions on abortion. Compelling revision of Agamben's theorizing of the state of exception, abortion in Côte d'Ivoire must be read in the context of the postcolonial state's attempts to encourage population growth and define its reproductive policies against prior and current French policies. Three other segments of *Gestures or Life* and the *AIDS in the City* 1, 2, and 3 (1995–96, 1997, and 2003, respectively) series attempt to contain the threat of nonprocreative female sexualities and to correct prior recommendations about abortion. In these segments, HIV-positive women are urged to test and, if they test positive, to obey the proscriptions of biomedical authorities. Women who submit to medical and paternalistic authority, adhere to prophylactic regimens, and carry their pregnancies to term are redeemed and rewarded by the promise of their further subsumption into the patriarchal family as metaphor and metonym for the nation.

Chapter 4, "The Melodrama and the Social Marketing of HIV Prevention," focuses on the telenovela, *AIDS in the City*, financed primarily by the United States–based nonprofit organization Population Services International (PSI) in Côte d'Ivoire, which receives significant funding from the U.S. government through the United States Agency for International Development (USAID). Focusing on two of the four segments from the 2003 *AIDS in the City* series, "Adams the Driver" and "The Story of the Fiancés," this chapter analyzes how the series relies on the melodramatic mode of the educational telenovela and on social marketing and its consumerist ethos to represent and promote the transformations that the series seeks to effect. The segments elide political and economic contexts to depict the HIV epidemic as the result of individual choices, a problem to be resolved through individual awareness, behavioral change, compassion, and reliance on NGOs. The series thereby promotes neoliberal approaches to dealing with the HIV epidemic: the self-disciplining and market participation of individuals persuaded through education to freely make correct, responsible decisions about their well-being. Issues generated by the global inequities underpinning differential access to HIV testing and treatment remain unanswered, as families are restored and heterosexual romantic love prevails through the constitutive exclusions of those both directly and indirectly dismissed in the series as unredeemable: drug users, "fags," and "prostitutes."

The last chapter, "'Stay away from unhealthy places': Sex Work, Condoms, and the NGO," examines a selection of HIV prevention media featuring and targeting female sex workers: Guinean-born director Henri Duparc's feature film, *Rue princesse* [*Princess Street* (1993)]; and Population Services International's *Amah Djah-Foulé* 1 (2002) and 2 (2005). All three productions celebrate monogamous, reproductively oriented marriage as the resolution for the central characters, and all three code gender empowerment as self-discipline and individual responsibility. However, while the earlier two productions refrain from condemning sex work as a survival strategy for women, the later *Amah Djah-Foulé* 2 reflects PEPFAR's approach to sex work as inherently exploitive and demeaning. Produced in ten-year intervals, *Rue Princesse* and *Amah Djah-Foulé* 1 and 2 are emblematic of a shift in HIV prevention approaches that center on the social marketing of condoms, female empowerment ("gender power"), and the promotion of the NGO as central source of support for sex workers.

As I note in the afterword, this book challenges some of the underlying presumptions of HIV prevention media and of their approaches: Behavior Change Communication; Information, Education, Communication; and social marketing, among others. The point is not to more effectively tailor HIV prevention messages to inaugurate better-behaving subjects but to engage in the perpetually unfinished, messy, and time-consuming tasks of thinking through convergences of pasts, presents, and futures in HIV prevention narratives that prescribe heteronormative gendered sexualities and families. In other words, the point is to interrogate and challenge how HIV prevention media works to bolster neoliberal postcolonial policies and restrictive conceptions of citizenship, and thereby to contribute to gendered precarity that in turn exacerbates the spread of HIV/AIDS, just as HIV/AIDS further intensifies conditions of gendered precarity. The point is to argue for the importance of anticipating and creating futures that are yet to come and that extend far beyond those that HIV prevention narratives have enjoined viewers to imagine.

CHAPTER 1

AIDS as an "Imaginary Syndrome"

*Humor as Negotiation of Racism,
Austerity, and the Single-Party State*

IN 1985, Director of the World Health Organization (WHO), Halfdan Mahler, dismissed the impact of HIV/AIDS in sub-Saharan Africa: "AIDS is not spreading like a bush fire in Africa. It is malaria and other tropical diseases that are killing millions of children every day."[1] While in hindsight, Mahler's comment reads as shockingly myopic, his perspective was shared by many political leaders in the United States as well as in sub-Saharan Africa. Ivorian officials essentially echoed Mahler to justify the government's own delays in taking action after the first two reported AIDS cases in the country in 1985. The Ivorian Health Minister did not publicly mention AIDS until 1987, when he reiterated that it was not as severe a health issue as many others confronting the country. The first governmental informational campaign began only at the close of the following year.[2]

In the absence of more formal responses, from 1985 to 1987, the popular humorous *Moussa* column emerged as the most consistently outspoken com-

---

1. As quoted in Iliffe, *The African AIDS Epidemic*, 68. United States President Ronald Reagan did not publicly acknowledge AIDS until September 1987, seven months after the Ivorian Health Minister did, and six years after the first report of a syndrome later termed "AIDS."

2. The Ivorian state weekly noted that the Rwandan Health Minister similarly commented that AIDS should not obscure other illnesses, like malaria and diarrhea, which, despite available treatment, killed many more people than AIDS, for which no treatment was available. Am Atta, "L'Afrique et le SIDA," *Ivoire Dimanche*, February 15, 1987, 6.

mentary on HIV/AIDS and on HIV prevention methods in the state press. Although purporting to represent the unmediated voices of uneducated urban male migrants, the fictional column was created by academics and published in the state weekly, *Ivoire Dimanche*. Moussa's column necessarily negotiated with the authority of the president since the country's independence, Félix Houphouët-Boigny, and with his political party, the Democratic Party of Côte d'Ivoire-African Democratic Rally [Parti democratique de la Côte d'Ivoire-Rassemblement démocratique africain (PDCI)]. Until 1990, the single-party state controlled all of the country's media, which was mandated to promote its interests, and in depictions of attempts to understand HIV/AIDS, *Moussa* complied with the state's definition of the instrumentalist function of the media. The column educated, informed, and entertained—and contained dissent. Leveling its crude humor at HIV/AIDS—a mysterious sexually transmitted disease about which so much was still unknown—the *Moussa* columns represented HIV/AIDS as a racialized crisis of modernity and development to be resolved by a reassuringly paternalistic and moral leader. The columns' attempts to grapple with HIV/AIDS conveyed information about a growing epidemic and at the same time worked in tandem with attempts by Houphouët-Boigny to consolidate his authority.

As Jean-Pierre Chauveau argues, after independence from the French in 1960, "The mode of colonial governance [used in the descriptive, not normative, sense] did not radically transform. There was still a 'peasant State' characterized by the combination of a bureaucratic power and a despotic power."[3] Houphouët-Boigny maintained French agricultural policies reliant on foreign capital and labor migration, which contributed to economic growth referred to as the "Ivorian miracle."[4] The first AIDS cases in Côte d'Ivoire were reported during a period of crisis that shattered the country's reputation as a regional model of economic and political stability. Steep declines in global prices of Côte d'Ivoire's primary export crops, especially coffee and cocoa, beginning in 1977, and the oil crisis in 1979 imperiled the country's tax revenues and, therefore, the financing of state budgets. As the burden of debt servicing became increasingly onerous, the government turned to the World Bank and the International Monetary Fund (IMF) for assistance. In response, the World Bank granted the country its first structural adjustment loans in 1980, for a total of twenty-six adjustment loans through 1999.[5] The general conditions of all adjustment loans included neoliberal economic restructur-

---

3. Chauveau, "Question foncière," 101. Toungara considers Houphouët-Boigny's exercise of power as informed by Akan models of leadership. Toungara, "The Apotheosis."
4. Akindès, "The Roots of the Military-Political Crisis," 9.
5. Easterly, "What Did Structural Adjustment Adjust?" 3, 5.

ing, which in Côte d'Ivoire as elsewhere, entailed the privatization of previously state-owned industries; export-oriented growth with market-based pricing and interest rates; and reduction of government expenditures, including on personnel, on education, and on health spending, which was reduced by 70% to 80%.[6]

Until the late 1980s, the World Bank considered Côte d'Ivoire a "model pupil."[7] The IMF characterized Houphouët-Boigny's response to the imposition of structural adjustment policies as highly cooperative—meaning that he generally complied with the demands of the IMF and the World Bank (known as The Bretton Woods Institutions).[8] The World Bank and the IMF's self-aggrandizing assessments affirmed the Bretton Woods Institutions' knowledge, expertise, and authority in dictating Ivorian economic policies, even as their affirmations of their own importance supported more critical interpretations of their neocolonial influence in much of sub-Saharan Africa.[9] However, as political scientists Bernard Contamin and Yves-A. Fauré have pointed out, from 1978 to 1980, before implementation of World Bank and IMF adjustment policies, Houphouët-Boigny had already initiated restructuring of the public sector to recentralize his political and economic control, especially over the country's powerful elites. The corruption and financial excesses of these "bosses" or "barons" jeopardized the country's economy, and, perhaps more importantly, the barons and their cultivation of their own fortunes and followers threatened Houphouët-Boigny's status as the biggest of the "big bosses." In the so-called President's Revolution beginning in 1978, Houphouët-Boigny justified implementation of reforms checking the power of the barons as necessary to stabilize the economy. These reforms, which became conflated with the later World Bank and IMF adjustment policies, secured the supremacy of Houphouët-Boigny's own authority. If Houphouët-Boigny later proved compliant to the World Bank and IMF, his responses were motivated at least in part by an alignment of his own political interests with the mandated reforms—and some have argued that far from submitting to structural adjustment programs, Houphouët-Boigny circumvented their implementation.[10]

---

6. Mahieu, "Variable Dimension Adjustment," 10; Barbé and Kerouedan, "Santé publique et privée," 18. From 1980 to 1985 alone, real government health expenditures decreased by 43%, from $114,658,000 to $64,925,000. Vogel, *Cost Recovery in Health Care,* 21. On the effects of retrenchment on health-care services, see also Nguyen, "Therapeutic Modernism in Côte d'Ivoire," 40–42.

7. Mahieu, "Variable Dimension Adjustment," 14.

8. International Monetary Fund, *External Evaluation of the ESAF,* 71.

9. Contamin and Fauré, *La Bataille des entreprises publiques,* 114–18.

10. Fauré, "Côte d'Ivoire: Analysing the Crisis," 70–72; Crook, "Multi-Party Democracy and Political Change," 13–14; Contamin and Fauré, *La Bataille,* 123; B. Campbell, "Political Dimensions of the Adjustment Experience," 164–65.

Moussa offered particularly productive insights into how Houphouët-Boigny, with characteristic canniness, curbed increasing strikes and demonstrations against implementation of many of the deeply unpopular measures, especially reductions in state subsidies, salaries, administrative jobs, and services, and attending increases in unemployment.[11] As indicated in the state press, Houphouët-Boigny repeatedly co-opted the rhetoric of austerity to urge a restive public to demonstrate maturity, sacrifice, and rigor and to submit not only to cutbacks but also to his command. As Houphouët-Boigny's rule extended into its third decade, *Moussa* echoed the president's figuring of austerity as impelled not by foreign funders or by powerful local elites—and therefore suggesting a potentially vulnerable single-party state—but by a strong and moral paternalistic leader responding forcefully to corruption and waste.

A naive villager in the big city of Abidjan, the *de facto* capital of Côte d'Ivoire and a major economic center in the region, Moussa ambivalently figured modernity and development as desirable and necessary but at the same time degrading and dangerous. He represented HIV/AIDS as emblematic of widespread urban economic and sexual corruption and of white modernity embodied in the figures of "homosexuals," "prostitutes," and "transvestites." Depicting HIV/AIDS as a moral issue to be resolved through individual sexual and economic self-discipline, the column endorsed compelled austerity measures that it cast as a uniquely Ivorian form of development. At the same time that *Moussa* affirmed the need for state cutbacks, it underscored the vitality of Houphouët-Boigny's leadership as paternal authority guiding the nation.

From its first identification as a "gay cancer," AIDS was associated with stigmatized identities and sexual practices. As Cindy Patton argues, the invention of "African AIDS" drew from and elaborated on a Western discourse of Africa as homogenous heart of darkness, the sign and site of absolute difference.[12] In South Africa, such representations helped to overdetermine the new post-apartheid state's responses to HIV/AIDS, including resistance to the provision of antiretrovirals.[13] In Côte d'Ivoire, early coverage of HIV in the state press likewise challenged racialized and sexualized definitions of Africa and African AIDS. However, in the column's counterdiscourse on AIDS, *Moussa* suggested that the epidemic was most effectively addressed not through

---

11. Mahieu, "Variable Dimension Adjustment," 12.
12. Patton, *Inventing AIDS*, 77–97.
13. The literature on what has been termed *AIDS denialism* and its consequences in South Africa is extensive. See, for example, Fassin, *When Bodies Remember*; Nattrass, *Mortal Combat*; Susser, *AIDS, Sex, and Culture*.

attempts to resist the terms of the country's incorporation into global capital but through compliance with structural adjustment policies.

Prior to the formulation of a formal global AIDS policy, early HIV prevention messages disseminated in the *Moussa* column promoted neoliberal conceptions of free individuals responsible for their own health and well-being. It produced HIV/AIDS as a crisis of white modernity and fused sexual and economic austerity as necessary to preserve and protect the nation. It thereby rationalized the abdication of state responsibility for social welfare and worked to facilitate the implementation of adjustment policies. At the same time, the column supported Houphouët-Boigny and his control of the single-party state. It promoted austerity as a specifically Ivorian version of development and of Ivorian identity, with sexual self-control as moral alternative to foreign models of development and as a solution for HIV.

"PHILOSOPHER AND GUIGNOL": *MOUSSA* AND THE STATE PRESS

The national boundaries of Côte d'Ivoire encompass speakers of more than sixty different languages, and Houphouët-Boigny fostered what W. Joseph Campbell terms "development journalism," which "sought to tap the perceived power of mass media to promote economic and social development and to forge a national identity in embryonic states where ethnic cleavages were often pronounced and potentially destabilizing."[14] For almost three decades, the government controlled all of the country's mass media, including the only daily newspaper, the French-language *Fraternité Matin*, as well as radio, television, film, and photography production.[15] Generally preferring co-option rather than direct repression to enforce his authority, Houphouët-Boigny viewed the media's principal functions as promoting the policies of the PDCI, facilitating economic development, and creating proper national subjects. The first edition of the state daily *Fraternité Matin*, the replacement for the colonial French *Abidjan Matin*, was printed on December 9, 1964, and did not significantly differ in its mandate from *Fraternité Hebdo*, the official newspaper of the PDCI, the country's sole legal political party.[16] During a February 1986 conference titled "The Role of the Press in Education of the Masses," the managing editor of *Fraternité Matin*, Auguste Miremont, emphasized that the

---

14. J. Campbell, *The Emergent Independent Press*, 76.

15. On May 11, 1987, *Fraternité Matin* began publishing the evening daily, *Ivoir'Soir*, which covered society, culture, and sports.

16. Moussa, *Les Médias et la crise politique*, 1; Tudesq, "Problems of Press," 293.

press's function was to serve the interests of the PDCI: "We have a very precise role to play; it is a political role, I don't have to hide it from you. We are activist journalists [des journalistes militants]."[17]

Created by professors at the state university, Moussa's column was published beginning in the first edition of the state culture and sports weekly *Ivoire Dimanche* in 1971. The column provides a useful archive not so much of early "popular" understandings of the virus but rather of how such understandings were produced in order to manage definitions of the virus and responses to it as a threat. Maintaining the fiction that the column transparently represented the marginalized urban migrant in Abidjan, Moussa's column was written entirely in "Moussa's French," a derogatory designation for the pidgin that was used by French colonists with immigrant labor imported from the Upper Volta (now Burkina Faso) that became creolized.[18] As journalist Abdoulaye Niang notes, Moussa's Popular Ivorian French (français populaire ivoirien, FPI), or Popular French of Abidjan (français populaire d'Abidjan, FPA), became known as a specifically Ivorian French, a "'French transcription' of our national languages."[19] Joseph Mianhoro, who organized courses on "Popular French" at the national university beginning in 1976, described it as "a spoken language," with its speakers using "French words based on the grammar of the speakers' maternal languages [mots français que sous-tendent les grammaires maternelles des locuteurs]."[20] In the 1980s, during economic retrenchment, Moussa's French transformed and became known as an urban slang, *nouchi*.[21] Its use in the official press generated controversy; Moussa's

---

17. Benita Ahossy, "'La Presse dans l'éducation des masses,'" *Fraternité Matin*, February 15–16, 1986, 11.

18. Hattiger, "Humour et pidgin," 182.

19. Abdoulaye Niang, "Le Français de Moussa: Substitut des langues nationales," *Fraternité Matin*, March 17, 1989, 22.

20. J.-B. Kouamé, "Le Français de Moussa à l'université: Une expérience pour montrer comment naît, vit et meurt une langue," *Fraternité Matin*, February 7, 1986, 10.

21. Abolou, *Les Français populaires africains*, 101–2; Akindes, "Playing It 'Loud and Straight,'" 92–93; Akindes, "Program: The Hip Hop Generation"; Newell, *The Modernity Bluff*, 50–51. Yacouba Konaté contrasts "Moussa's French," which became popular during the 1970s "Ivorian miracle," with nouchi, the urban slang deployed by the young that became popular starting around 1984 during a period of economic retrenchment. Konaté, "Génération Zouglou," 783. See also Konaté, "Abidjan," 324–25. For a perspective from the period on "nouchi," see B. A. and A. C., "Nouchi: Langage branché d'origine inconnue," *Fraternité Matin*, September 3, 1986, 3. Moussa continued to epitomize the gendered "everyman" Dioula immigrant in HIV prevention efforts. *The Adventures of Moussa the Taxi Driver* [*Les Aventures de Moussa le taximan*], directed by Henri Duparc, was the title of a 2000 series of seven humorous shorts on HIV prevention that were centered on a character also named Moussa (though not the same Moussa as the character in the column). Televised in France in 2003, *The Further Adventures of Moussa the Taxi Driver* targeted African immigrants in France.

column was suspended in 1973 because of intense criticism about its use of "popular French," but it resumed printing in 1983.[22]

Moussa's French established Moussa and his column as the authentic and defiant voice of the marginalized. Popular idioms enabled the columns' educated writers to express dissenting opinions that could be published—and dismissed—precisely because of Moussa's use of Popular French. As one of the coauthors of *Moussa*, Diégou Bailly, noted in a 1984 interview, "The Moussa column is a way to dodge to get things by [un moyen biaisé de faire passer les choses] that we could not say in academic French without getting ourselves beaten up [sans se faire taper dessus]. Readers are perhaps more tolerant of Moussa than of Diégou Bailly or someone else."[23] The use of Moussa's French further flouted Houphouët-Boigny's insistence on the primacy of French and his repeated chastisements not to mix French with other national languages.

The first constitution of Côte d'Ivoire declared French the country's official language, and Houphouët-Boigny's vision of modern nationhood was inextricably tied to French as a unifying force. As Sasha Newell argues, nation-building was a top-down process in Côte d'Ivoire, "replicating French colonial institutional structures and ushering in an explicitly Francocentric worldview in which many central social distinctions oriented around proximity to the standard of French culture."[24] Ironically, although the nonliterate poor majority whom Moussa was supposed to represent could not read the column, the educated creators of Moussa's column claimed to speak on their behalf. The column creators imagined Moussa and his "Moussa's French" as rudely resisting official language and culture. As *Ivoire Dimanche* noted, "Moussa, philosopher and Guignol, [is] also the spokesperson of a majority who are recognized—and who recognize themselves—in this flipping of the middle finger to the ardent supporters of academic French."[25]

In an analysis of Ivorian comedies, Sélom Komlan Gbanou identifies the Guignol, a character in early nineteenth-century Lyon puppet shows, as a significant "figure and genre" in popular Ivorian theater and radio shows. Gba-

---

22. Tallon, "Le Français de Moussa," 149.

23. As quoted in Tallon, "Le Français de Moussa," 153. As an August 24–25, 1985, *Fraternité Matin* column on satiric comics noted, "We see how humor is an educational element that has the benefit of expressing a political, economic, social or cultural message. . . . Everyone knows that in our cities and villages, a smart man [sic] can't say certain truths without accompanying them with jokes." A. Bassolé, "Au Fil du temps: Humour et rire," *Fraternité Matin*, August 24–25, 1985, 13.

24. Newell, *The Modernity Bluff*, 222.

25. "Moussa, philosophe et Guignol [est] aussi le porte-parole d'une majorité qui se retrouve dans ce bras d'honneur aux inconditionnels du français académique." As quoted in Lafage, "'Français façon là . . . !,'" 179.

nou traces the adaptation of the Guignol in television programs and video recordings of Cameroonians Daniel Ndo's Uncle Otsama, and especially Jean-Michel Kankan's skits. Such shows inspired further comic acts throughout Francophone West Africa, including the popular television show created in 1993, *The Guignols of Abidjan*.[26] In the shows, as in the Guignol puppet performances, characters directly address the audience and, as Paula Amad describes, "turn[] the spectators into witnesses of an often ironic commentary between characters."[27]

Gbanou views the Guignol as subversive and shifting, "above all a language of audacity and demystification, animated by a consciousness of history and a keen concern for contemporary events that requires, over time, alterations in the genre and the original figure."[28] However, the Guignol represented a more ambivalent figure than Gbanou suggests, entangled as he was—and he was gendered male—in colonial, as well as postcolonial, histories.[29] Identifying Moussa as a Guignol, Moussa's creators situated him within the very French cultural traditions that he purportedly critiqued. At the same time, *Moussa* adapted and revised the Guignol for publication in a weekly created to advance the interests of a single-party state.

In a well-known essay, "The Banality of Power and the Aesthetics of Vulgarity in the Postcolony," later incorporated into *In the Postcolony*, Achille Mbembe offers a productive theoretical framework for beginning to consider how *Moussa* might actually work to reinforce, rather than demystify, state authority.[30] In the essay, Mbembe challenges Mikhail Bakhtin's account of popular vulgar humor as site of popular or "plebian" resistance and subversion of ruling authorities. Mbembe insists on an interpretation of popular humor that does not focus on an evaluation of its vulgarity based on aesthetic or ethical principles but that instead examines how the state, in order to reinforce its domination, relies on a vulgarization or popularization of itself, a spreading and rendering accessible of

---

26. An Uncle Otsama skit from the early 1990s by Daniel Ndo mocks AIDS prevention messages. In the skit, the village bumpkin, Uncle Otsama, enters a restaurant and refuses all offers of French food. He insists on monkey meat but then, out of fear of AIDS, refuses it, as well as offers for a wash basin and towel. The skit satirizes theories of the origins of AIDS as well as fears of contamination. But it concludes with a long rant about AIDS as a disease of publicity [maladie publicitaire] and about how AIDS prevention has explicitly served as a political weapon [arme politique] benefiting the political elite. Uncle Otsama also decries the complicity between doctors and pharmaceutical companies who profit from AIDS diagnoses.

27. Amad, "Visual Riposte," 69.

28. Gbanou, "De la Planche," 48.

29. In "Visual Riposte" (68) Paula Amad describes the children filmed in *Christian Dahomey* (Société des Missions Africaines, 1930) who watch a Guignol puppet show.

30. Mbembe, "The Banality of Power," 27; Mbembe, "Notes provisoires"; Mbembe, *On the Postcolony*.

its own power. As Mbembe later clarified, his broader project was to challenge what he considered simplistic theories of resistance and to address some of the shortcomings of alternative explanations. In so doing, he drew from Gramsci's writings on hegemony about how elites rule without violent coercion and how subaltern classes not only accept their own oppression but also naturalize the worldview of the dominant as "common sense."[31]

Drawing most of his examples from public ceremonies and festivities from Cameroon, Mbembe is interested in how the sovereign [commandement] reinforces its rule, as well as how, in deconstructing its rituals through often humorous and satiric renderings of its displays of power, "subalterns" re-ratify that rule. Reworking readings of Baktin, Mbembe proposes that these seemingly contradictory—but widespread to the point of banality—practices constitute "the prosaics of servitude and authoritarian civilities."[32] This "banality of power" is constitutive not only of unofficial culture, as Bakhtin would have it, but also "at the same time of any regime of domination and of every method of its deconstruction or ratification [à la fois de tout régime de domination et de toute modalité de sa déconstruction ou de sa ratification]."[33]

Moussa adds another layer to Mbembe's account of the state's vulgarization of its own authority. In representations of Moussa and his friends discussing HIV, *Moussa* staged the popularization of official, especially biomedical, knowledge and instruction. Through its publication in the state weekly (with an estimated 1987 circulation of 665,000 of a total population of about 11 million), the column simultaneously recuperated the voice of the uneducated and poor urban male migrant whose elevation and inclusion in official discourse in itself provoked laughter—and ratified the domination of the state.[34] In a typically convoluted defense of censorship never identified as such, during a 1988 conference on the Ivorian press, *Fraternité Matin* political writer Alfred

---

31. Mbembe notes that Gramsci's approach does not account for how the power operates in the postcolony, how "coercion and the quest for legitimacy, rather than being opposed, go hand in hand." Nor does it explain the uneven and contradictory processes in which "'dominated groups' . . . accept and reject their position in the social hierarchy. They accept and reject parts of the definition of the world as common, and parts as exceptional, sense. They collaborate in their oppression and they fight against it, simultaneously. . . . The 'ruled' define their subjective identities through the ruling myths and superstitions. Simultaneously, they transform these myths and superstitions in the process." Mbembe, "Prosaics of Servitude," 128. See Bernard's "On Laughter" for a useful critique of Mbembe's reading of Bakhtin. For additional comments, see the special edition of *Public Culture*, which includes essays by Butler, "Mbembe's Extravagant Power"; Cohen, "The Banalities of Interpretation"; Coronil, "Can Postcoloniality Be Decolonized?"

32. Mbembe, "Prosaics of Servitude," 128.
33. Mbembe, "The Banality of Power," 1; Mbembe, "Notes provisoires," 76.
34. Lafage, "'Français façon là . . . !,'" 176.

Dan Moussa, an Ivorian journalist and president of the International Francophone Press Union, maintained that "the Ivorian press is at the same time a press in support of the Government and the Party and press of criticism." As examples of the openness and freedom of the state media, he cited *Moussa* among other comedic productions circulating in state media that were free to use "humor [to] denounce society's shortcomings [les travers]."[35]

Moussa column writers highlighted the negative impact of foreign-funder and state policies, especially structural adjustment and accompanying austerity measures, on the poor.[36] Their depiction of Moussa's blundering vulgarization of official pronouncements—including on HIV—at times mocked, subverted, and demystified. However, as a Guignol, Moussa, and the friends whom he cited, represented educated elites' renditions of simple and ignorant rubes commenting on the venality of modern urban life. The monologues and dialogues in the state weekly co-opted and erased the perspectives that the writers claimed to represent. The sketch accompanying the column, and the given name *Moussa,* identified Moussa as a Muslim Northerner and villager. Enlisting colonial tropes of backwardness and primitiveness and displacing them onto a caricature of the Muslim Northerner as outsider, the column affirmed the superiority of the reader as well as the need for a paternalistic state to guide its childlike subjects (figure 1.1).[37] This production of the Muslim Northerner would take on additional signification as struggles continued to deepen around land tenancy and voting rights.

Houphouët-Boigny actively cultivated his role as patriarch, father, and, later, grandfather of the nation, and as elder wise man [le vieux or le sage] leading the country to its maturity.[38] A characteristic column conveying Moussa's best wishes to the president positioned Moussa in the role of child and follower happily subservient to the benevolent and beloved "Plesident": "Happy birt'day Plesident Fouphouet Boigny, Your Li'l Moussa's Still and Always a Fan of Yours [Bon niversaire Plésident Fouphouet Boigny, ton pitit Moussa i l'è toujours fan

---

35. Jean-Paul Abissa, "La Presse ivorienne, un rôle de soutien et de critique," *Fraternité Matin,* August 18, 1988, 5. In a conference titled "Single Party and Freedom of the Press [Parti unique et Liberté de la Presse (capitals in original)]," *Fraternité Matin* journalist Jean-Pierre Ayé insisted that discussions and disagreements exist "so freedom of expression is therefore a reality." Léon Francis Lebry, "'Les Journalistes ne sont pas des extra-terrestres,'" *Fraternité Matin,* February 28, 1990, 6. An accompanying article pointed out that press freedom in "developed or developing countries always serve the controllers of capital or of political choices [sera toujours function des puissances d'argent ou des choix politiques]."

36. See, for example, "Walaï la vie dans Abidjan la, c'est plis que caillou a l'ère actièle," *Ivoire Dimanche,* February 22, 1987, 48. Léon Francis Lebry, "La Liberté de presse existe chez nous," *Fraternité Matin,* February 28, 1990, 6.

37. Lafage, "'Français façon là . . . !,'" 177.

38. Toungara, "The Apotheosis," 23.

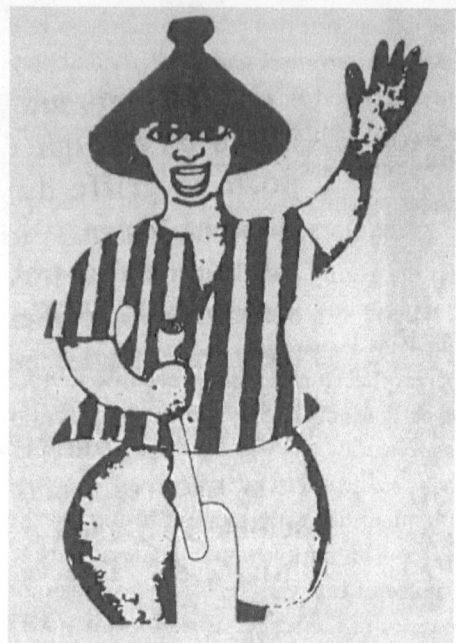

FIGURE 1.1. Sketch of "Moussa" accompanying each weekly column in *Ivoire Dimanche*.

de toi]."³⁹ Playing on the depiction of Moussa as childlike, the column portrayed Moussa expressing his naive astonishment and disgust about what he represented as the corruption of Abidjan. Even before his first responses to AIDS, Moussa repeatedly expressed anxieties about modernity, development, and the economic crisis as they were articulated as issues of sexual morality. His depiction of the need for austerity measures—especially individual sexual self-restraint—as a response laid the groundwork for his later columns on HIV/AIDS.

"WHITES HAVE TOO MANY WEIRD DISEASES": CONTESTING THE ORIGINS OF HIV

State media such as Moussa's column participated actively in the production of "homosexuals" through a counterdiscourse of "AIDS" as foreign. As Neville

---

39. "Bon niversaire Plésident Fouphouet Boigny," *Ivoire Dimanche*, October 18, 1987, 47. See also "Très bon anniversaire, Plézident Fouphouet, premier nandjelet de Codivoire," *Ivoire Dimanche*, October 20, 1985, 48.

Hoad has traced, ambivalent constructions of "Africa" and "homosexuality" were intertwined in nineteenth-century colonial narratives of evolution, progress, and development. One strand of those productions imagined "Africa" as indexing a backward sexual depravity. Reversing the terms of such productions, Moussa's column and state reporting on HIV/AIDS in Côte d'Ivoire sought to ascribe the signs of African depravity—promiscuity, sexual perversion, and disease—to "Whites." Central to their efforts was the establishment of an identitarian sexuality—"homosexual"—articulated through racialized national identities. The reversal relied on another strand of colonial imaginings of "Africa" not as primitive and depraved but as primitive and innocent, corrupted by modern practices imported from elsewhere.[40]

After the first published report of five cases of a rare form of pneumonia among young, white, gay men from the West Coast of the United States in 1981, intense anxieties began to circulate around certain individual and collective bodies marked as sources of contagion.[41] References to the condition first as Gay-Related Immune Deficiency (GRID) and, more informally, as the "gay plague" or "gay cancer" signaled the conflation of certain stigmatized sexual identities and bodies with disease. Reflecting shifting understandings of the condition, the term *AIDS* replaced *GRID* in 1982, and in 1983 the U.S. Centers for Disease Control identified the so-called 4-H's, the four groups at "increased risk" for AIDS: homosexuals, heroin users, Haitians, and hemophiliacs.[42] The identification of Haitians in particular drew from racialized European colonial geographies linking blackness with contagion and with deviant sexual practices—associations that theories about the origins of HIV in Central Africa only reinforced.[43]

---

40. As Megan Vaughan notes, colonial conceptions of primitive, dangerous, uncontrolled African sexualities coexisted with their production as "innocent," and these representations were never uniform. Vaughan, *Curing Their Ills*, 129–30. Neville Hoad focuses on late nineteenth-century Buganda, but his analysis of colonial narratives of development applies in this context as well. Hoad, "Arrested Development," 139; Hoad, *African Intimacies*, 4–5. What Ato Quayson describes as an "obsession with the structure of obverse denomination" of "Africans" is also at work here. Quayson, "Obverse Denominations," 586. On the contested status of the modern in scholarship on Africa, see Thomas, "Modernity's Failings."

41. "Epidemiological Notes and Reports," 250–52.

42. Farmer, *AIDS and Accusation*, 211; Treicher, *How to Have a Theory in an Epidemic*, 20.

43. See Pourrut, Galat-Luong, and Galat, "Associations du singe vert" (47–58) for discussion of cross-infection between green monkeys and patas monkeys. Also see Bibollet-Ruche et al. for discussion of such cross-infection as evidence for cross-species transmission of HIV from primates to humans. Bibollet-Ruche et al., "Simian Immunodeficiency," 773–81. See Hahn et al. for discussion of cross-species transmission of HIV-1 and HIV-2 to humans from primates through contact with blood, possibly through vaccinations or possibly through butchering of meat. Hahn et al., "AIDS as a Zoonosis," 607–14.

Shortly after identification of the HIV virus, scientists theorized that HIV originated from viral cross-infection between nonhuman primates from West Africa and humans.[44] Speculation about African origins of HIV and the discovery in 1986 of a different strain of HIV in West Africa that was closely related to what were later named Simian Immunodeficiency Viruses (SIVs) contributed to the construction of "African AIDS" as the product of a primitive, bestial, and promiscuous "African sexuality."[45] As UNAIDS reported, during the first international conference on AIDS held in Atlanta, Georgia, in 1985, an American journalist asked an African doctor if AIDS in Africa could be spread through Africans having sex with monkeys.[46]

Marc Epprecht analyzes how, in seeking to contest such racist conceptions of African sexualities and "African AIDS," many African leaders and scholars reinforced another stereotype about the absence or nonexistence of homosexuality in Africa.[47] In the context of Côte d'Ivoire, in 1984, French anthropologists Marc Le Pape and Claudine Vidal noted that African "male homosexuals" in Abidjan designated the networks they formed as the "*milieu.*" According to Le Pape and Vidal, in implicit contrast to Michel Foucault's account of the emergence of "homosexuality" as a "species" in nineteenth-century Western Europe and to self-identified "male homosexuals" in the United States and France, the *milieu* in Abidjan did not form separate communities in particular neighborhoods or claim a separate "gay" culture or identity: "Up to the present, claiming of 'differences' and panegyrics to identity have failed to take. No trace either of the theme 'discovery of oneself through understanding of the other.'"[48] Anthropologist and medical doctor Vinh-Kim Nguyen traces how Abidjan became a self-consciously modern and cosmopolitan city where a discourse of sexuality linking sexual behavior with sexual identity emerged only after the economic crisis of the 1970s and 1980s and after HIV became a major health issue.[49] More recent adoption of the public health category MSM (men who have sex with men) by gender and sexual minorities underscores how identity categories based on sexualities continue to shift over time and

---

44. Doolittle, "The Simian-Human Connection," 338–39.
45. Sharp and Hahn, "Origins of HIV," 2; Fassin, *When Bodies Remember,* 148–49; Dozon and Fassin, "Raison épidémiologique," 21–36.
46. Knight, UNAIDS: *The First Ten Years,* 13–14.
47. Epprecht, *Heterosexual Africa?* 11, 14, 25.
48. Le Pape and Vidal, "Libéralisme et vécus sexuels," 116, 118. Le Pape and Vidal neither clarify what they mean by their use of the term *homosexual* nor note the contradiction in their reliance on a category that they at the same time insist does not apply.
49. Nguyen, "Uses and Pleasures," 246.

how they have been appropriated, modified, and redefined in response to HIV prevention efforts.[50]

Moussa's column actively participated in the linking of sexual acts with racial and national identities, as it persistently explored central contradictions in representations of AIDS. In a September 8, 1985, column, "AIDS iz More Danzerous than the Clap [Sida c'è plis danzéré que gono]," Moussa depicts the confusion ensuing from inconsistent and racist accounts about the origins of AIDS. He describes how AIDS first appeared in the United States and is now in France, which his friend Poussanaka notes with alarm is very close to Côte d'Ivoire. The column conveyed information about HIV in a parody of AIDS education where the ignorant instructs the even more uninformed. The Popular French is untranslatable, but in their dialogue Moussa attempts to inform his friend Poussanaka about AIDS: "I'm not a doctor but journalists say it's a disease of homo—homo homosess, yes, homosexuals [homossessuels]." When his friend does not understand the term, Moussa elucidates: "It's said that they are boys who do the thing among themselves." In a caricature of enlightenment, his friend exclaims, "Oh! Fags [Pédés]!"

Satirizing the translation of "scientific" to "popular" terminology, the column stages AIDS education as clearly inadequate and ineffective, a debased process, with the column both representing and reproducing its failures. Moussa's information proves no less reliable than that of the journalists who cite doctors, who in turn cannot provide answers to many questions about the virus. In response to his friend's question, Moussa says that he does not know if "women who make love-love among themselves" can get AIDS. Even if AIDS is a disease of "boys who do the thing among themselves," Moussa nevertheless further explains that a "man that gets that, he can give that quickly to a woman." Confirming the possibility of transmitting AIDS by kissing, Moussa refers to the newspaper coverage of the American actress Linda Evans playing "Kristelle" in the popular television show *Dynasty*, who he says has filed charges against Rock Hudson for having kissed her on the mouth during the show when he was sick with AIDS. In any event, Poussanaka concludes that AIDS is a disease of white people: "Really, Whites [Blancs] have too many weird diseases. Cancer, that's them. Now AIDS that's them."[51]

---

50. Thomann, "HIV Vulnerability"; Thomann, "Zones of Difference."

51. "Sida c'è plis danzéré que gono," *Ivoire Dimanche*, September 8, 1985, 48. Linda Evans never actually filed charges against Rock Hudson. Poussanaka's comment could be read as a kind of dramatic irony: While the conditions termed *cancer* were produced and defined as such by "Whites," their effects are also legible as such on bodies in Côte d'Ivoire, as are the conditions that fall under the name *AIDS*.

By insistently identifying AIDS as a health crisis of "Whites," primarily "homosexuals," in the United States, early journalistic coverage of HIV in the Ivorian state press, like *Moussa,* contested racist theories of Africa as source of AIDS. In a November 17, 1985, article in the first extensive series on AIDS in *Ivoire Dimanche,* the Chief of the Immuno-Hematology Department at the University Hospital Center in Cocody, Abidjan, noted that "the reservoir" for HIV "could be a monkey." Nevertheless, he reassured the public "NO PANIC": Those "most exposed" to HIV were homosexuals, drug users, and people who have had blood transfusions.[52] Insisting that AIDS affected mostly "homosexuals" in the United States, accompanying articles challenged accounts of African AIDS. After summarizing one account of macaque monkeys in Angola as the source of AIDS, another article, "AIDS Is Not Anything New for Medicine," asked, "Did AIDS research just establish new close **ontological** relationships [nouvelles parentés **ontologiques** étroites (emphasis in original)] between the monkey and the African?" The author condemned such accounts as racist and asked how then to explain the large numbers of people living with HIV in the United States, 96% of them homosexual.[53] An accompanying article criticized accounts of AIDS originating in Zaire and reminded readers that during the colonial period, all Africans were considered syphilitic, when, in fact, of four strains, only one was sexually transmitted. The writer implied that AIDS could prove a similar error based on racist assumptions about African sexualities and sexual practices.[54]

In the same issue of *Ivoire Dimanche,* Moussa's column responded to the official medical research and journalistic coverage on AIDS. The column titled "AIDS: Imazinary Syndrome to Dizcourage Lovers [Sida: Syndrome imazinaire pour décourazer les amoureux]" cites the widely circulating joke that puns on the French acronym for AIDS (Sida) and on the Molière play *Imaginary Invalid* [*Le Malade imaginaire*]. In the column, Moussa describes "Hollywood Americans" using drugs and engaging in uncontrolled anal sex. He observes that Hollywood is known as the "world capital of cinema" and as "super capital of the world in the asshole business [affaires de cui (*sic*)]. Ah yeah, the people live at 100 mph in rough rides of butts mixed with drug

---

52. Atta, "Pas de panique," *Ivoire Dimanche,* November 17, 1985, 16. A year and a half later, the paper qualified the headline, "AIDS: No Panic, but . . ." Ahua, "SIDA: Pas de panique, mais . . . ," *Fraternité Matin,* April 15, 1987, 3.

53. Ado Désiré, "Le SIDA n'est pas une nouveauté en médecine," *Ivoire Dimanche,* November 17, 1985, 17.

54. De Campos, "Méfions-nous des conclusions hâtives," *Ivoire Dimanche,* November 17, 1985, 19–20. On misdiagnosis of yaws and endemic syphilis as venereal syphilis, see also Vaughan, *Curing Their Ills,* 129–54.

business."⁵⁵ However, Moussa continues, Hollywood has recently suddenly quieted down: "You know why? All that there that began with the death of an actor named Rock Hudson. It seems that the Guy, his love-love business with boys is not a joke! Up to the point that he caught AIDS."⁵⁶

In vulgarizing medical authorities' association of homosexuals and drug use with AIDS, Moussa further delineates a racialized sexual identity based on sexual acts—anal sex—performed in the United States. Although Moussa describes AIDS as a disease of drug-using homosexuals engaging in anal sex, Rock Hudson's death from AIDS-related illnesses has frightened heterosexual men in Hollywood: "All the skirt-chasers have stopped their goings on." Hollywood has become "world capital of the fear of AIDS." In contrast, despite reports of increasing numbers of cases of AIDS in Africa, "people, they don't care about all that, they just party hard. They think that in increasing their good life 100 times, they will discourage doctors' campaigns. . . . The guys [doctors], they have increased their severe warnings. Currently, they are talking about the serious consequences of AIDS and then they say to people to be very very careful." According to Moussa, people in Abidjan laughingly disregard medical authorities' repeated warnings. His untranslatable French and nouchi read, "The guys, they just laugh then they say: 'Ha! Ha! Ha! Who is it whose asshole's going to play a joke on you? AIDS means only one thing: Imazinary Syndrome to Dizcourage Lovers. Dizcouragement in love-love, that exists in Wollywood now, here where we are, we don't care about AIDS.'"⁵⁷

The *Moussa* column quotes a fictional character, Moussa, quoting generalized male Africans in Abidjan who punningly refigure medical authority as the asshole (*cui* in nouchi) that in Hollywood has led to the spread of AIDS. Their joke about AIDS as an imaginary syndrome mocks as hypocritical pretext the ongoing attempts to control the sexual behavior of Africans, who in contrast to white skirt-chasers in Hollywood get the joke and rather than be deterred, attempt to deter such doctors' campaigns. The column quotes laughing responses to warnings about HIV as suggesting not so much

---

55. "Les zens i vivent à cent à l'hèr dans gazoil [a footnote translates *gazoil* as *turbulences*] de fesses milanzé avec affair de drogue."

56. "On paraît que le Type son affair de l'aime-l'aime avec garçon c'è pas bouche [a footnote translates *bouche* as *blague*, or *joke*, but the phrase also puns on the French for mouth]!" "Sida: Syndrome imazinaire pour décourazer les amoureux," *Ivoire Dimanche*, November 17, 1985, 48.

57. "Les gars eux i rigolent selment é pis i dit: 'Ah! ah! ah! . . . C'è qui son cui vous va blagué! Sida ça vé dire in chose selment: Syndrome Imazinaire pour Décourazer les Amoureux. Décourazement dans l'aime-l'aime ça existe à Woliwoud actielement, chez nous ici on s'en fout de Sida.'" "Sida: Syndrome imazinaire pour décourazer les amoureux," *Ivoire Dimanche*, November 17, 1985, 48.

ignorance about AIDS but rather resistance to theories about African origins of AIDS, as well as about African sexual practices.

At the same time, Moussa suggests that such responses are in fact ignorant and potentially dangerous. The column openly confronted the contradiction between attempts to redefine AIDS as homosexual and white and the rejection of sexual austerity and self-discipline that such a redefinition might seem to imply. In the context of the economic crisis, refusing to curb sexual behavior and continuing to "party hard" defied state admonishments to submit to austerity measures. To resolve the contradiction, the column conflated "homosexuality" with anal sex as signs of sexual corruption attending white development and proposed austerity as the solution, as the sign of Ivorian morality.

"ALL MEANS ARE GOOD TO EARN SOME G'S IN LIFE": DEVELOPMENT AS CORRUPTING SEXUAL ECONOMIES

The French colonial state had funded social services through direct taxation, and under Houphouët-Boigny, a sprawling central state bureaucracy continued to focus on delivering these services, especially education and health care. High expectations about the state's provision of social welfare precipitated predictable frustration and resentment during state retrenchment.[58] In columns, Moussa regularly voiced support for the austerity measures urged by Houphouët-Boigny. Sending his best wishes for a new year to Houphouët-Boigny in early 1985, for example, Moussa echoed the president's calls for "courage and hope"—and for compliance to necessary belt tightening. Citing a white foreigner [toubabou] who observed no signs of economic crisis during a visit to Côte d'Ivoire, Moussa recounts, "Me I responded that yeah, it's true: there is a crisis but we Ivorians we don't sit holding our heads crying like children: we work in courage and hope and then we calculate before spending. If you don't have enough money to buy something you stay quiet, that's all."[59] Dismissing ongoing protests against austerity measures as the whining of spoiled children, Moussa characterized compliance not as mandated by foreign funders but as uniquely Ivorian, that is, individual moral response, a sign of maturity and a shared national identity rather than submission to the development policies that the column depicted as degrading.

---

58. Maclean, *Informal Institutions and Citizenship*, 143–44, 147–48.
59. "Bon nanée Plézident!" *Ivoire Dimanche*, January 13, 1985, 48.

A glimpse at some of the headline news in *Fraternité Matin* around the time of the first reported AIDS cases in the state press later in 1985 provides a sense of some of the paternalistic injunctions to demonstrate calm, rigor, discipline, and maturity during tightly controlled single-party elections, continuing state cutbacks, and ensuing strikes of civil service workers. A September 9, 1985, front-page headline described and simultaneously urged "Calm and Discipline" during general secretary elections. In October 1985, Houphouët-Boigny, as usual as the only candidate, won the presidential elections, and in November, the PDCI, the only legal political party, won 175 out of 175 legislative seats (although the elections were competitive). From October 9 to 12, Houphouët-Boigny oversaw the "Congress of Maturity" that named him sole presidential candidate and suppressed rumors that he might name a vice president and, therefore, a potential successor.[60] Warnings to behave with "maturity" echoed throughout the press with municipal elections proceeding with "Calm and Discipline," "Under the Sign of Maturity," and with "Vigilance."[61] During festivities celebrating the twenty-five years of independence at the end of the eventful year, Houphouët-Boigny proclaimed "Pride and Austerity" and condemned the waste that he declared required the enlistment of the nation in "an enormous sanitization [un vaste assainissement]."[62]

Houphouët-Boigny deployed the terms of austerity and maturity not only to rationalize mandated structural adjustment but also to legitimize his control of the single-party state. *Moussa* reproduced and reinforced this agenda. The column consistently described the economic crisis in racialized terms as the result of dissolute white sexual economies that paradoxically compelled austerity not as a sign of a state destabilized by economic crisis and forced to submit to World Bank and IMF measures, but as an assertion of Houphouët-Boigny's firm paternalistic leadership. As a childlike subject, Moussa required this guidance to be shepherded to maturity.

A March 1986 column quotes a conversation with a friend, Barakrou, in which Moussa described very young girls selling sex, taking drugs, and drinking with Whites [Blancs]. Barakrou observes that since the "hard [economic] times came, people do too much crap [i déconnent trop]" and that "we in Côte d'Ivoire here we should not want to do a forced imitation of bad things that happen among Whites [Blancs]." Moussa further remarks that "it seems

---

60. "Le Congrès de la maturité," *Fraternité Matin*, October 13, 1985, 14.

61. "Élections municipales: Calme et discipline," *Fraternité Matin*, November 25, 1985, 1. "Élections municipales: Sous le signe de la maturité," *Fraternité Matin*, November 25, 1985, 26. "Élections municipales à l'intérieur: Vigilance," *Fraternité Matin*, November 25, 1985, 28.

62. A. Dan Moussa, "Le Message présidentiel: Une société forte et sereine," *Fraternité Matin*, December 9, 1985, 17.

that there are little boys too who whore themselves [i font bordel]. If this is true, what a big shame for us! Where are we going like that? Really, in Abidjan now there are too many stupid things." As in his column critiquing the influx of porn theaters in Abidjan, Moussa emphasizes the need for both parents and the government to assert their authority over the young. In other words, he proposes enforcement of (hetero)sexual morality as alternative to white development to which he attributes national sexual and economic crises: "The authorities along with parents are going to have to take action to block all this bullshit [I faut que les autorités avec les parents i vont agir pour bloqué tous ces coronis-là]."[63]

An especially popular October 19, 1986, *Moussa* column, "There Are Too Many White Women Who Are Doing Prostitution in Plateau at the Moment," reprinted in January 18, 1987, "at the request of loyal I-D [*Ivoire Dimanche*] readers," ambivalently centers on homosexuality and homosexuals as tropes for contaminating economic and sexual transactions and links them to white "prostitutes" as signs of corruption, development, and modernity. In the column, Moussa comments on the increase of white female "prostitutes" in the business district of Plateau in Abidjan. When his friend Pouncrac notes that these women were not as visible in the past, Moussa replies, "There are those who say that prostitution of White women, that means that our country begins to make good development." Pouncrac jokes, "Development from and of behind(s), yeah [an untranslatable pun: développement de derrières, ouaih]! In any case, me Pouncrac, I'm not at all okay with this new way [cette nouveau mode-là]. We have already gotten [gagné] a lot of Ghanaian prostitutes in Côte d'Ivoire here. The Whites mustn't come mess us up [Faut pas que les Toubabous i vont veni nous emmerdé] with their prostitutes also." Prostitution is not just a sign of development; Pouncrac's crude joke personifies development itself as white female prostitute to invert an evolutionary narrative that would situate white Europe as its telos and Africans as "behind."

The English translation does not adequately convey how the use of Moussa's French clearly excludes Moussa and Pouncrac from the "development" they condemn. Nor does it capture how their French violates grammatical rules to combine the masculine (especially the adjective *new* [nouveau]) with the feminine (the noun *way* [cette mode]). Like the "development from and of behind(s)" associated with white female "prostitutes," the disruption of gendering in "this new way [cette nouveau mode-là]" rewrites the terms and the temporality of narratives of development. The promise of white modernity

---

63. "Y'a trop de filles minairs i déraillent dans Abidjan-la!" *Ivoire Dimanche*, March 9, 1986, 48. "Y'a trop de flims porno ça passe dans les cinémas, a l'hère actiele," *Ivoire Dimanche*, June 8, 1986, 48.

and progress, its "new way," contravenes proper gendered sexualities, as does the white prostitute who embodies the modern as actually "behind." Anal sex, "the asshole business," condenses the deviant sexualities and practices of the "new way" that entice in the form of white "prostitutes" but prove a ruse, like that deployed by transvestites and drag queens to dupe their clients. Moussa's warning to Pouncrac that people must be careful since AIDS has become increasingly common among whites abruptly transitions. This section of their dialogue is worth reproducing:

> MOUSSA: With this AIDS thing that is heating up a lot there, I think people have to be really careful to not fall into that. And then, me Moussa, I think of something that happens a lot among Whites [Blancs] over there, it's the business of boys who wear woman's dress to trick those searching for prostitutes [c'è affair de garçons que i porte boubou de femme pour trompté les cherchairs de toutous]. Their name is called Transvestites or tranny [Ler nom s'appelle Travestis ou bien travelo].
> POUNCRAC: Really, the Whites they are going to kill man with the asshole business [Vraiment, les Toubabous i vont tier l'homme dans affair de cui]. That means there are all kinds of ways [tous les façons modes], huh!
> MOUSSA: That's what the Whites [Toubabous] they themselves say: "**all means are good to earn some g's in life [tous les moyens sont bons pour gagné pognon dans la vie** (emphasis in original)]." In any case, it's not me Moussa that I am going to go waste my money on white women whores [femmes blanches bordels]. Better that I save that to do something good, man [*man* written in English].[64]

Achille Mbembe writes that "the postcolony's patriarchal traditions of power are founded upon an originary repression" whose "central figure" is the anus, which "in the symbolic universe of many pre-colonial African societies . . . was considered an object of aversion." The site of excrement and danger, in "contrast to the buttocks, the anus is the accursed organ and the sign *par excellence* of abjection."[65] I cannot directly address the "symbolic universe" to which Mbembe refers except via its production as a fantasy in Moussa and Pouncrac's dialogue, which represses anal sex by naming and attributing it to "White" and foreign female prostitutes, transvestites, and drag queens. The "asshole business" and "the business of boys who wear women's dress" serve as

---

64. "Y'a trop beaucoup blanches i font toutous au Prateau a l'hère actièle," *Ivoire Dimanche*, January 18, 1987, 48.

65. Mbembe, "*On the Postcolony*: A Brief Response," 166–67. See also, Mbembe, "Le Potentat sexuel."

metaphors and metonyms for commercial sex as a depraved foreign practice imported to Côte d'Ivoire from "over there." As figures of gender and sexual transgression, prostitutes, transvestites, and drag queens index what Moussa describes as white immorality regarding the economy generally: "All ways are good to earn some g's in life."

Development itself has proven a trick, a scam of whites, evidenced by and analogous to white transvestites and drag queens' greedy money-making sexual scams targeting unsuspecting male clients. The critique pointedly revises coverage in the same weekly and on television of the legendary Oscar, a Malian immigrant, and of members of the *milieu*'s popular drag performances in Abidjan.[66] Although Moussa refers to the threat of AIDS, he says that the primary reasons why he will avoid white female prostitutes are to decline participation in what he figures as an immoral and deadly racialized sexual economy and to refuse the terms of "White" development. His withdrawal from this economy assures his heterosexual masculinity, as he will thereby avoid being deceived by "this new way" into having sex with a "transvestite or tranny."[67]

Through the productions of the homosexual, the transvestite, and the female prostitute as foreign and white, Moussa's column depicted "White" economic development as fatally corrupting sexual economies, creating the "asshole business," the cause of the spread of AIDS. *Moussa* thereby contested not only theories of the origin of AIDS but also foreign-lender policies. Moussa depicted his decision not to frequent white prostitutes as principled rejection of this sexualized, pathologized economy and its terms of degradation. However, significantly, what he framed as necessary individual response—self-discipline, rigor, refusal to "waste ... dough," "sav[ing] to do something good"—deployed the same state rhetoric justifying implementation of the development policies that he and Pouncrac critique. In critiquing prostitution, homosexuality, and AIDS as consequences of white development, the column positioned the state as an indispensable, paternalistic authority overseeing austerity as a moral alternative to rather than manifestation of the very economic policies it contested.

---

66. "Oscar, imitateur d'Aïcha Koné," *Ivoire Dimanche*, October 24, 1982, as quoted in Le Pape and Vidal, "Libéralisme et vécus sexuels," 116–17. See also Nguyen, "Uses and Pleasures," 249.

67. "Transvestites" were associated with criminality and duplicity in recent media stories, including in a story about a transvestite prostitute who robbed her male clients. See "Le travesti-voleur arrêté pour la 15e fois," *Fraternité Matin*, January 15, 1985, 3; "Deux ans de prison pour le travesti-voleur," *Fraternité Matin*, January 30, 1985, 4. "Male prostitution" was also associated with scams directed at clients who were blackmailed by Johns. Am Atta, "Prostitution au masculin," Ivoire Dimanche, June 8, 1986, 6.

After the Ivorian Health Minister Alphonse Djédjé Mady first publicly commented on HIV/AIDS on state television and in articles published in the state press in early 1987, *Moussa* generally mirrored his messages. The minister attempted to reassure a panicking public by contextualizing HIV/AIDS in relation to the many other endemic and epidemic diseases in the country and increasingly shifted to disseminate inconsistent and contradictory information about condoms as a means of prevention. As in previous columns, Moussa's rejection of condom usage as an affirmation of "African" identity nevertheless reinforced messages that sexual self-discipline and self-control constituted the most effective responses to the epidemic.

"NOT ... THE EVIL OR THE ILLNESS OF THE CENTURY": *MOUSSA*'S AND THE HEALTH MINISTRY'S RESPONSES TO HIV/AIDS

The earliest coverage in the Ivorian press of condoms as a means of prevention against sexual transmission of HIV recounted resistance to their usage. On December 3, 1985, *Fraternité Matin* published an article from L'Agence France-Presse (AFP), the French news agency, describing how in Central Africa "the use of condoms faces obstacles [se heurte] because of the population's prejudices against them and because of financial constraints."[68] Although Laurent Vidal dates the first explicit reference to condoms in the state daily to late 1988, *Moussa* first mentioned them almost two years earlier in *Ivoire Dimanche*.[69] In the first reference to condoms in the Ivorian context that I could locate in the state press, a February 1, 1987, *Moussa* column enacted widespread resistance to condom usage.

Moussa opened the column by again brushing aside theories identifying green monkeys in Central Africa as the origin of AIDS: "Let's just drop all that. Whites are going around making accusations against Africans [On n'a qu'à laissé tout ça-là. Les Toubabous i vé metté aquizations sir les Africains]."[70] Moussa continued quoting a friend, Djéprou, deciding that given the danger of AIDS, "from now on, I will use an English rubber [capote anglaise, the French term for *condom*] to do business [fait les affaires]; that way, AIDS, even

---

68. AFP, "Le Sida en Afrique: Des études alarmantes," *Fraternité Matin*, December 3, 1985, 26.

69. Laurent Vidal dates the first explicit reference to condoms in *Fraternité Matin* to November 29, 1988. Vidal, "Images du SIDA," 158–64.

70. "Moussa: A condé de SIDA, Djeprou i l'a gagné trop pèr des gos mainant!" *Ivoire Dimanche*, February 1, 1987, 48.

if it's tough, it can never block me up." As Moussa describes, Djéprou consults his friend Barakrou who advises him that condoms are not reliable: "It seems that they lied about the condom business and all that, because the AIDS virus can pass through that no problem." Fretting that his sperm will accumulate in his groin, Djéprou concludes that he will "only look" at women no matter how beautiful they are, but remain faithful: "'Until a vaccine is discovered against this bad AIDS, me, Djéprou, I am staying at home to hit on my wife only [pour dragué mon femme selment].'" In other words, he proposes sexual self-discipline—fidelity—as the most effective prevention method, given the unreliability of condoms. Moussa concludes the column in an ambiguous direct address to readers: "Is Djéprou right or wrong? You yourselves have to reflect on that."[71]

Health Minister Djédjé Mady did not publicly comment on reports of AIDS cases in the country until a week later, in a February 9, 1987, interview on the monthly state television program, *Right to Health* [*Droit à la santé*].[72] Noting the recording of 118 AIDS cases and of 9 deaths attributed to AIDS-related infections in the country, he tried to calm fears about the epidemic by pointing out that measles killed many more children and tuberculosis many more adults than did HIV/AIDS: "I do not consider AIDS the evil or the illness of the century [comme le mal ou la maladie du siècle]." Djédjé Mady advised Ivorians to implement individual behavior change: limit their sexual activity, not change partners too frequently, and avoid what he described as high-risk partners, like prostitutes. He further suggested the avoidance of blood donations from infected donors and encouraged the use of sterile, ideally disposable, needles for medical purposes.[73] The program was supplemented by coverage of the show in *Fraternité Matin*, as well as in a February 15, 1987, *Ivoire Dimanche* issue headlined "Africa and AIDS."[74] The lengthy main article reiterated Djédjé Mady's message of reassurance as well as his figuring of self-restraint as sanitization. The discourse of hygiene explicitly underscored the state's insistence on the importance of sanitization of the corrupt and bloated state civil service: "There is no cause to be alarmed. The fight requires in particular a sanitization of sexual morals and special precautions at blood transfusion centers [La lutte passe notamment par un assainissement

---

71. "Moussa: A condé de SIDA," *Ivoire Dimanche*, February 1, 1987, 48.

72. Critics later accused the Health Minister and the Ivorian government of minimizing the threat of HIV and cited the two shows on which he appeared as evidence. Koné and Agness, "La Communication," 304.

73. Bernard Ahua, "Le Ministère Djédjé Mady: Le Sida ne doit pas nous affoler," *Fraternité Matin*, February 12, 1987, 2.

74. "Face à face dramatique: L'Afrique et le SIDA," *Ivoire Dimanche*, February 15, 1987, 1.

des moeurs sexuelles et des précautions particulières au niveau des centres de transfusion sanguine]."[75]

Essentially parroting—and parodying—Djédjé Mady's messages, Moussa two weeks later blamed the spread of HIV and sexually transmitted diseases on female migrants who leave their villages for Abidjan, even though "there is a lot a lot of work in the plantassions over there." These girls "bother all the boys. Just to try to earn a little money." Like other migrants to Abidjan, the girls refuse to contribute the labor necessary for proper economies: "Currently, everyone knows that the economic crisis, that prick! is continuing to beat up Ivorians. So, since there are people who don't like to work, to earn good money, they do all kinds of bullshit: steal, do prostitution, sell drugs, do fags. . . . You'd say that these bunch of lowlifes [ces bandésalauds-là] don't know about AIDS which the whole world talks about!"[76] Gendered rural-to-urban migration, an improper work ethic, and inadequate sexual discipline create a morally and physically contaminating sexual economy in which "dirty" or "bad" money circulates alongside and as a metaphor for diseases. The column concludes with Moussa's friend weeping as he realizes that he has contracted HIV or another sexually transmitted disease from a prostitute with gonorrhea and AIDS.[77]

The following week, Moussa vulgarized the Health Minister's messages advising the reduction of sexual partners and condoms: "In sexual affairs, don't have a multiplication of girls or men. Those that get around at all costs are doing sessual promiscuity, they must have protection and then put on their dicks before sex that rubber way that is called French letter or condom."[78] Moussa expressed skepticism about condom education as a foreign method of HIV prevention: "But the way that this thing is talked about works with the Whites [Blancs] over there, that's not going to work here." In addition, Moussa repeated his doubts about the reliability of condoms themselves: "I don't trust in that rubber business [affaire de capotes] that the Whites talk about so much now. Me, I think that to not earn problems in Abidjan, don't do sexual promiscuity. It's better than to make a bursting of rubbers and then get AIDS,

---

75. "L'Afrique et le SIDA," *Ivoire Dimanche*, February 15, 1987, 4.
76. Moussa uses the phrase "a fa kaya," an untranslatable Dioula vulgar term for male genitalia.
77. "Moussa: Les djancals que i n'ont pas gagné rien a fait dans Abidjan ici, i n'ont qu'a retourné au village," *Ivoire Dimanche*, March 1, 1987, 48.
78. "Dans affair de cognement i faut pas que on va fait miltiplication de gos ou bien de l'hommes. Ceux que i vé, coûte que coûte, fait vacabondage sexiel, i doit fait protection e pis metté sir lèr zob avant les affairs, in façon caoussou on pélé capote anglais ou bien priservatif." "Moussa: Actielement, les Toubabous i dit que c'è capotes selment ça moyen bloqué SIDA," *Ivoire Dimanche*, March 8, 1987, 48.

stupidly to die for nothing [i faut pas fait vacabondage sixiel. C'è plis mié que de fait éclatement de capotes pour gagné SIDA, bêtement pour mouri cado]."[79]

Nevertheless, a month later, *Ivoire Dimanche* quoted Djédjé Mady as announcing, "'Condom use must enter into the habits of Ivorians,' especially if they have multiple partners." The article cited people interviewed in Abidjan about their attitudes about AIDS, and observing that 50,000 deaths in Uganda had already been attributed to AIDS, it urged readers to avoid such an outcome in Côte d'Ivoire. The article countered the journal's own earlier coverage to remind readers that "AIDS is not an illness only among homosexuals and drug addicts from the West." Echoing Djédjé Mady, the article exhorted, "Let's slip on rubbers! [Enfilons les capotes!]."[80]

However, the following evening, in a second interview on the March 16, 1987, television show *Right to Health*, Djédjé Mady contradicted his own messages. He sought again to reassure viewers: "I never minimized AIDS. I situate AIDS in its place in our African country. . . . In the last program, I said, almost word for word this: that I did not find justified the cries of Africans about a few cases of AIDS deaths against which we can do nothing once the illness has manifested [déclarée] in contrast to their indifference and their silence in front of thousands, even millions of deaths due to illnesses against which we can do something." The state daily reproduced Djédjé Mady's contradictory messages of assurance on April 9, 1987. It republished a photograph from *Jeune Afrique* of an alarmingly emaciated person identified as "suffering from AIDS" but also included an interview with the regional director of the World Health Organization who commented that "here, in Africa, we have numerous epidemics. . . . For us, AIDS is one illness among others."[81]

When pressed by a journalist from the International Press Association and the founder of *Our Health* magazine, Samba Koné, Djédjé Mady underscored the seriousness of the situation: "We must take AIDS seriously and the Ivorian government takes AIDS seriously." But for Djédjé Mady, the solution to the "problem of public health" of high HIV rates among sex workers was "individual sexual self-control [maîtrise de la sensualité de quelqu'un]." As he stated, this approach was preferable to condom usage, since condoms proved unreliable: "I say, the best solution is first, individual: one can use male condoms. We have advised them—everyone is now aware [au courant]—but I

---

79. "Moussa: Actielement, les Toubabous i dit que c'è capotes selment ça moyen bloqué SIDA," *Ivoire Dimanche*, March 8, 1987, 48.

80. Venance Doudou, "Les Ivoiriens face au SIDA: Entre la capote et la fidélité," *Ivoire Dimanche*, March 15, 1987, 8–9.

81. B. A. [Bernard Ahua], "SIDA: L'offensive de l'OMS commence," *Fraternité Matin*, April 9, 1987, 28.

think that if one can abstain from frequenting those people supposed to be AIDS carriers, that would be better because male condoms have been tested. They are not absolutely guaranteed against ripping. . . . Better avoid all risks or minimize them as much as possible [minimiser au maximum]."

In yet another follow-up interview in the April, 12, 1987, edition of *Ivoire Dimanche*, Djédjé Mady sounded almost exasperated about having to repeat his message: "The best plan of action, since you want us to talk about AIDS again, is first, on the level of personal behavior and in sensitization, in sanitary education that must be able to be given to each citizen male and female, so that he [sic] can avoid to the utmost contaminating himself." He refused to consider implementation of any measures that he deemed ineffective and draconian, such as enforced quarantines of people who tested positive for HIV or compulsory medical exams for prostitutes.[82] The Health Minister's assurances effectively located the solution for HIV not in the state, which Djédjé Mady associated with harshly punitive and excessively intrusive measures, but in individual Ivorians educated to recognize the gravity of the epidemic and to demonstrate necessary self-discipline, primarily through changing their sexual behavior. The Ivorians addressed by HIV prevention messages were defined as citizens not through the services provided to them by the government that ensured their well-being but by the exercise of individual will demonstrating their national belonging.[83]

In an April 19, 1987, column a week later, *Moussa* depicted widespread misunderstandings about HIV prevention messages. According to Moussa, some have responded to the threat of AIDS by obeying governmental injunctions and are refraining from sex or are using condoms. Fearing that condoms will break, he advises readers to double-layer them, one on top of another, for added protection. Others laughingly dismiss the threat of AIDS: "AIDS or the clap, we don't care. . . . AIDS or another illness, we're all going to die all the same one day." Moussa recounts the story of a friend, Moucharafou, who meets a woman whose "super ass" makes his penis, or "John Thomas," burst out of his pants. After Moucharafou arranges to meet the woman in a hotel that night, another man warns him that she is known as the "super banger [siper cogneuse]" for having had sex with many men in the neighborhood, so Moucharafou should "take precautions."[84] Moments later, Moucharafou stum-

---

82. Raphaël Lakpé and Kouassi Lambert, "SIDA: Paroles de ministres," *Ivoire Dimanche*, April 12, 1987, 4–7, 5.

83. Lakpé and Lambert, "SIDA," 6.

84. There is no adequate English translation for "siper cogneuse." A footnote translates "cogner," the verb form of the noun "cogneuse," as "faire l'amour," or to have sex, so "siper cogneuse" would translate as someone defined as female who has a lot of sex.

bles upon a vendor of herbal aphrodisiacs who recommends expensive salves and powders. When Moucharafou finally meets the woman, he administers the treatments, which prevent him from attaining an erection. The woman leaves in disgust to go "bang elsewhere [cogné ailleirs]."[85]

The column depicts as comical the urban heterosexual male rivalry and anxiety about women with multiple sexual partners, as well as the failure to understand and correctly put into action HIV prevention messages. The depictions of misinterpretations of HIV prevention messages as sources of entertainment rely on and affirm the superior knowledge of the literate and presumably better-informed readers who understand proper condom usage (e.g., not thinking that doubling condoms would increase their effectiveness) and the references to "precautions." The column represents emasculation and humiliation as hilarious and deserved consequences for the rural bumpkin, or gaou, who does not practice sexual discipline or grasp correct HIV prevention methods and who instead relies on traditional medicines.[86] Much of the humor of the column derives from the irony that the herbal remedy did in fact serve as protection against HIV—it prevented Moucharafou from having sex at all.

Perhaps not surprisingly, the press noted that the public was not responding to HIV prevention messages. Using the mispronounced English term to underscore perceptions of the condom as unfamiliar technology from the United States or Europe, a *Fraternité Matin* article noted in early 1988 that in Africa, "AIDS is transmitted primarily through sexual relations and blood transfusion. The first cause has not much changed couples' sexual behavior, and the 'Koudom' (condom) is still not accepted."[87] The state daily figured "public information and education" as the "new hobbyhorse," in the fight against AIDS, a metaphor that provides some insight into what the article describes as skeptical responses to sexual behavior change, despite USAID's

---

85. "Moussa: Attentionnez-vous beaucoup avec les vendairs de demarairs," *Ivoire Dimanche*, April 19, 1987, 48.

86. The comic strip *Monsieur Zézé*, created in 1978 and also written in nouchi, centered on a poor urban male migrant and similarly portrayed lack of awareness of HIV as a sign of the lack of sophistication of village bumpkins, manual laborers, and Abidjan hoods [loubas d'Abidjan]. S. Bamba, "Les Nouchis," *Ivoire Dimanche*, October 25, 1987, 50; S. Bamba, "Les Nouchis," *Ivoire Dimanche*, November 8, 1987, 49.

87. Léon Francis Lebry, "Lutte contre le Sida: Comment établir un diagnostic fiable?" *Fraternité Matin*, January 19, 1988, 2–3, 2. See also Déniaud, who notes that condoms in Côte d'Ivoire were considered European or American. Déniaud, "Jeunesse et préservatifs," 94.

promise of 3 million condoms: "It will be necessary to convince Ivorians about the systematic use of such a 'cure [remède].'"[88]

CONCLUSION

As early as April 1987, Djédjé Mady had firmly rebuked those who mocked HIV prevention efforts as mere pretexts to control sexual behavior, those who said "that AIDS is an 'imaginary syndrome to discourage lovers.'" As Djédjé Mady responded, "That is unfounded and is spread [fait] just to clown around as it's said [pour amuser la galerie comme on dit]."[89] In 1987, WHO's Global Programme on AIDS funded Côte d'Ivoire's National Committee for the Fight against AIDS [Comité national de lutte contre le Sida (CNLS)] and its National Program for the Fight against AIDS [Programme National de Lutte contre le Sida (PNLS)], and Côte d'Ivoire put the country's first Short-Term Plan into effect.[90] At the end of 1988, the first AIDS prevention poster campaigns enlisted scare tactics to rebuke those who continued to fail to take AIDS seriously. The brightly colored posters with a screaming man clutching his head presumably portrayed the response they hoped to incite: "AIDS is there . . . It kills."[91] At the bottom of the poster, the national symbol, an elephant, literally stamped out AIDS (SIDA) (figure 1.2).

After USAID funded the distribution of 3.5 million free condoms, beginning in late 1988, mostly in Abidjan, the written press increasingly mentioned condoms as essential for HIV prevention and renewed its efforts to

---

88. The article continues: "It is this sexual behavior that it will be necessary to put into action. To know how to choose partners with full knowledge of the facts [C'est sur ce comportement sexuel qu'il faudra mettre l'action. Savoir choisir ses partenaires en connaissance de cause]. In other words, love but taking precautions nevertheless." Lebry, "Lutte contre le Sida: Information et éducation du public: Le nouveau cheval de bataille," *Fraternité Matin*, February 12, 1988, 5. As the director of the CNLS told a convention of religious leaders in August of 1988, to limit the spread of HIV, "it will be necessary [il s'agira] to reduce partners, especially casual partners, avoid anal sex, and maybe above all using [sic] condoms correctly." Lebry, "Convention nationale des Églises baptistes méridonales à Daloa: Vaincre le sida par les enseignments de la Bible," *Fraternité Matin*, August 2, 1988, 6.

89. Raphaël Lakpé and Kouassi Lambert, "SIDA: Paroles des ministres," *Ivoire Dimanche*, April 12, 1987, 4–7, 5.

90. Announced in June 1987, the PNLS Short-Term Plan had as its principal objectives to manage the national institutional and legal response to AIDS, to create an HIV epidemiological surveillance system, to prevent HIV transmission through sexual contact and contact with blood products, and to improve care of people living with HIV/AIDS. Kerouedan, "Lutter contre le sida," 207.

91. The poster echoed the language of a 1986 prevention campaign in Uganda: "Beware of AIDS. AIDS kills." Kaleeba et al., *Open Secret*, 12.

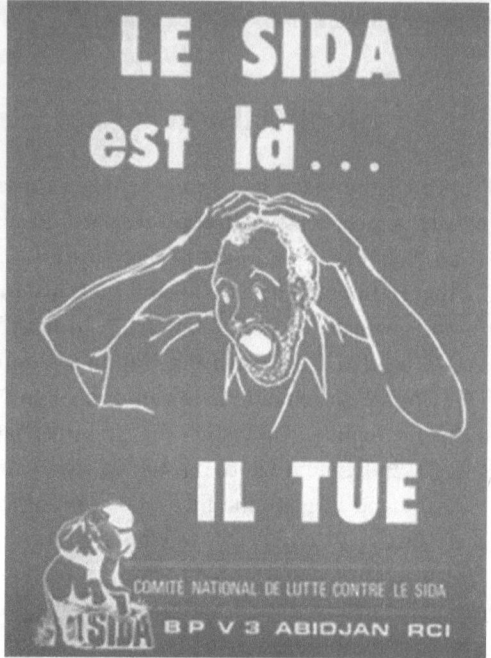

FIGURE 1.2. AIDS is there . . . IT KILLS.

convince the public to stop viewing AIDS as a joke.[92] As virologist Mireille Dosso warned *Ivoire Dimanche* readers, "Until now the illness [AIDS] was in its incubation phase. It could be said that it was imaginary. Now, people are dying of it, whether in our houses, our villages, or our workplaces."[93] As part of the PNLS medium-term AIDS prevention plan, in 1989, the CNLS launched its first official government HIV prevention television campaign, including a special half-hour state television program featuring Ivorian athlete Gabriel Tiacoh. In the program, Tiacoh, seated in front of a television, plays the role of elder brother to young people posing him questions in interviews on the street. Directly addressing the camera, Tiacoh chastises both the young people who pose questions and the television viewers: "You must never say that [AIDS] stands for 'Imaginary Syndrome to Discourage Lovers'" (figure 1.3).

92. Nazaire Breka, "Un Soutien appréciable de l'étranger," *Fraternité Matin*, November 29, 1988, 25. See also Séry and Gozé, "Jeunesse, sexualité et le SIDA," 85. Koné and Agness write that USAID funded distribution of 6 million condoms from 1989 to 1990. Koné and Agness, "La Communication," 322.

93. Yasmina Pauquoud, "Mme Mireille Dosso, agrégée de biologie: En ligne de front contre le Sida," *Ivoire Dimanche*, June 25, 1989, 19.

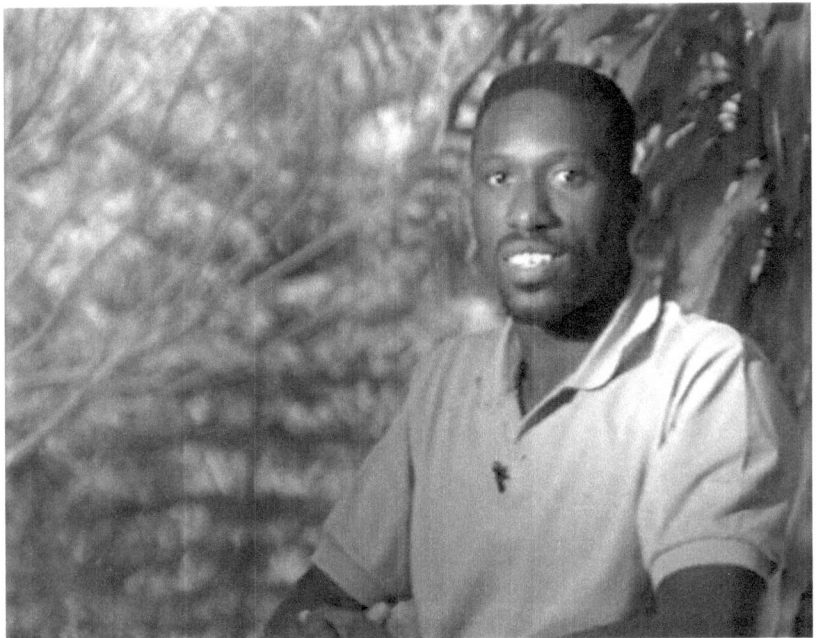

FIGURE 1.3. Ivorian athlete Gabriel Tiacoh.

Images of suffering, emaciated bodies index the truth of AIDS: "Of course AIDS exists. It is a terrible, frightening disease" (figure 1.4).

Additional short television spots broadcast that year feature a young man walking on-screen and then facing the camera. Wagging his finger, he rebukes young male viewers and directs them to stop joking about AIDS: "AIDS is not a joke. It exists. Me, I have to protect myself [Moi, il faut me protéger]. There's no other solution. I use condoms, rubbers, until a vaccine is found. Man, you're warned! [J'utilise les préservatifs, les capotes, en attendant qu'on trouve le vaccin. Man, tu es averti!]" (figure 1.5). A young woman in another spot offers advice to her peers: "AIDS exists. For me, the only solution to protect myself is abstinence." In a third spot, a woman embracing her male partner addresses the camera: "For us, our way of protecting ourselves is trust." Her male partner adds, "And fidelity."

Injunctions such as these presume that jokes about AIDS indicate ignorance about the reality of the virus and the gravity of its effects. A 2005 African Center for Research and Action in Development [Centre Africain de Recherche et d'Intervention en Développement (CARID)] report on behavior change and HIV/AIDS in Côte d'Ivoire similarly attributes the high HIV

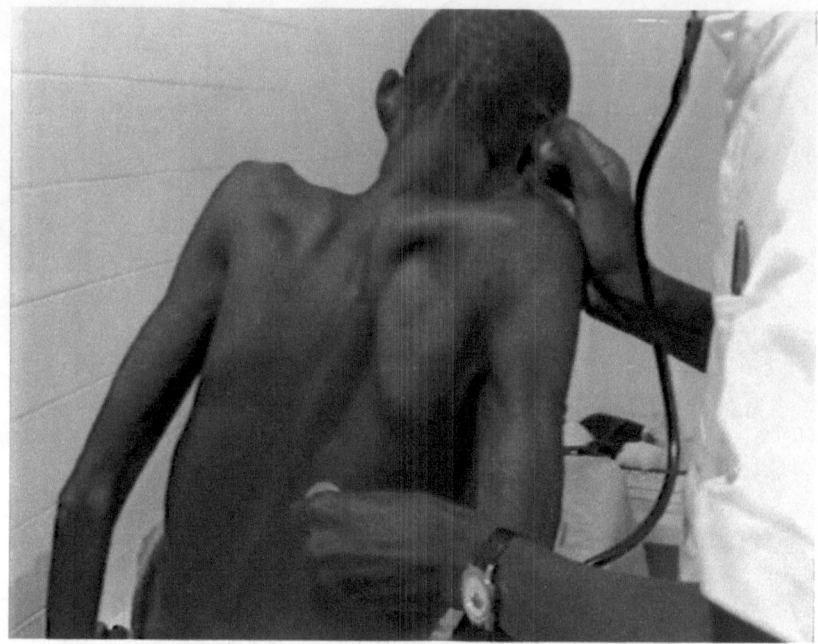

FIGURE 1.4. Emaciated bodies as index of the truth of AIDS.

prevalence in Côte d'Ivoire to the Ivorian government's disengaged response to the epidemic in the early years and to its HIV prevention approach, which emphasized information rather than behavior change. As the report reads, this government response "convinced a significant part of the population of the nonexistence of the illness [HIV/AIDS]. In the popular conscience, AIDS was considered as an imaginary syndrome to discourage lovers. Thus, young people continued to adopt high risk sexual behavior that exposed them to higher risk of HIV infection."[94] The report operates as a morality tale to blame the Ivorian government for the high rates of HIV in the country, with the joke cited about AIDS as "imaginary syndrome to discourage lovers" epitomizing state and public heedlessness and the dire need for implementation of behavior change education.[95]

Like the state's own early AIDS education campaigns, the report does not acknowledge the state press's ambivalent and shifting representations of jokes

---

94. The French "syndrome imaginaire . . ." is a pun on the French for AIDS, *Sida*. Centre Africain de Recherche et d'Intervention en Développement, "Communication pour le changement," 1.

95. Not coincidentally, behavior change communication education is a primary focus of the Johns Hopkins Bloomberg School of Public Health/Center for Communications Programs, a major recipient of USAID funding.

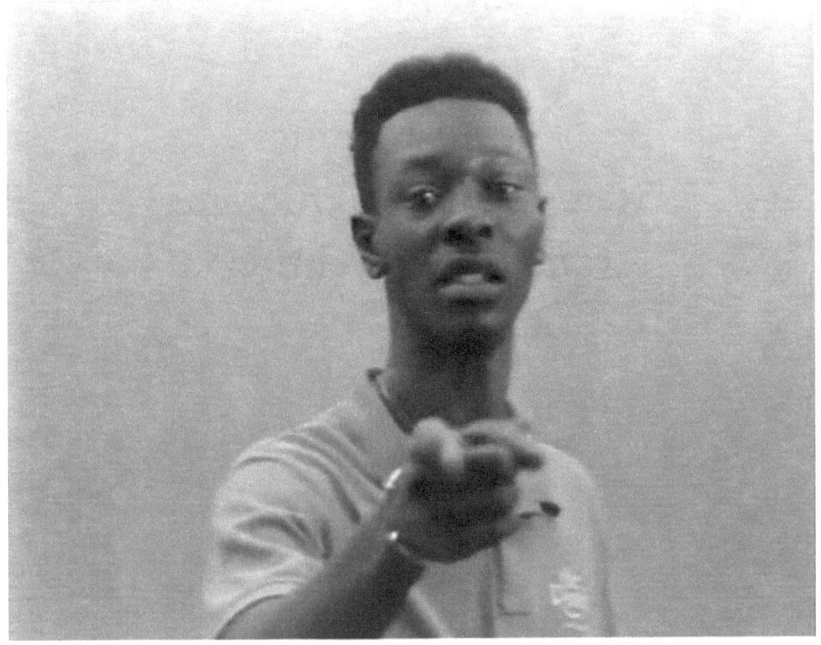

FIGURE 1.5. Television spot: "AIDS is not a joke. It exists."

about AIDS as challenging racialized definitions of the disease and of African sexualities, as well as responding to ongoing debates centered on the terms of modernity, development, and national belonging. *Moussa* represented multiple scenarios in which AIDS and misunderstandings about the virus and methods of prevention were treated as sources of humor rather than alarm. The humor instructed through negative example, with the column's recalcitrant subjects' wayward sexualities evincing the need for individual discipline and paternalistic guidance rather than increased social services. *Moussa* thereby reinforced the production of HIV/AIDS as an issue to be resolved by proper sexual self-management, a moralistic response reflecting the state's own calls for austerity and maturity as solution to economic and political crises. Conformity to austerity measures demonstrated racialized national belonging of responsibilized subjects incorporated into a national narrative of development and progress under the leadership of Houphouët-Boigny. HIV prevention, and jokes about it, did not index ignorance and denialism so much as attempts to negotiate with state and foreign-funder policies and authority. These negotiations similarly extended into humorous television programs, as I discuss in the following chapter.

CHAPTER 2

Popular Satiric State Television Programs and HIV Prevention

LIKE THE humorous *Moussa* column in the state press, satiric programs on state television provided information about HIV/AIDS and commented on HIV prevention campaigns. Treating AIDS as the dire consequence of the failure to take prevention warnings seriously, and as the inspiration for jokes and pranks, shows from the late 1980s to early 1990s veered wildly, contradicting their own messages. Satiric television shows initially coded resistance to HIV prevention as resistance to state policy and threatened AIDS as a punishment. After the country's first president, Félix Houphouët-Boigny, was compelled to hold multiparty elections and to liberalize the state-controlled media in 1990, programs shifted, depicting resistance to HIV prevention as a comically effective strategy to manage female sexual availability. Whether they urged submission to austerity measures or celebrated unruly males' manipulation of HIV prevention campaigns, the shows, like their satiric newspaper counterparts, contained and deflected rising political and economic instability and popular unrest.

This chapter centers on two popular satiric shows that aired on state television: *How's it going?* and *Wintin Wintin and Old Headscarf.* The 1989 "AIDS: The Illness of the Century" episode of *How's it going?* rendered laxity and corruption in the state bureaucracy in sexual terms to emphasize the need for cutbacks and to underscore the dramatic negative consequences of the failure to comply with mandated sexual and economic austerity. In contrast, the

1990 "Joke to Kill" episode of *How's it going?* and the "500 CFA If You Don't Come" *Wintin Wintin and Old Headscarf* skit from the early 1990s depict as hilarious male protagonists (played by Alain Djédjé Tiébé and Léon N'Cho Assamoi, respectively, discussed later in this chapter) who subvert and openly defy HIV prevention messages. Significantly, in the later episodes, the men's defiance was directed not against the state or foreign funders but against their female sexual partners represented as dictating the terms of economic and (hetero)sexual exchanges with their male partners. Effectively displacing any resistance to state policies, the later shows' comic staging of gender conflict defuse any suggestion that humorous or defiant responses to HIV prevention messages might challenge government policies and, therefore, the authority of the state. The later shows identify women as ultimately unsuccessful agents of HIV prevention and affirm a recalcitrant male heterosexuality at the expense of female characters, who serve as the target of the episodes' humor.

In their satiric approach to contemporary social issues, shows such as *How's it going?* and *Wintin Wintin and Old Headscarf* might productively be read as examples of koteba performance. Accounts of koteba differ in their descriptions of the performances, which vary across time and region, but some of the most relevant attributes for this discussion include its central focus on satire.[1] According to anthropologists working primarily in Mali, koteba performances with masks and marionettes representing mythical figures feature in large public festivities. However, another strand of performance (accounts differ as to whether they are performed for the same or for different occasions) include satiric sketches with stock characters: the Cuckold, the Unfaithful Wife, the Foreigner, and the Con Man; and, beginning in the colonial period, the Corrupt Police Officer, the Interpreter, the Boastful City Boy, the Arriviste, and so forth.[2] The plays provide popular entertainment but also often serve instructional and mediating purposes, resolving conflicts or chastising community members for improper behavior. As Anny Wynchank writes, "The objective [of koteba] is to entertain [divertir] but also to teach; in making fun [faisant rire aux dépens] of the ridiculous and of social vices, koteba fulfills didactic, moral, and social functions."[3]

The various targets of koteba are specifically gendered: According to one account, through satire and parody in koteba performances, young men (who acted, drummed, and danced, while women served in the chorus) expressed frustration about rigid age hierarchies and their social status relative to the older men in the community. In another account particularly relevant for this

---

1. Haffner, *Essai sur les fondements*, 63.
2. Okagbue, *African Theatres and Performances*, 136.
3. Wynchank, "Persistance du théâtre populaire."

chapter, laughter, satire, and mocking are aimed at women through a "certain at times cruel, often disparaging 'vulgarity.'"[4] In neither case, however, did the lampooning disrupt larger societal frameworks. As Alioune Sow argues about the incorporation of koteba theatrical traditions into Malian television, in koteba, "Satire and derision are acceptable and privileged ways of dealing with critical or tragic moments in history."[5] Rather than challenge the status quo, koteba performances represent the restoration of a social order that they hope through the productions themselves to initiate. Osita Okagbue describes koteba plays he attended in Markala, Mali, as following the same structure: "Harmony and a state of equilibrium, but in the course of the action this state was severely threatened by the actions of some of the characters—disharmony and dis-equilibrium reigned momentarily—but in the end a state of harmony and equilibrium was restored."[6] Recognizing the potential usefulness of koteba in health education, the United States–based Population Services International in 1993 produced a three-part koteba television series promoting family planning services in Mali.[7]

Koteba performances have also been incorporated into the dramatic arts in Côte d'Ivoire. The well-known Koteba Theater, founded by the late Souleymane Koly in Abidjan in 1974, was part of a rich tradition of public performances that educated through humor. Like other playwrights in the 1970s, including Bernard Dadié, Germain Coffi Gadeau, and Bernard Zadi Zaourou, Koly viewed language itself as central to his performances and incorporated "Moussa's French" and, later, nouchi into productions.[8] Such approaches were also incorporated into television in Côte d'Ivoire, especially as the state ramped up its more formal educational programming. The producer and lead actor of *How's it going?*, Léonard Groguhet, was the most prominent early star of humorous educational programs produced to promote state policies. In a 1975 interview published in the state weekly journal *Ivoire Dimanche*, Groguhet explicitly aligned himself with the country's only television station at the time, the state-controlled Ivorian Radio and Television (RTI), and there-

---

4. Haffner, *Essai sur les fondements*, 63.
5. Sow, "Alternating Views."
6. Okagbue, *African Theatres and Performances*, 137, 168.
7. Kane et al., "The Impact of a Family Planning Multimedia Campaign." See also Pagézy, "Le Théâtre *koteba*."
8. Kwahulé, *Pour une Critique*, 208–9. The use of nouchi in the theater provoked debate. A 1989 conference organized by the Ivorian Committee of the Alliance Française centered on the theme, "What Aspects of the French Language in the Ivoirian Theatre dans l'univers du théâtre ivoiren." A round table at the conference focused on the question: "Moussa's French, for or against? [Le français de Moussa, pour ou contre?]." Jusu K. K. Man, "Alliance française: Des Journées culturelles pour promouvoir le français," *Fraternité Matin*, March 17, 1989, 20.

fore with the state itself: "My objectives are joined [s'intègrent] with those of RTI. Nobody is unaware of the power of audiovisual media on populations. In exploiting the possibilities of this mass media, one can play a leading educational role."[9] *Ivoire Dimanche* similarly described *Wintin Wintin and Old Headscarf* in August 1985: "Wintin Wintin and Old Headscarf propose to entertain television viewers even as they hope that the viewers will also perceive the deeper meaning of the issues tackled [tout en espérant qu'ils sauront aussi percevoir le sens profond des thèmes abordés] . . . education and public-spiritedness, for example. . . . They tear down the delusions of grandeur of certain of their fellow citizens . . . and make people laugh while at the same time they moralize [faire rigoler tout en moralisant]."[10]

Houphouët-Boigny allowed the airing of satiric sketches that never explicitly targeted him or his party, the Democratic Party of Côte d'Ivoire-African Democratic Rally [Parti democratique de la Côte d'Ivoire- Rassemblement démocratique africain (PDCI)], just as he orchestrated "days of dialogue" to demonstrate his openness. He was able to point to satiric shows as evidence of freedom of speech under his reign and of his responsiveness to popular demands. In a conference criticizing foreign journalists, Auguste Miremont, the director of the editorial office of the state daily, *Fraternité Matin*, acknowledged that the Ivorian press served the interests of the PDCI. However, he pointed to Groguhet's *How's it going?* to underscore that the Ivorian media enjoyed "wide latitude in the assessment of social phenomenon [grande marge de manoeuvre dans l'appréciation des faits de société]."[11] Although cited as proof of the openness of the Houphouët-Boigny regime, the satires never openly targeted Houphouët-Boigny and the PDCI. Airing on state television, satiric programs were entangled with the state and actively promoted state policies—or faced the threat of repression.

Satiric shows such as *How's it going?* and *Wintin Wintin and Old Headscarf* were part of state educational television programming, which historically had been integral to nation-building projects. From its inception, television in Côte d'Ivoire promoted agendas determined not only by a single-party state under Houphouët-Boigny but also by bilateral and multilateral funders, especially the French government. In Côte d'Ivoire, the institution of the Educational Television Program [Programme d'Éducation Télévisuelle (PETV)],

---

9. "Léonard Groguhet: Un retour fracassant," *Ivoire Dimanche*, May 11, 1975, 2.

10. Am Atta, "Wintin-Wintin Pierre et Vieux-Foulard: Rire à tout casser," *Ivoire Dimanche*, August 25, 1985, 4–7, 7.

11. Paul Bouabré, "La Presse a un rôle de levier dans les pays en voie de développement," *Fraternité Matin*, February 7, 1989, 4. See also Jean-Paul Abissa, "La Presse ivoirienne, un rôle de soutien et de critique," *Fraternité Matin*, August 18, 1988, 5.

which broadcast for more than a decade (from 1971 to 1982), served as particularly important precedents for the country's later educational television efforts centered on HIV prevention. As an example of uneven state and foreign funder collaborations to educate the public, PETV and the controversies that it engendered informed later educational programming even after the program's demise. Before discussing the satiric shows, I will therefore provide some background on PETV and the conflicts it generated.

PETV

As in most of the continent, television and film in Côte d'Ivoire were instituted to serve primarily educational purposes in order to further national development.[12] In 1965, Houphouët-Boigny had announced that "the advancement and education [la promotion et la formation] of men [sic] must be understood as simultaneously method and goal [fin] of development."[13] The 1968–70 national plans identified televised educational planning as integral to national development and modernization inseparable from the formation of national identity. In 1968, the Ivorian Minister of Information outlined the mission of the media:

> The overall current mission of the informational media [La grande mission actuelle de l'information] in our country is to contribute to:
>
> 1. the development [la progression] of national identification [du sentiment national] in contrast to atavistic regionalism;
> 2. the transformation of the mentality of citizens;
> 3. the overall [globale] education of the masses.[14]

Côte d'Ivoire had been one of the first countries in Africa to install television stations and had made national coverage a priority. With French support, the Ivorian government established a radio and television service, Radiodiffusion Télévision Ivoirienne (RTI), in 1962.[15] By 1963, RTI had begun broadcasting to a small radius in Abidjan five and a half hours a week. A third of the Western region had television reception by 1965, and educational television programming further expanded television viewership throughout the country, with almost 70% of villages receiving service by 1972. By 1983, when a second national channel, TV2, began broadcasting, 60% of the country had television

---

12. Tudesq, "La Télévision," 242; Tozzo, "La Réforme des médias publics," 101.
13. République de Côte d'Ivoire, et al., *Actualisation du programme*, 18.
14. Laurent, "Formation, information et développement," 430.
15. Land, "Ivorien Television," 12.

reception, and by 1990, 90%.[16] Early educational television in Côte d'Ivoire included workers' literacy programs initiated by factories, Chambers of Commerce, and the Ministry of Education, with French technical assistance (and most funding from UNESCO and UNICEF, as well as France). Literacy programs from 1963 to 1966 included closed-circuit television programs broadcast on RTI. In 1967, the Ministry of Youth and Popular Education produced a program for rural populations. The program addressed health, among other issues, and in 1968, the Ivorian government began airing what became known as Radio-Télé-Bac, a television and radio program designed to prepare students who had failed high school examinations.[17]

The government's efforts corresponded with global projects enlisting television as an educational technology. In an updated version of colonialism's civilizing mission, in 1960, UNESCO declared that "a substantial mass of illiterates is incompatible with the development of civilization and the maintenance of peace" and that education constitutes "the most urgent and vital need in Africa today."[18] UNESCO encouraged "the use of mass communication techniques in education" and "the use of audio-visual materials in education, science and culture" in Africa, as well as in Latin America and Asia.[19] In 1964, UNESCO funded programs in Niger, American Samoa, and El Salvador, all of which became models for Côte d'Ivoire's PETV. Multilateral funders viewed the founding of PETV as by far the largest and most ambitious such undertaking in the world: USAID considered PETV a "unique venture" in television education programming, part of a pedagogical television project that UNESCO touted as a global model, and the World Bank, as a "pilot effort."[20] With funding from UNESCO, the World Bank, and the French and Canadian governments, the Ivorian government in 1969 constructed a Complex for Televisual Education [Complexe d'Education Télévisuelle (CETV)] in Bouaké, which UNESCO claimed was the best-equipped educational television center in the world.[21] Technologically, administratively, and pedagogically, educational television simultaneously facilitated and signified the attainment of modernity and modernization for Côte d'Ivoire.[22] It was the instrument whose

16. Tudesq, "La Télévision en Côte d'Ivoire," 244–45. Tudesq, *Les Médias en Afrique*, 122.
17. Yao, "Communication Technology Transfer," 135, 139–40.
18. UNESCO, 11th Session of the General Conference Resolution 1.2322.
19. UNESCO, 11th Session of the General Conference Resolution 5.131; 5.132.
20. Evans and Klees, *ETV Program Production*, 53; Égly, *Télévision didactique*, 60; World Bank, *Republic of Ivory Coast*, 10.
21. Égly, "L'Utilisation de la Télévision Scolaire," 242.
22. Aghi Bahi details how new information technology and education continue to inform young people's imaginings of modernity in Abidjan. Bahi, "Jeunes et imaginaire." See also Land, "Ivorien [sic] Television."

implementation, almost as much as its actual effects, represented what the state and its funders framed as the country's progress toward and achievement of development.[23]

PETV began broadcasting to first-year primary school students in the fall of 1971, initially to 447 schools (about 20,000 students) but added additional schools and grades each year until by 1977, 2,268 schools were receiving daily instruction in French in six to eight 5- to 10-minute segments, first in French, math, and social studies and, later, in civics, geography, physics, history, and biology.[24] In primary school especially, French received particular emphasis, since it was not the first language of most students.[25] Teachers also acquired training via television programming, and new printed school textbook materials were developed to complement the telelessons. Initially run by the Ministry of National Education, PETV in 1972 was incorporated into a new Ministry of Primary and Televisual Education, the first such ministry in the world.[26]

PETV, THE FRENCH, AND *TV FOR ALL*

In 1969, Côte d'Ivoire devoted around 3.7% of the gross domestic product to education (a proportion increasing to around 6.6% by 1970), an education that was aimed at producing a loyal, technocratic elite and encouraging economic development defined as "modernization of agriculture, promotion of rural areas, and Ivoirization of the economy."[27] Through PETV, the Ivorian government further sought to decrease wide gaps in quality of instruction and in school exam passing rates in rural and urban areas, as well as to redress

---

23. The goals of Ivorian radio and mass media did not differ so radically from other national media. Stuart Hall's comments about the impact of the BBC are strikingly relevant: "It was an instrument, an apparatus, a 'machine' through which the nation was constituted. It produced the nation which it addressed; it constructed its audience by the ways in which it represented them." Stuart Hall, as quoted in Morley and Robins, *Spaces of Identity*, 32.

24. Tudesq, "La Télévision," 244. The World Bank notes that among the programs that its evaluators viewed in early 1979, only one program lasted nine minutes; all others lasted less than five. World Bank, *Project Performance Audit Report*, 10.

25. In Côte d'Ivoire during the broadcast of PETV, the educational system followed that of the French: six years of primary school followed by competitive exam for secondary school admission. Secondary school was divided into a four-year first cycle and then a three-year second cycle, terminating in the baccalaureate exam.

26. Le Président de la République, Decrèt no. 72-555 du 28 août 1972 fixant les attributions du Secrétaire d'État chargé de l'enseignement primaire et de la télévision éducative et portant organization du Secrétariat d'État. Égly, *Télévision didactique*, 61.

27. République de Côte d'Ivoire et al., *Actualisation du programme*, 19; Akindès, "La Côte d'Ivoire," 8.

gendered differentials in schooling.[28] Another of PETV's central mandates was to impart "cultural unification," a national identity through a shared mode of communication, which the 1960 Ivorian constitution's first article succinctly defined: "The official language is French." PETV's creation and operation were financed by external funders: primarily France, and UNESCO, the World Bank, Canada, the United States, Belgium, and Germany.[29] The French government provided more than half of total PETV funding and the majority of financing for all production and reception equipment produced in France and exported to Côte d'Ivoire.[30] All televisions, as well as their batteries for use in non-electrified rural areas, were imported from France by a private Franco-Ivorian company, African Television Company (Compagnie Africaine de Télévision [CATEL]).[31] French investment in Ivorian educational television, in terms of provision of personnel and equipment and in the promotion of French language and education, helped to secure the continued cultural and economic dominance of the former colonial power, even as PETV promoted national identity and development.[32]

---

28. République de Côte d'Ivoire et al., *Actualisation du programme*, 1.

29. The French (through the Fund for Assistance and Cooperation [Fonds d'aide et de coopération (FAC)]) provided technical assistance for TV production, maintenance, evaluation, out-of-school assistance, and administration, as well as of initial receiver installation and production equipment. UNESCO, UNDP, and UNICEF provided technical assistance for administration, teacher training, data processing, and evaluation of out-of-school education, as well as funding for some initial studio facilities and equipment. The World Bank provided technical assistance for evaluation and management, loans for half the cost of the new TV complex, and funding for studies of the program. The Canadian government through the Canadian International Development Agency provided technical assistance in the development and printing of written materials and in administration, and funded some equipment and operations expenses. The United States (through United States Aid for International Development [USAID]) provided technical assistance for program evaluation. West Germany and Belgium provided study grants (also provided by the UN, France, and Canada) and backup academic support. Kaye, "Ivory Coast Educational Television Project," 156. From 1969 to 1980, the French contributed by far the most foreign funds: 10.1 billion CFA francs out of 17.2 billion CFA francs total foreign funding. The Ivorian government contributed 45.1 billion (all in 1980 CFA francs). Ivorian contributions to ETV financing increased steadily from 22.9% in 1969 to 1970, to 58.1% in 1974, to 90.6% in 1980. Service centrale de l'organisation de la gestion de l'éducation (SCOGE), "Coût de l'enseignment primaire du PETV," as quoted in Koné and Jenkins, "The Programme for Educational Television," 88.

30. Koné and Jenkins, "The Programme for Educational Television," 80; Via FAC, France provided 1.5 billion CFA of 2 billion CFA, or about three-quarters of funding for equipment between 1969 and 1973. République de Côte d'Ivoire et al., *Actualisation du programme*, 170; Benveniste, "Côte-d'Ivoire," 476.

31. Yao, "Communication Technology Transfer," 252.

32. Koné and Jenkins, "The Programme for Educational Television," 87, 89; Benveniste, "Côte-d'Ivoire," 476; Yao, "Communication Technology Transfer," 260–61.

In the early years of PETV, foreigners composed more than half of total PETV civil service personnel—27 versus 14 in 1970—but those numbers shifted by 1975 when 107 foreign technical assistants (a significant number were young French men fulfilling military obligations by working at the complex) and 179 Ivorian functionaries constituted the nonlaborer personnel.[33] Foreign assistants produced, directed, and wrote the majority of PETV programs until 1974, when the numbers were almost even, although rough estimates indicate only about half of the French technical assistants had any formal training in their area of specialization.[34] Only 35 of 105 total educators and trainers [animateurs] involved in the training of teachers at the Center of Educational and Teacher Training [Centres d'Animation et de Formation Pédagogique] for primary school teacher training in 1973 were Ivorian nationals.[35] Significantly, regardless of how the actual make-up of PETV staff shifted since its founding, PETV was perceived as run by outsiders, and *TV for All* as "white people's business [une affaire des blancs]."[36]

Televisions sets themselves were expensive, with individual ownership limited to the relatively wealthy, and the Ivorian government distributed over 17,000 sets to schools and community centers throughout the country.[37] By 1980, teleclasses reached 651,743 students, or 80% of schoolchildren.[38] To maximize use and justify the expense of television distribution, RTI; the ministers of Primary Education and Educational Television, Health and Agriculture; and the National Office of the Promotion of Rural Areas [L'Office national de la promotion rurale] all collaborated to use the school televisions to broadcast out-of-school television [télévision extrascolaire] programming produced by CETV. Out-of-school education began as part of teacher training in 1972, but in 1973, *Télé pour tous* [*TV for All*] for adults and young people not attending school began broadcasting mostly in rural areas.[39] *TV for All* had as the central

---

33. Evans and Klees, *ETV Program Production*, 16, 62.

34. However, in 1974, almost seven times more funding was spent on foreign personnel (there were 188 foreign personnel in 1975, mainly French) and lodging than on Ivorian personnel (64 versus 418 million CFA). Evans and Klees, *ETV Program Production*, 16, 62; Hawkridge, *General Operational Review*, 2. Ivorian producers earned about 1.5 million CFA compared to the 5 million CFA that a French producer earned (including housing and traveling allowances). Evans and Klees, *ETV Program Production*, 16, 62. The proportion of foreign personnel began to shift from 1977 to 1978, when French technicians constituted eight, and Ivorian national civil servants eighteen, of the CETV management. Evans and Klees, *ETV Program Production*, 10.

35. République de Côte d'Ivoire et al., *Actualisation du programme*, 211.

36. Benveniste, "Côte-d'Ivoire," 473.

37. Yao, 133. Of households in Abidjan, 24% had televisions in 1977, 13% in other cities, and very few in the villages. Tudesq, *Le Télévision*, 244.

38. Pauvert and Egly, *Le "Complexe" de Bouaké 1967–1981*, 20.

39. Pauvert and Egly, *Le "Complexe,"* 25; Lenglet, "Educational Television," 157–59.

objective of its "educational message" the promotion of economic development or, as the Secretary of State of Primary Education put it, "to emphasize information and education [la sensibilisation] of the entire population about development policy, to participate in the improvement of their conditions and in the better distribution of the fruits of economic production [fruits économiques]."[40]

The once- or twice-weekly half-hour evening programs aired Wednesday and Fridays after the evening news and provided instruction on subjects related to economic and social development, including tourism, coffee and cocoa production, and filtering water.[41] The programs were considered a tool of various government ministries and were linked to governmental development projects (e.g., on rice production and on farming cooperatives) and to campaigns, including those related to health.[42] In 1974, *TV for All* administration was relocated from Bouaké to Abidjan for closer collaboration with relevant ministries and development agencies. In rural areas, the programs were broadcast in the schools equipped with televisions, and though the shows were in French, "animators"—generally male primary schoolteachers—translated the shows and facilitated discussion on-site.[43] From 1975 to 1976, 899 television schools had animators. Accounts of the actual number of adult viewers vary, with about 15,500 per broadcast with animators to 300,000 regular viewers.[44]

DEMISE OF PETV

Criticism of PETV from both teachers and parents began almost immediately after its first broadcast.[45] Former UNESCO advisers to PETV dismiss the criticism as reactionary resistance, "irrational negative factors that always accompany new undertakings [les entreprises novatrices]."[46] They accuse the union

---

40. Secrétariat d'État à l'Enseignment Primaire, as quoted in Benveniste, "Côte-d'Ivoire," 467. These objectives shifted annually and were modified in 1975 to state that the programs should familiarize Ivorians "with the economic, political and administrative structure, and to motivate them to make use of the services these structures offer" and "to promote awareness and analysis of existing situations and to search for solutions to the problem of integration into the modern world, without abandoning certain traditional values." Lenglet, "Educational Television," 159.
41. Touré and Munier, "Primary Education by Television," 309.
42. Benveniste, "Côte-d'Ivoire," 468.
43. Tudesq, "Le Télévision," 244; Klees, *Cost Analysis*, iii; Lenglet, "Educational Television," 157, 159.
44. Klees, *Cost Analysis*, iii, iv, 84.
45. Koné and Jenkins, "The Programme for Educational Television," 90.
46. Pauvert and Egly, *Le "Complexe,"* 38.

of secondary schoolteachers and the parents who protested against PETV of misunderstanding both programming costs and the role of foreigners in PETV administration.[47] However, criticism of PETV, which exploded in *Fraternité Matin* in August and early September of 1980, signified more than just unhappiness with televised education. Debates about PETV were entangled in broader struggles around education as a vehicle for upward class mobility, the role of the French in the country, and Houphouët-Boigny's control over teachers' unions.

While the Houphouët-Boigny regime controlled most of the country's professional associations, including those of journalists, doctors, and primary schoolteachers, the union of secondary schoolteachers (Syndicat National des enseignants du Second Degré [SYNESCI]) and the union for teachers in higher education (Syndicat national de la recherche et de l'enseignement supérieur [SYNARES]) proved more intractable.[48] The primary schoolteachers' union had historic links to the PDCI even before independence, but in 1970, both SYNESCI and SYNARES had outright rejected PDCI control, and Houphouët-Boigny ordered the arrest and imprisonment of their secretary-generals. Laurent Gbagbo, an opposition leader who became president after contested boycotted elections in 2000 and who was finally forced from office in 2011, was a leader of SYNARES and among those imprisoned in the early 1970s. University students supported the associations' independence, and escalating conflicts between the Houphouët-Boigny regime, SYNESCI, and SYNARES throughout the 1970s provided the backdrop for formal protests against PETV during SYNESCI's tenth annual congress in late July 1980.[49]

On August 5, 1980, *Fraternité Matin* published SYNESCI's denouncement of PETV for its failures in educating children despite its high costs. As the paper reported, during its congress held the week before, SYNESCI moved to decide that PETV be suppressed "before generations of Ivorians are culturally and intellectually sacrificed."[50] Responding angrily to the SYNESCI declara-

---

47. Pauvert and Egly, Le *"Complexe,"* 24.

48. Jeanne Maddox Toungara reads Houphouët-Boigny's assimilation of dissent as a tactic deployed by Akan chiefs. See Toungara, "The Apotheosis." Marcel Amondji criticizes Houphouët-Boigny's concessions to the French as inaugurating neocolonialism in Côte d'Ivoire. Amondji, *Côte d'Ivoire*.

49. Woods, "The Politicization of Teachers' Associations," 117.

50. "Motion relative au système de l'enseignement télévisuel," *Fraternité Matin*, August 5, 1980, 3. See also Désalmand, "Une Aventure ambiguë," 94. "Sacrificed Generation" later became the title of a popular 1997 Zouglou song and album by Les Salopards that aired students' protests about the failures of the education system and the effects of the economic crises following structural adjustment in the 1980s on young people. For a discussion of the song, see Schumann, "A Generation of Orphans," 540–41.

tion, a group of primary school inspectors invited public debate on television education.[51] Dwayne Woods argues that the debates over PETV were particularly significant because they demonstrated the PDCI's waning control over dissident organizations such as the teachers' unions that were able to mobilize public opinion and force the government to change its education policy.[52] But the outpouring of public criticism of PETV as solicited and published by the state media did not in itself instigate the government to take action. During one of his "Days of Dialogue" in September 1978, Houphouët-Boigny had already posed the question, "I wonder whether schools television ought not be done away with," and, significantly, foreign investors were scheduled to withdraw all financing from PETV in 1980.[53] As Paul Désalmand argues, the Ivorian government, confronting economic crisis after the fall of prices of its primary export crops, was increasingly burdened by PETV costs (almost 90% of total funding in 1980) and used the public discontent as a pretext to clear itself of responsibility to international funders.[54] The publication of hostile responses to PETV and the curtailing of televised lessons in October (by 30%) further evidenced Houphouët-Boigny's carefully orchestrated "new democracy."[55]

In 1980, the government had instituted a series of political and economic reforms, including the closure or privatization of a number of state-owned companies and the organizing of the country's first competitive legislative elections (though all candidates were still members of the PDCI), as well as the fifth presidential election, with Houphouët-Boigny once again the sole candidate.[56] The publication of the protests against PETV also coincided with the publication of students' secondary school entrance exam results. By permitting and even instigating the debates in the country's sole daily newspaper, the state signaled its apparent openness both to SYNESCI and to parents frustrated by their children's failure to pass the exams or to obtain places in secondary school. The cutbacks of televised lessons in 1980, and the demise

---

51. "Les Inspecteurs de l'enseignement primaire: Un système aux qualités reconnues," *Fraternité Matin*, August 5, 1980, 3.

52. Woods, "The Politicization," 118–19.

53. As Joseph W. Campbell notes, dissenting opinions could not be articulated in the state-owned press, but only through the days of dialogue whose "grandiloquent, if contrived and unwieldy mechanisms" managed and co-opted opposition. However, Campbell argues that such dialogues could not quite manage the opposition that they sought to control; they created the conditions of possibility for what eventually became independent journalism in Côte d'Ivoire. J. Campbell, *The Emergent Independent Press*, 78; Koné and Jenkins, "The Programme for Educational Television," 90; Yao, "Communication Technology Transfer," 141.

54. Désalmand, "Une Aventure," 94.

55. Yao, "Communication Technology Transfer," 129, 150–51.

56. Fauré, "Democracy and Realism," 315–16.

of PETV at the end of the following school year in June 1982, represented seeming concessions in response to the public protest.[57] The publication of the debates could be characterized, then, not so much as gains by a strengthening opposition but as what Jeanne Maddox Toungara describes as part of Houphouët-Boigny's strategy of negotiation and reconciliation: the initiation of dialogue to gauge and manage public opinion in order to better consolidate his power.[58]

In any event, critiques leveled against PETV did not necessarily index critique of the government. Laurence Proteau maintains that educational television became so contentious an issue because SYNESCI teachers sought to preserve benefits, such as free housing and higher salaries than those granted to other government employees (though in *Fraternité Matin*, SYNESCI complained that secondary schoolteachers received less pay than their primary school counterparts[59]). Threatened downgrading of special advantages reflected an overall degradation of their status further damaged by their having been implicated in a high school exam cheating scandal from 1979 to 1980.[60] Similarly, parents protested against PETV because it threatened their children's attainment of coveted government posts. From the colonial period, the mostly male African elite achieved and maintained their privileged status as *évolués* [the evolved] through education, especially university degrees. As Basile Ndijio notes, during the colonial period, the term referred to the "educated natives" of Francophone Africa who adopted the language, culture, and values of the West.[61] After independence, the state was able to exercise its control over social stratification and class formation through differential educational resource allocation and access that created and perpetuated deep social and economic inequalities. Proteau describes how educational capital enabled accumulation of critical economic and political capital, and lower-middle-class parents perceived PETV as threatening their "access to educational resources as a privileged mode of social reproduction."[62] The protests, then, articulated not so much opposition to a single-party state but objections to its failure to better incorporate them into its civil service and to provide the financial, material, and social benefits that historically had accrued to the formally educated.

---

57. Yao, "Communication Technology Transfer," 151.
58. Toungara, "The Apotheosis," 36–37.
59. R. Diodan, "Fin du 10ᵉ Congrès du SYNESCI: Les Enseignants du secondaire demandent le relèvement du salaire des décisionnaires," *Fraternité Matin*, August 1, 1980, 4.
60. Proteau, *Passions scolaires*, 77–78.
61. Ndjio, "Evolués and Feyman," 207.
62. Proteau, *Passions scolaires*, 75.

After the implementation of PETV, promotion to successive grades in primary school became essentially *pro forma* rather than reliant on annual exams. However, an average of only 15% of students passed the required secondary school entrance exam to gain admission to public school sixth class (middle school) throughout the 1970s.[63] Even students who passed the initial secondary school entrance exams were not guaranteed a place, as the government did not commit necessary resources to accommodate the influx of students and had in fact halted all construction of postprimary schools after 1978.[64] Hugues Koné and Janet Jenkins note that one of the "unspoken goals" of PETV was to restrict secondary school and university to the elite.[65] The elite sent their children abroad or to local private schools, thereby avoiding televised lessons entirely. That these children performed much better on selective secondary school entrance exams only reinforced the perception that PETV was part of a conspiracy to exclude the aspiring lower-middle classes from accessing educational credentials that in the past had essentially guaranteed civil service posts and attendant upward class mobility.[66]

Perspectives from rural villages were, significantly, never represented in debates around PETV published in *Fraternité Matin*, although USAID and the World Bank did conduct a number of detailed studies of PETV and the out-of-school program, *Télévision extra-scolaire*. Their assessments were harshly critical of the inability of *TV for All* producers to recognize the needs and realities of the peasants in the programs that were meant to educate them.[67] A World Bank report appraised PETV in stinging terms: "Although evaluation studies showed some positive outcomes, the project has 'sunk without a trace' and educators say that never was so much wasted, including Bank funds, on such poor television broadcasts with so little effect. This project coloured attitudes towards distance education throughout the international aid and lending community."[68]

---

63. Again, Ivorian schools followed (and continue to follow) the French system. At the time of PETV broadcasting, primary school encompassed the following: Cours préparatoire (preparatory class) 1, CP2; Cours élémentaire (elementary class) 1, CE2; Cours moyen (middle class) 1, CM2. Lower secondary school began with the sixth class. At the end of the six years of primary school, students were required to take an exam to obtain a primary school certificate (Certificat d'Études Primaires Elementaires [CEPE]) and an additional exam to continue to lower secondary school (concours d'entrée en sixième).

64. Proteau, *Passions scolaires*, 74.

65. Koné and Jenkins, "The Programme for Educational Television," 87.

66. Désalmand, "Une Aventure," 95. Proteau, *Passions scolaires*, 75.

67. Interestingly, a 1975 survey of animators and of participants in *TV for All* indicated that participants were particularly interested in programming on health. Evans and Klees, *ETV Program Production*, 8, 10.

68. Hawkridge, *General Operational Review*, 2.

PETV ended broadcasts in 1982, but educational television itself had become a source of contention not only over educational policy but also over broader questions of national identity, modernity, and development. Educational television further generated debates over allocation of resources, the role of the French in the country, increasing economic inequalities, and Houphouet-Boigny's dictatorship. French, the language supposed to maintain national unity, was the language of the former colonizers, but rather than unify the rural and urban and the diverse linguistic groups within the boundaries of the new nation, it exacerbated divisions between those able to speak French, in other words, those with formal schooling, and those without.[69] It also aggravated distinctions between the South, where children tended to attend school and leave rural areas for administrative positions in the cities, and the North, where children tended to be incorporated into traditional family production as traders, sharecroppers, and apprentices.[70] Television, the instrument of modernity intended to communicate and maintain Ivorian cultural identity and convey the state's vision of development in effect exacerbated dependence on French and American technology and further enabled the dissemination of American and French television programs to Ivorian audiences.[71] Significantly, the first AIDS cases in Côte d'Ivoire were reported in 1985, only three years after the termination of PETV. The larger questions and controversies that PETV generated did not merely evaporate but persisted and extended into television programming promoting HIV prevention.

"EDUCATED THROUGH LAUGHTER": "AIDS"

At the same time that PETV broadcast its school programming, the state channel aired humorous programs that conveyed educational messages. The

---

69. Benveniste, "Côte-d'Ivoire," 476–78. On French schooling during the colonial period and its emphasis on the teaching of the French language, see Suret-Canale, *French Colonialism*, 381.

70. Dembélé, "La Construction," 142.

71. The government controlled RTI until December 27, 1991, when it became a public company with independent financing, and in 1992 it became a semipublic company, with the state still controlling 98%. Tudesq, *Les Médias en Afrique*, 117. In 1993, Comstat, a U.S. company, financed 85% of the renovation of existing satellites and the construction of additional satellites to extend the reach of television in the country, thus creating a shift from technical dependence on France (122). In 1985, 38.15% of programs broadcast on Channel 1 were produced abroad, but 77.8% of entertainment shows and films and 22% of cultural programming were imported, 54.6% from France and 30.65% from the United States. In 2000, 50.5% of television programming on Channel 1 on RTI was produced in Côte d'Ivoire. On Channel 2 (created in 1983), only 27.6% of programs were Ivorian productions. Tudesq, "Télévision en Côte d'Ivoire," 249–50.

satiric shows mocked the solemnity of the didactic mode of the more formal educational televisions but also reinforced their lessons. By 1975, a program Groguhet had created, *We Won the Case* [*On a gagné affaire*], had become *How is it going?*—a title that echoes that of Roger Gnoan M'Bala's 1972 humorous short film, *Amanie*, which translates from Baoulé as "How is it going?" or "How are you? [Comment ça va?]." The series offered extended comic fictional scenarios, rather than just gags or sketches, and drew authorities' attention. From May 1978 to February 1979, the show went off the air, a long hiatus that Groguhet explained in a 1979 *Ivoire Dimanche* interview as a holiday, and then as the result of restructuring of the state radio and television, RTI.[72] The unnamed interviewer explicitly posed questions about censorship, presumably to address the more reliable rumored reports that Groguhet's show had been silenced by the state. Reinforcing state authority at moments when he seems to critique it (though it is worth repeating that he never directly leveled critiques at either Houphouët-Boigny or his party), and justifying his critiques by appealing to the state, Groguhet responded, "Am I in the service of the authorities [le pouvoir]? Yes and no. I put things in perspective. Since as much as I deplore disastrous management, the laxness of certain administrative authorities, I work for these authorities [ce pouvoir] when I educate citizens about citizenship." Groguhet described himself as a "useful tool" of the state who has at the same time been given a tool—a television show—to work in the service of the authorities.[73] The state in turn embraced Groguhet and his show.

After a 1979 episode on unhygienic conditions at one of the large outdoor markets in Abidjan, funding for cleaning the markets that had been long delayed was suddenly made available, and Groguhet was summoned to the Presidential Office. Houphouët-Boigny praised Groguhet and *How's it going?* in front of various government officials, and from that point on, the show was known to television insiders as "'Houphouët-Boigny's show." After struggling for years with shifting time slots, *How is it going?* [*Comment ça va?*] was granted a prime-time spot: Saturday nights at 8:30 p.m. after the evening news.[74] In case viewers might have missed a broadcast or failed to grasp its central message, *Ivoire Dimanche* articles regularly summarized, praised, or sharpened the critiques leveled during a particular episode.[75] It also fre-

---

72. Bahi, "Narration, tradition et modernité," Appendix 2, 13.
73. "Interview," *Ivoire Dimanche*, March 4, 1979, 28–29.
74. Bahi, "Narration, tradition et modernité," Appendix 2, 13.
75. One *Ivoire Dimanche* commentator endorsed Groguhet's critique of people who take in young students and mistreat them. D. B., "Le Drame de Léa," *Ivoire Dimanche*, June 16, 1985, 13. Another praised Groguhet for "shedding light" on hotel clients' thefts. Am Atta, "Les Pil-

quently published letters, purportedly from fans. One such letter to the editor of the state sports and entertainment weekly, *Ivoire Dimanche*, noted the show's wide popularity in neighboring countries: "Groguhet's secret is simple. During his sketches, he describes, weighs the pros and cons [le pour et le contre] of a societal problem and always concludes with a cleverly administered moral [une morale savamment dosée]. The television viewer is thus educated through laughter."[76]

The official endorsement of *How's it going?* coincided with openly expressed dissatisfaction with PETV and suggests the state's flexibility in enlisting the media to communicate messages. In a period when rappers educated the public about issues such as reversing rural to urban migration, popular state entertainment television programming— including *How's it going?*—consistently complemented government campaigns, including those centered on health.[77] In 1989, a three-part *How's it going?* series on illicit drugs corresponded with an intensification of coverage on the prevention and repression of drug usage and distribution and a national campaign against drug addiction.[78] The show

---

leurs d'hôtels," *Ivoire Dimanche*, February 1, 1987, 7. Yet another underscored the importance of not littering. Even though Groguhet declared mayors "not to blame [non coupables]" for the open sewage canals lining streets, the article insisted that the local governments were, in fact, responsible. Fidèle Djessa, "*Comment ça va?*: Abidjan: Des poubelles pour rien," *Ivoire Dimanche*, May 17, 1987, 8. See also "*Comment ça va?*: Rumeur qui ment, rumeur qui dit vrai . . . ," *Ivoire Dimanche*, February 22, 1987, 13; "*Comment ça va?*: Profession: Mendiant," *Ivoire Dimanche*, March 8, 1987, 14. In a characteristic example of intertextual references in the state media, Moussa's column cited Groguhet as his inspiration for commentary on outdoor bars [maquis] near schools. "Moussa: A fa kaya! I faut que on va kpatara tous les maquizards que i sont devant écoles," *Ivoire Dimanche*, November 22, 1987, 47.

76. Joséphine Gohourou, "Mieux étoffer: 'Comment ça va?'" Letter to the editor, *Ivoire Dimanche*, March 9, 1986, 8.

77. In a eulogy to rapper R. F. K. (Roger Fulgence Kassy), *Fraternité Matin* praised the singer and his television show, *Podium*, which "aimed not just to entertain or to influence young artists; the program was also educational: With its topical themes [thèmes imposés, with connotations of *imposed on*] ("return to the earth," "rural exodus," etc.), it subscribed perfectly to the educational policies of the Party and the Government [il s'incrivait parfaitement dans la politique de sensibilisation du Parti et du Government (capitals in original)]." Jusu K. K. Man, "R. F. K.: Adieu l'artiste!," *Fraternité Matin*, January 29, 1989, 15.

78. A front-page headline on March 15, 1988, announced that parents of students had organized a march against drug use. "Drogue à l'ecole: Les parents d'élèves se mobilisent," *Fraternité Matin*, March 15, 1988, 1; Koblan Avoni, "La drogue à l'école: Un fléau à endiguer," *Fraternité Matin*, March 15, 1988, 23; Léon Francis Lebry, "Lutte contre la drogue: 14 comités départementaux bientôt installés dans les régions d'infiltration," *Fraternité Matin*, March 22, 1989, 2; J. B. Akrou, "Oui à la vie, non à la drogue," *Fraternité Matin*, April 5, 1989, 2; "Death to drugs! [Sus à la drogue!]" screamed an April 6, 1989, front-page headline. "Education and Repression to Counter this Plague [Sensibilisation et répression pour contrer ce nouveau fléau]," *Fraternité Matin*, April 6, 1989, 1; J. B. Akrou, "Campagne nationale contre la toxicomanie: Vivement la sensibilisation, activement la répression," *Fraternité Matin*, April 6, 1989, 24–25; J. B. Akrou,

similarly reproduced state messages around HIV. The episode "AIDS: The Illness of the Century" served as an explicit corrective to the Health Minister's earlier comments that AIDS was NOT the "illness of the century" and reinforced messages about partner reduction and condom usage. It broadcast on April 29, 1989, shortly after a special program on AIDS (*AIDS, The Big Meeting* [*SIDA, le grand rendez-vous*]), on April 20, 1989, and two months after a special episode on AIDS urging condom usage aired on the state television show *The Big Questions* [*Les Grandes questions*].[79] Three months earlier, a radio program had broadcast an interview with a young man talking about his AIDS diagnosis, which was transcribed in the state press.[80] A few weeks after the interview, huge outpourings of grief had followed the death of popular singer, entertainer, and television show host Roger Fulence Kassy, known as R. F. K., at age thirty-three after what *Fraternité Matin* described as "a long period of illness," widely understood but never officially acknowledged as AIDS-related.[81]

A clip from the song "AIDS" by former boxer-turned-singer Waby Spider plays as the "AIDS" episode opens: "The National Committee for the Fight against AIDS [Comité national de lutte contre le Sida (CNLS)] presents . . . Let's fight against AIDS." By visually demonstrating the existence and consequences of AIDS, the episode replicates the scare tactics of governmental information campaigns, which repeatedly warned the public not to take AIDS as a joke, and enacts the costs of ignoring their warnings. The "AIDS" episode conspicuously incorporates media from the CNLS's HIV education campaign and from prior programs, such as *The Big Questions*' representations of HIV prevention efforts. Portraying characters who have successfully adopted suggested HIV prevention measures, the "AIDS" episode centers on the disobedient office worker in need of proper disciplining.

The "AIDS" episode opens with Groguhet's wife worrying because Groguhet is late for dinner, and because she suspects that he is having affairs.

"Campagne nationale contre la toxicomanie: Drogue ou la mort à petites doses," *Fraternité Matin*, April 6, 1989, 26; Youssouf Sylla, "Le Grand Nord dit non à la drogue," *Fraternité Matin*, April 9, 1989, 2.

79. RTI, *The Big Questions: AIDS in Question* [*Les Grandes questions: Le Sida en question*], February 21, 1989.

80. Brigitte Obrou, "J'ai 26 ans et j'ai le SIDA." *Ivoir'soir*, January 17, 1989, 4–5.

81. Justin Kassy, "Un Homme de coeur," *Fraternité Matin*, January 29, 1989, 17. Alpha Blondy addressed such rumors in an interview: "The memory of my friend Fulgence Kassy was a little sullied by talk that he had died of AIDS [On a un peu sali la mémoire de mon ami Fulgence Kassy, en disant qu'il est mort de Sida]. . . . . Ful was a person with malaria, not a person with AIDS [Ful était un paludéen, pas un sidéen]." Diégou Bailly Paulus and Jérôme Carlos, "Alpha Blondy parle de R. F. K.," *Ivoire Dimanche*, April 16, 1989, 6.

Confronting him in his office, Groguhet's wife refers to prior educational programming on HIV: "There are too many diseases! You didn't see the show [film] that was on TV?" Groguhet responds that he has seen the show and has learned to fear the consequences of infidelity: "You can come to my office anytime you like, and you will always find me here among my papers. Haven't I seen the people who are infected, who scratch themselves everywhere, who have tumors everywhere? They are sick. Ah, no. Calm down." Groguhet and his wife represent the properly educated who, after having viewed HIV prevention media about the dangers of AIDS, are taking proper precautions, including changing their sexual behavior.

The scene then cuts to a young man, Badoté, behind his desk in his office where two girlfriends come in quick succession to complain that he is seeing other women and not meeting them as promised. After extracting money from him, the first woman leaves, and Badoté's officemate Bagnon, who has witnessed their exchange, warns him, "You're playing the pretty boy [Tu joues au beau gosse] without thinking of the consequences." In a scene of heavy-handed dramatic irony, a laughing Badoté brushes him off: "Consequences! When there's life, there's hope!" Another girlfriend comes into the office to complain to Badoté that she knows he has other girlfriends. Citing HIV prevention campaigns, she cautions, "Be careful! Don't give me diseases, you understand. . . . Photos . . . I learn things. Don't give me diseases." After she has also demanded money from him and then left, Bagnon again instructs Badoté: "Look at this magazine. Are you thinking about that? [Tu penses en ça?]." Bagnon holds up a copy of the monthly *Our Health* magazine with the word "AIDS" on the cover and a photograph of a gaunt seated woman, a black rectangle covering her eyes to preserve her anonymity. A laughing Badoté dismisses his concerns: "Bagnon, those are just stories [histoires]." In a quote later cited in the state newspaper as evidence of "irresponsible carelessness," he brushes off the danger of AIDS: "We have to die of something! [Il faut qu'on meure de quelque chose!]."[82]

The scene of Badoté dismissing warnings about the dangers of AIDS cuts to a woman at a clean, well-stocked pharmacy,[83] where in the French of the formally educated, she asks for "the thing that protects against AIDS." The pharmacist enunciates carefully: "Condoms [les préservatifs]? . . . Miss, it's

---

82. As an August 13–14, 1989, *Fraternité Matin* article noted, "In fact, no one likes to live with fear. It happens then that it is said reflexively with a kind of irresponsible carelessness, 'We have to die of something.'" Marcellin Abougan, "Les Préservatifs doivent faire partie des choses de la vie," *Fraternité Matin*, August 12–15, 1989, 6.

83. An April 18, 1986, ministerial decree limited condom sales to pharmacies. "Sida en Côte d'Ivoire: Faits et gestes," *Fraternité Matin*, July 11, 1990, 3.

for men, not for women." The woman insists: "Exactly. I am going to propose that to my boyfriend. If he doesn't want it, I won't go forward [S'il veut pas, je marche pas] because my father gave me advice, and I follow his advice." In the next scene, a different woman seated on a bed in medium close-up shoves a shoulder away from her: "Do you have the thing? . . . The condom? . . . I don't want to die." Offscreen, Badoté's officemate, Bagnon, responds, "I don't want to die either." The camera cuts to Bagnon seated on the bed as he takes a condom from his pocket and displays what he describes as "a really strong [solide]" condom. "Put it on properly [Il faut bien mettre]," says the woman who begins to undress while Bagnon, promising that he will, walks offscreen.

After the CNLS began distribution of 3.5 million condoms provided by USAID at the end of 1988, the Ivorian government increased its prevention messages centering on condoms, including on the February 21, 1989, news and current events program, *The Big Questions,* when the president of the CNLS Odehouri Kakou emphasized, "Condom usage must be advised. The disease [la maladie] kills." The "AIDS" *How's it going?* episode underscores the state's attempts to encourage condom usage as a means to prevent the spread of HIV. Scenes of female characters' demonstrating proper assimilation of messages about the importance of condoms contrast vividly with what the episode portrays as Badoté's heedlessness, for which he is dramatically punished. In the very next scene after the two women purchase and insist on the use of condoms, Badoté, his face shiny with fever, begins to scratch his skin and must repeatedly race from his restaurant table to the toilet where he suffers from bouts of uncontrollable diarrhea. While he is in the bathroom, his two dinner companions speculate, "I am convinced. It is not diarrhea." "I saw a dark sore." "A dark sore? It's a symptom!" Under the pretext that they have to attend a meeting, Badoté's friends rush away from the table.

When Badoté goes to Groguhet to ask for time off because of his sores and diarrhea, Groguhet tells him to take off his shirt so that he can have a look (figure 2.1), and the camera zooms in on the dark sores on his face (figure 2.2). The shot recalls the episode of *The Big Questions* devoted to AIDS which incorporated long takes lingering on emaciated body segments and extreme close-ups of sores and skin growths as a voiceover intoned, "This is Kaposi in its florid, aggressive form." Recoiling from Badoté in horror, Groguhet tells him not to scratch in his office and to leave immediately. In response to Badoté's questions, Groguhet says that he is not a medical expert but confirms that Badoté suffers from the same maladies depicted in prior prevention programming: "All I know is what I have seen in shows [films]." A wailing Badoté departs from the office.

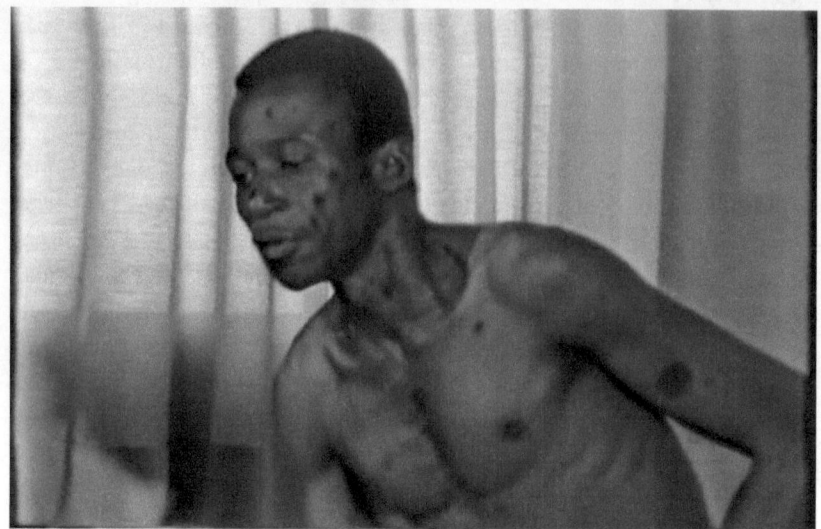

FIGURE 2.1. Badoté's body marked by sores.

The episode's punitively moralistic narrative depicts Badoté as rightfully abandoned by all his friends and acquaintances who in the next scene conclude that he has AIDS and refuse to sit next to him. In a tearful close-up, Badoté looks pathetically at his friends as they quickly leave him. The camera cuts from the people filing out of the room back to Badoté, sores visible on his skin, tears streaming as he laments, "I am screwed [foutu]. I am screwed, screwed. I am doomed [condamné]. I didn't want to listen to people. . . . I am screwed." The scene cuts to Groguhet seated behind his desk as he faces the camera to recap the message of the episode. The long monologue is worth quoting at length:

> I bet that he has AIDS! It is what the doctors tell you [vous dit]! It's what the Minister of Health hasn't stopped repeating to you [vous] since: We have to change our behavior [Il faut qu'on change nos comportements]! You [tu] had ten girlfriends [camarades]. You have to [il faut] reduce them to just one girlfriend! You [tu] have a chance of not catching AIDS! If you keep 1, 2, 3, 4, 5, 10, you [tu] have a chance of getting AIDS! You [Vous] are married? You leave your [votre] office, go home. From the house to your office, from the office to your house. You [Vous] also, you are engaged? Well, go get married! That way, you have a chance of not catching AIDS! Don't go try to go get [conquérir] anyone, anyhow! It's in your [votre] interest. You saw? He is in my department [Il est dans mon service]. Today, he introduces you to

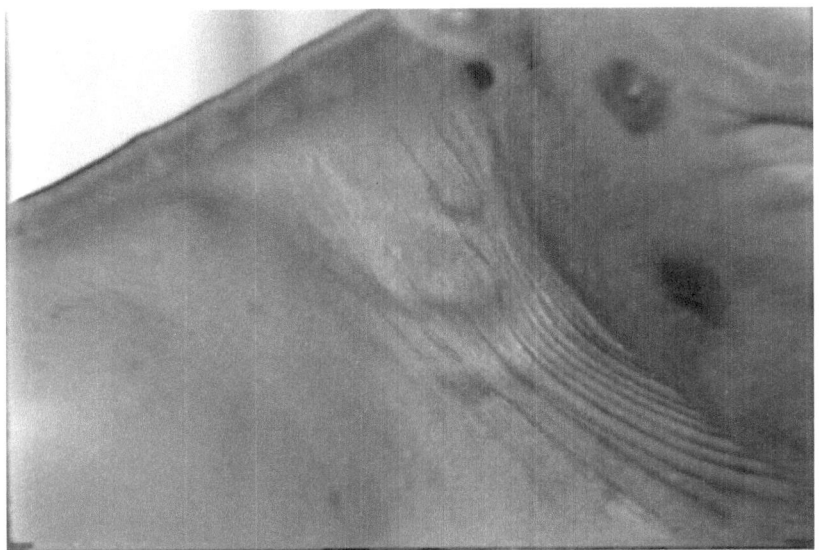

FIGURE 2.2. Sores on Badoté's face.

one girl, he introduces you to another because he's a good-looking guy [beau gosse]! [*Laughs*]. That's what he says. [*Laughter turns to half sob*]. No, it's terrible. How [Comment]? Well, the ball is in your court. [*Cut to pharmacy with condom packages on the counter, then to a bright red poster with a man clutching his head and screaming. The poster reads in white lettering: "AIDS is there. It kills." Groguhet continues in a voiceover*]: You have all the opportunities, all the chances to escape this thing. There are some who say, [*cut back to Groguhet at his desk*] oh, you're going to die of something. You've seen the films? [*Groguhet points to his eye. Then the scene cuts to a photograph of a man, seated in a wheelchair, head cropped off, sores on his arms; then it cuts to a photograph of an emaciated woman with sores on her skin. In voiceover, Groguhet continues*]: You've seen in the newspapers? You've seen what happens in the world? [*Cut back to tighter medium close-up of Groguhet pointing to his eye*]. So protect yourself!

Directly addressing the camera, Groguhet both parodies and affirms the authority of the boss and of the host of educational television shows to admonish spectators to trust AIDS prevention campaign materials, including the "AIDS is there . . . It kills" campaign—"You have seen? [Vous avez vu?]" (figure 2.3). The boss refers first to the transformation of Badoté after he has contracted HIV and then to the cutaways that serve as both warning and proof, as photographic "evidence" of the seriousness of AIDS and of how it

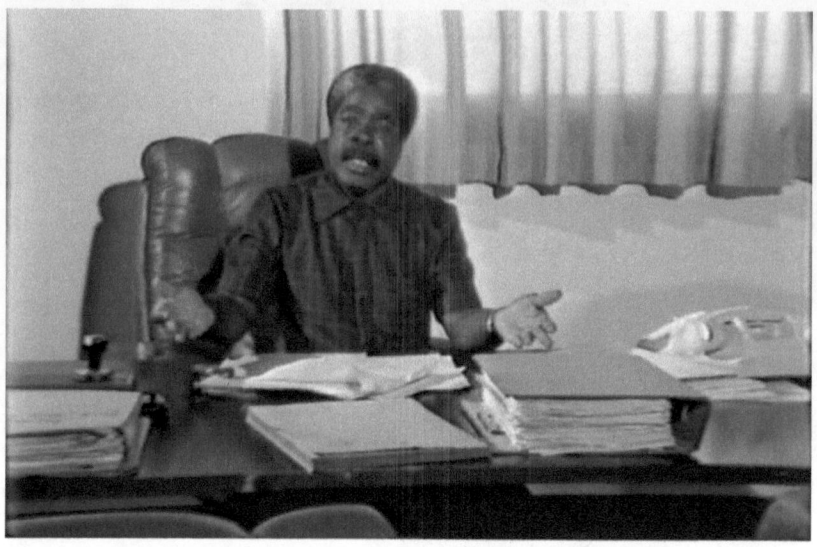

FIGURE 2.3. Kaloua as boss lecturing viewers.

manifests. He then refers to "programs" and "newspapers," the multiple media used for the first time in Côte d'Ivoire to raise awareness about HIV—the three television shows and news articles—and, finally, to "what happens in the world."[84] The episode supplements the media campaign that it cites, and through its direct references to and incorporation of national AIDS prevention campaigns, it derives its authority from and fortifies that of the state. The fictional show, like the "real" photographs and other mass media, depicts the consequences of the failure to take AIDS seriously and to implement the behavioral changes that the boss represents as required: reducing the number of sexual partners, getting married, and practicing monogamy.

As Kaloua addresses the audience, he slips from the formal and plural "you," *vous,* to the informal and singular "you," *tu.* His advice about how to prevent HIV is directed at the middle-class male, presumed heterosexual, the civil servant and office worker [functionnaire]. In depicting the disease as a justified punishment for sexual excess, the "AIDS" episode reiterates moralistic approaches to AIDS and to HIV prevention familiar from humorous *Moussa* columns in *Ivoire Dimanche*. But it further imparts an implicit lesson about gender and class, the threat of HIV and of unregulated sex signaling

---

84. The Minister of Health had appeared on two episodes of the program *Right to Health* [*Droit à la santé*], one on February 9, 1987, the other on March 16, 1987. He also had appeared on the program *The Big Questions: AIDS in Question* [*Les grandes questions: Le Sida en question*], February 21, 1989.

more generalized threats to the status of the elite male in need of discipline and in danger of losing his office job. The show effectively translates state demands for economic austerity into sexual terms, even as it offers justifications for the deterioration of the status of the middle-class male.

"DYSFUNCTIONS IN OUR ADMINISTRATIONS": AIDS IN THE OFFICE

As part of mandated structural adjustment, cuts were directed at the enormous civil service, which had traditionally incorporated the formally educated, especially men, for whom it secured middle-class status. These cuts from November 1983 to December 1984, and again in 1985, were rationalized as necessary measures of austerity, rigor, and self-sacrifice. As Minister of the Civil Service [Fonction Publique], Jean-Jacques Béchio reminded the public in a 1985 television interview also published in the state daily, "When it is a lean period [période de vaches maigres], each person must make necessary sacrifices, even if it's difficult, to enable Côte d'Ivoire to get out this bad patch [pour permettre à la Côte d'Ivoire de sortir de cetter mauvaise passé]."[85] In January 1988, Béchio warned prefects [préfets] that 73% of the government's administrative budget was spent on paying the salaries of 115,000 civil servants and that further restructuring was pending. He repeated "his favorite refrain": "Rigor, competence, punctuality, honesty" are required for public servants and agents of the state,[86] and "men of firmness and rigor are wanted."[87] In September 1988, Béchio announced that to save 4 billion francs, all further civil service appointments were suspended and transfers frozen until 1990.[88] A March 1989 Ernst and Young study of the public service published in November 1989 found massive absenteeism (50%) and inadequately trained administrators (60%), both of which were a result of nepotism and clientelism.[89]

As the state daily reported, during days of meetings in November 1989 about privatizing and renovating the civil service, Béchio blasted civil servants as "undermined by 'derailing indiscipline, revolting absenteeism, obvious complacency, and in short, blatant disrespect for public affairs [indiscipline

---

85. "Fonction publique: Accepter les sacrifices nécessaires," *Fraternité Matin*, January 25, 1985, 2–3, 3.

86. Jean-Baptiste Akrou, "Jean-Jacques Béchio aux préfets: Soyez les contrôleurs du personnel de l'État [sic]," *Fraternité Matin*, January 26, 1988, 6.

87. Jean-Baptiste Akrou, "Souplesse," *Fraternité Matin*, January 26, 1988, 6.

88. "Fonction publique: Affectation suspendue," *Fraternité Matin*, September 10–11, 1988, 1.

89. Mariam C. Diallo, "La Fonction publique face à la crise: Béchio fait le ménage," *Ivoire Dimanche*, February 4, 1990, 4–6.

déroutante, un absentéisme révoltant, une désinvolture caractérisée et en somme, un mépris souverain de la chose publique]."' In response, the civil service had to be modernized and renovated: "Now more than ever in the past, the key word will be to responsibilize men to administer and monitor well [le maître-mot sera de responsabiliser les hommes pour bien gérer et pour bien contrôler]."[90] A month later, Béchio announced another round of World Bank–mandated cutbacks, including of salaries, in the civil service. He gave directors until the end of the year "to clean up their departments [assainir leurs services, which has connotations of rendering more healthful]" of "disorder [la pagaille] and laxity," a process that will be overseen by "foreign technicians."[91]

All of the *How's it going?* episodes opened with cartoon explosions following the words *Laziness, Dishonesty, Crime,* and *Corruption,* and in previous episodes, Groguhet had criticized public officials for their absenteeism. An *Ivoire Dimanche* article linked his September 1986 representation of a minister who made appointments and never showed up in his office to Béchio's announcement the day after his nomination as Minister of the Civil Service that he was engaging in a fight against such "wrongdoings [agissements]."[92] The "AIDS" episode of *How's it going?* figures the state's call for vigilance against corruption and laxity and the need for "rigor and austerity" in the civil service as encompassing and articulated primarily through regulation of sexual behavior.[93] Groguhet's lecture to the audience attributes the elite male's degradation in class status and privileges to lack of sexual discipline—and not to state cutbacks and failures of the educational system—that requires as solution the exercise of individual restraint. The office functions as metonym for the class status that attracts the women, *deuxième bureau* [second office, and also a reference to France's intelligence services], common slang for men's female sexual partners outside marriage. A 1986 *Ivoire Dimanche* article noted that after the economic crisis of 1983, "second offices" were closed down but now were beginning to reopen.[94] As a 1989 *Fraternité Matin* article blaming the spread of the epidemic on "easy sex" notes, "Mistresses, or 'sec-

---

90. "Journées d'études sur la modernisation de l'administration: Rénovation des structures et des mentalités." *Fraternité Matin*, November 14, 1989, 1; Léon Francis Lebry, "Modernisation des administrations africaines: Place à la rénovation," *Fraternité Matin*, November 14, 1989, 30.

91. L. Patrice Douh, "Fonction publique: Le personnel journalier sera réduit aux 2/3 de son effectif: Bientôt un nouveau recensement des fonctionnaires et agents de l'État [sic]," *Fraternité Matin*, December 20, 1989, 2.

92. "L'Absentéisme qui tue," *Ivoire Dimanche*, September 28, 1986, 14.

93. The December 21, 1989, *Fraternité Matin* huge front-page headline reads "Rigor and Austerity [Rigueur et austérité]."

94. Am Atta, "Les 'Deuxièmes bureaux' sont ouverts," *Ivoire Dimanche*, April 20, 1986, 4. Moussa's column insisted that such offices never closed down. "Qui a dit que larzent è fini dans Côte d'Ivoire?" *Ivoire Dimanche*, June 23, 1985, 48.

ond offices' are numerous and are even the rule."⁹⁵ By March 1990, another article observed, "Despite the economic crisis that runs across Côte d'Ivoire, 'second offices' have never reached as high a level as today [les 'deuxième bureaux' n'ont jamais autant eu la cote qu'aujourd'hui]."⁹⁶ The metaphor of second offices figures sexual transgression through the language of bureaucracy—and vice versa—a sign of the corruption and absenteeism of the state administrators and of refusals to heed government mandates, including those imparted via television.

Groguhet's message, "We have to change our behavior," produces the community he addresses, with women depicted as carriers, or vectors, of disease against which the community must protect itself. Women in the show had already incited viewer condemnation for their purported sexual immorality. In two episodes that aired in May 1986, a pregnant Delta successfully convinced each of her two lovers—office colleagues—that he was the father of her child. Terrified by threats of her enraged father, the men gave her housing, a car, and other presents that she demanded before they discovered her scam. In the following episode, another woman, Léa, claimed to be pregnant by each of her three lovers whom she compelled to support her until her fraud was discovered and she was sent to the police. *Ivoire Dimanche* described Delta and Léa as similar to many other women in Abidjan: "shrews, without morality, who sell their bodies from office to office for payment [qui font commerce de leur corps de bureau en bureau, moyennant rétribution]. Really depraved women, arrogant, and full of effrontery and disrespectful, who pass most of their time blackmailing [rançonner] men."⁹⁷ The "AIDS" episode depicts economic insecurity as resulting from female sexual extortion and corruption and urges the elite male rendered powerless in a market controlled by women to reassert proper self-discipline and thereby protect himself against both AIDS and his economic vulnerability. Creating a more industrious and responsible public service then implies transformations in the sexual commerce of the

---

95. Léon Francis Lebry, "La Maladie des villes," *Fraternité Matin*, October 31–November 1, 1989, 2.

96. After a brief period of calm following the onset of the economic crisis in the early 1980s, the article continues, "The race to the 'second offices' is increasing nowadays [La course aux 'deuxième bureau' s'amplifie de nos jours]." Eugène Kadet, "Trompe qui peut et qui veut," *Fraternité Matin*, March 17–18, 1990, 16. Cautioning against generalizations about a sharp rise in male infidelity, sociologist Yéo Ouattara Souleymane notes that the phenomenon of the "second office" is unique to cities; it "does not exist in rural areas [dans les milieux ruraux]." "La Monogamie n'explique pas l'infidélité," *Fraternité Matin*, March 17–18, 1990, 17.

97. Am Atta, "*Comment ça va?*: Les Léa sont légion à Abidjan, les idiots aussi," *Ivoire Dimanche*, June 1, 1986, 13.

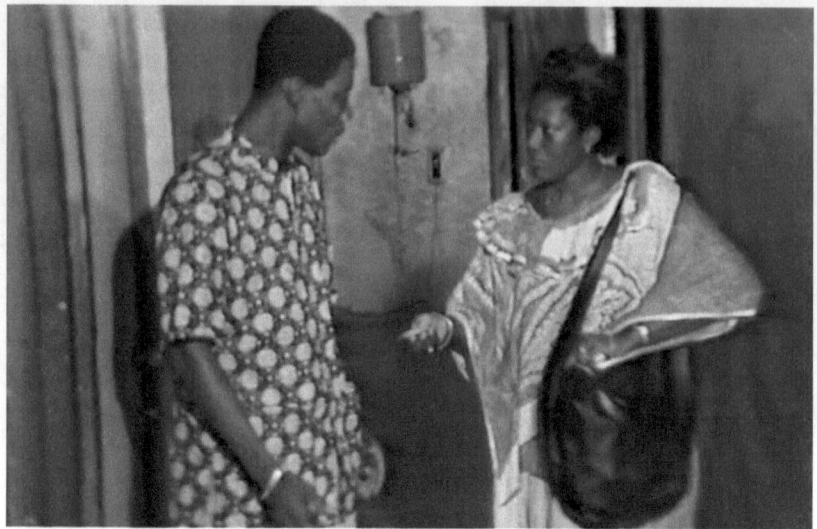
FIGURE 2.4. Woman handing her partner the condom she demands that they use.

office, transformations that if successfully accomplished would restore an elite heterosexual masculinity under economic and sexual threat.

Even though women both initiate and embody the corruption that must be corrected, they simultaneously serve as exemplars. In the "AIDS" episode, Kaloua does not direct his advice at women who are depicted as having already adopted HIV prevention measures. Both of Badoté's girlfriends—one of whom is named Léa—demand that he reduce his sexual partners, as Kaloua's wife demands Kaloua, so that they can avoid diseases. Although Kaloua never mentions condoms, both Bagnon's girlfriend and the woman at the pharmacy take the lead by insisting that their male partners use them. The woman at the pharmacy purchasing condoms quickly reassures the pharmacist, and viewers, that by obtaining condoms and insisting on their usage, she is merely conforming to proper gender roles, obeying her "father's" "advice"—the paternal authority of both the government and the head of the family, embodied in Houphouët-Boigny, who was commonly referred to as the "father of the nation." Rather than threaten, women's insistence on condom usage then affirms patriarchal authority even as it positions women as the voice of discipline and denial. In the closing scene, the woman who had purchased condoms in the pharmacy stands in a hotel hallway with her boyfriend. As he turns to open the door, she grabs his arm and says, "Wait, do you have it? [Attends, est-ce que tu as ça?]." When her boyfriend does not understand her question, she clarifies, "The condom! [Le préservatif!]." After he says that they have been together for a long time and do not need one, she pulls one out of her purse. Handing the condom to him, she insists she will not have sex without it (figure 2.4).

The closing scene of the "AIDS" episode cuts abruptly to a voiceover warning: "Do not risk your life as I did . . . [Ne risquez pas votre vie comme moi . . .]," as the camera zooms into the word: "AIDS" in red lettering. The graphic cuts to a gaunt, seated man whose face is obscured by shadows as he continues: "For only one moment of pleasure. Protect yourself [Pour un seul moment de plaisir. Protégez-vous]. Protect your life and that of others." The shadowy figures of an individual woman and an individual man, and of a man and a woman together, cut to the word "AIDS" in red lettering with the logos for the CNLS and the National Institute of Public Health [Institut national de santé publique (INLS)] underneath. As the camera cuts back to the seated man, he continues: "This is the advice of a sick man. [C'est le conseil d'un malade]." The word "AIDS" with the logos underneath fills the screen again before the episode cuts back to the credits for *How's it going?* By essentially narrativizing the government prevention message, the show blurs the woman's insistence on condom usage and fidelity, the "advice of a sick man," and the country's HIV prevention campaign. HIV serves as the threat to enforce compliance to state policies, and implicitly, also submission to women as exemplars and mouthpieces of prevention. It represents the elite male under threat from his own lack of sexual self-control. Just a year later, *How's it going?* addresses the ambivalence and anxieties generated by heterosexual men compelled to submit to the directives of their female sexual partners. The later episode depicts resistance to HIV prevention as resistance to women's attempts to control the terms of heterosexual exchanges.

"JOKE TO KILL" ["BLAGUER TUER"]

Shortly after the broadcast of the "AIDS" episode, the Ivorian government declared that it was no longer keeping silent about HIV/AIDS, and in July 1989 it announced that it was organizing prevention and greater transparency of information as part of its Medium-Term Plan for AIDS prevention funded by foreign funders and the World Health Organization.[98] On July 6, 1990, the

---

98. Am Atta, "Sida: Septième plaie d'Afrique?" *Ivoire Dimanche*, June 25, 1989, 29. On July 1, 1989, the Minister of Public Health and of the Population accepted 583 million francs to fund its medium-term plans for stronger prevention efforts. The announced campaign included two films and a clip on AIDS to be televised, a telephone hotline "AIDS Live [Sida en direct]," and a quarterly bulletin of information on AIDS. Am Atta, "Sida: 3 milliards pour cinq ans de lutte," *Ivoire Dimanche*, July 2, 1989, 29.

government announced plans to decentralize the National Program for the Fight against AIDS [Programme national de lutte contre le Sida (PNLS)] and its struggle against AIDS. It further noted that Côte d'Ivoire had the fourth highest number of reported AIDS cases—3,467—among fifty-two countries tracked by WHO, with Abidjan's HIV prevalence rates higher than those among males older than fifteen in New York.[99]

The AIDS education campaign was immediately obscured by almost-constant strikes throughout the country, including by transport and hospital workers, students, and teachers, and by a mutiny of security forces. Global prices for the country's primary export crops, coffee and cocoa, decreased even further, and Houphouët-Boigny's government could no longer afford to subsidize farmers as it had in the past.[100] Despite Houphouët-Boigny's convening of "days of dialogue" from September 21 to 23, 1989, after months of strikes and demonstrations, for the first time since independence, on April 7, 1990, the Ivorian government invalidated the entire academic year [une année blanche (literally a *white year*)] for all universities and schools. Under increasing pressure, including from foreign creditors, on April 30, 1990, Houphouët-Boigny agreed to hold multiparty elections and liberalize the media.

Without directly alluding to any of the history of AIDS prevention or to the ongoing economic and political turbulence, the *How's it going?* episode "Joke to Kill," which aired on September 15, 1990, responded to the conflicted history of AIDS prevention education, social and economic crises, and ongoing struggles for political authority, in part through revisions of *How's it going?*'s own prior representation of HIV prevention in the "AIDS" episode. By imparting a moral lesson about the downfall of a character who failed to heed HIV prevention campaigns, the 1989 "AIDS" episode participated in and strengthened attempts to counter perceived public indifference to the spread of HIV and to correct the state's own inconsistent messages about the epidemic. Echoing the rhetoric rationalizing major cutbacks in the country's enormous public service sector, the earlier "AIDS" episode represented HIV/AIDS as a symptom of a bloated and sexually corrupt state bureaucracy and of the failure to comply with directives around discipline and austerity. Through its stridently didactic plot, the episode illustrated the calamitous costs of not taking the threat of AIDS seriously and of not acquiescing to measures dic-

---

99. Nathalie Filion, "Séminaire de lutte contre le Sida: L'Ignorance, facteur de propagation," *Fraternité Matin*, July 6, 1990, 2.

100. In June 1989, Houphouët-Boigny cut producer prices for cocoa from 400 to 250 CFA, and then to 200 CFA in 1990. He cut the prices for coffee from 386 to 200 CFA during the same period. Cogneau and Jedwab, "Commodity Price Shocks," 510.

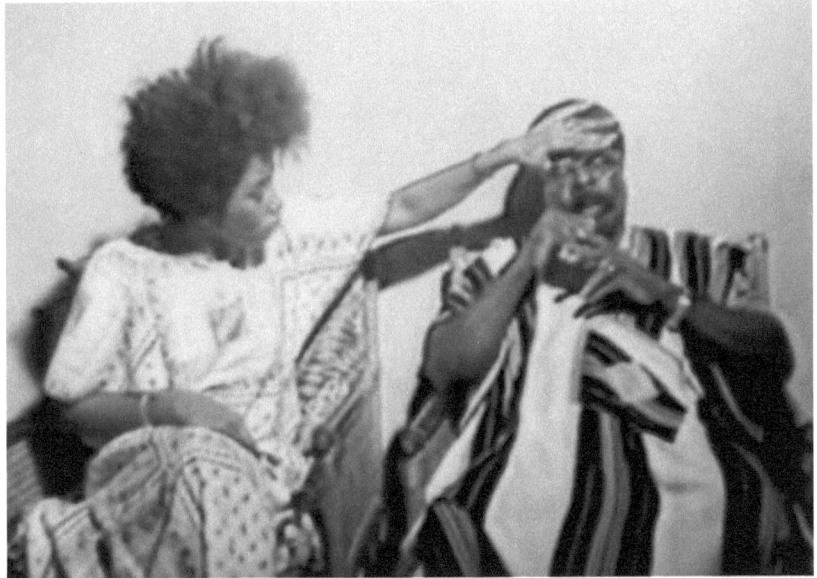

FIGURE 2.5. Kaloua to Delta: "Do you see the tears that flow?"

tated by state educational television, which ironically, through PETV, had promised greater access to that very bureaucracy.

In contrast, the 1990 episode "Joke to Kill" depicts jokes denying the existence of AIDS as enabling the punch line of the joke itself. The subversive approach to HIV prevention articulates not a critique of austerity measures, as the earlier episode would imply, but rather co-option of resistance to HIV prevention depicted as facilitating assertion of control over female sexuality—and the humor of the episode. In the episode, Groguhet plays the recurring character of the boss, Kaloua, who overhears his wife, Delta, played by Delta Akissi, planning to meet with her lover. He strides down the hall of his office, shrieking at and slapping his subordinates, slamming doors, and crumpling letter after letter to the minister before he finally concocts a plan. As Delta combs her hair to prepare to go to the market, or so she claims—Kaloua is well aware that she is planning to see her lover—Kaloua tells her that he has diarrhea and a rash and that he has lost 20 kilos (figure 2.5): "I am sick. Do you see the tears that flow? They're a symptom.... I have AIDS... I don't have to go to the hospital. I know.... Do you see the tears that flow? They're a sign."

While the earlier "AIDS" episode had referenced the show *The Big Questions* and its representations of symptoms of AIDS-related infections, here the weight loss and rash do not render "AIDS" legible on the body so much as the

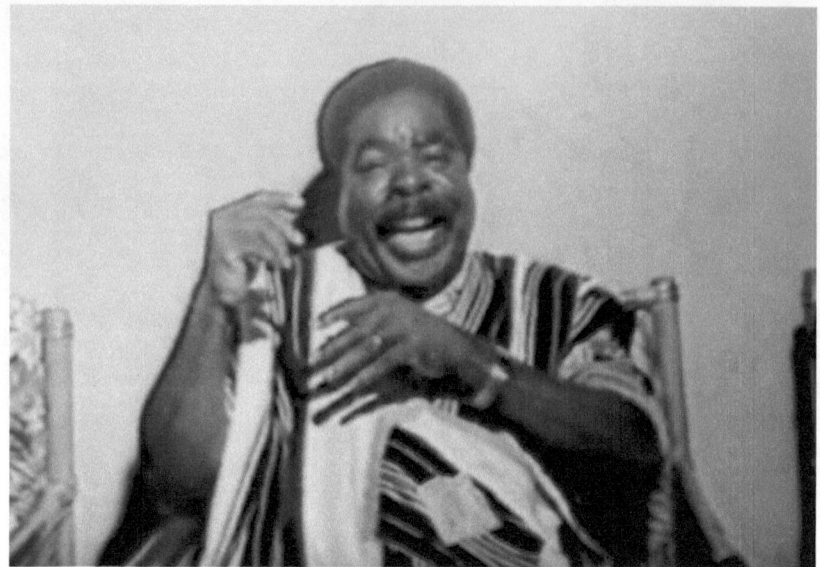

FIGURE 2.6. Kaloua's tears convert to laughter as Delta weeps offscreen.

tears, which link the AIDS narrative to the melodramatic mode as it has been enlisted in HIV prevention efforts, including in the prior "AIDS" episode.[101] The show lampoons the tears, overdetermined melodramatic representations of suffering, and the moral lesson implied by them. If the function of tears is, as Silvan Tomkins has proposed, to instigate "negative motivation" or, as Brian Larkin has argued about Nollywood cinema (the Nigerian film industry), to launch critique by provoking moral outrage, the tears in "The Betrayed Husband" represent a challenge to the didactic mode itself.[102] While Delta wails offscreen, Kaloua tries to suppress his laughter by turning it into a cough and then gagging (figure 2.6). Through his performance of "illness," Kaloua converts the melodrama of the emaciated, pitiful male body into a satire that enables the revenge of the cuckold.

The following scenes track what have more recently come to be termed "sexual networks" and some of the affective and financial ties underpinning them,[103] or what in a different register a March 18, 1990, *Fraternité Matin*

---

101. For a reading of how Kaposi's sarcoma signals AIDS on gay male bodies in the United States, see Yang, "Speaking of the Surface." For more on the melodrama, see chapter 4, "The Melodrama and the Social Marketing of HIV Prevention."

102. As quoted in Lutz, "Men's Tears and the Roles of Melodrama," 188; Larkin, *Signal and Noise*, 186.

103. "Sexual networks," or multiple, concurrent sexual partners, has become one of the current theories accounting for the high rates of HIV prevalence in sub-Saharan Africa. See Thornton, *Unimagined Community*.

spread on infidelity described as the "extramarital affairs of Ivorians." The newspaper article declaims, "We cheat [On trompe]. We cheat again. We always cheat on our partner [On trompe toujours son partenaire]. Man just as much as woman [Homme comme femme]. New couples just as much as old. All are doing it [Tous s'y mettent]."[104] Reinforcing the government's identification of sexual promiscuity as the cause of the spread of the epidemic, the *How's it going?* characters in the "Joke to Kill" episode blame Kaloua and what they describe as his "wandering" as the source of contagion. As Kaloua stands up, pretending to cough and clutching his stomach, the scene cuts to Delta's lover weeping into his hands as he and Delta bicker about who will die first. The lover demonstrates his awareness of the government campaign that "AIDS kills," as he laments, "It's Kaloua who has ruined everything [qui a tout gâté]. He gets around too much [Il se promène trop], Kaloua who has killed us, Kaloua!" In the following scene, Delta weeps, telling her husband's friend Bagnon about her husband's disclosure about his HIV-positive status. Delta tries to confirm that her husband has been using condoms that she has provided for him for his business trips when he "sees lots of girls," but a stammering Bagnon avoids her questions.

In the next scene, Delta's lover meets with another of his lovers. Although he had not told his other lover about his fears about contracting HIV, he had asked her to move out of his house and refuses to give her as much money as he has in the past. After she angrily storms away, the show undermines its own warnings when it reveals the threat of AIDS as in fact non-threat. Talking with Bagnon, Kaloua laughs uproariously, kicking his leg in the air:

> It's a stratagem that I dreamed up [inventé] so that my wife doesn't cheat on me [ne me trompe] because I know, I was told [on m'a dit] that she has liaisons with a certain bed your beard, enough beard soon, soon no beard [pieu ton barbe, barbe bientôt, tôt barbe bien[105]], doesn't matter what his name is. So I said, like this, one evening, I said, "My jewel [bijou], you know, I am infected [atteint]."
>
> [*In high-pitched voice, imitating Delta*] "Infected how?"
>
> I said, "I have the illness of the century! I have AIDS!"
>
> [*In high-pitched voice, imitating Delta*] "You have AIDS? Since when? And you didn't tell me that? You said nothing to me and I'm right here [on est là]. Since when have you had AIDS? So, so I am going to poison him!"
>
> I said, "What? What did you say?"

---

104. Eugène Kadet, "Trompe qui peut et qui veut," *Fraternité Matin,* March 17–18, 1990, 16.

105. These are untranslatable puns, in which *barbe,* or "beard," is a metonym for a man and also in slang signals "enough!" or "boring!" "Bed your beard/boring, beard/boring soon, soon beard/boring enough (with a pun: "All will be well")."

[*In high-pitched voice, imitating Delta*] "I am poisoned, I mean."

I said, "Speak well, speak little and say it well." [*laughter*] The face she made! [*laughter*] "It's a stratagem [stratagème] that I dreamed up! It's a strategy [stratégie]."

[*Men slap each other's hands.*]

Laughing, Bagnon congratulates Kaloua and says that he will use the same strategy with his girlfriend. In the stridently didactic mode of the earlier "AIDS" episode, characters in "Joke to Kill" reiterate the importance of obeying health authorities and their calls to change sexual behavior and use condoms. While the "AIDS" episode offers as models women insisting on condom usage, the "Joke to Kill" episode mocks those who have actually heeded medical authorities and prevention campaigns. Rather than represent the success of HIV prevention education, in "Joke to Kill," Delta's knowledge and propagation of information about HIV as much as her actual sexual transgression cause her downfall.

In the closing scene, Delta surprises her lover, who exits, briefcase in hand, outside his villa. She tells him she has dressed in a nice outfit for him. He recoils from her in horror:

LOVER: You told me your husband has AIDS! Go with him.
DELTA: Wait . . . we can always work things out [s'arranger]. We can use condoms for example.
LOVER: Condoms? With what you told me? Never! Never! Never! I may as well commit suicide! Please, you have to leave. Even now, I expect my death [Jusqu'à ici, j'attends ma mort]. I can't do anything intentionally to die [Je peux pas faire exprès pour mourir]. . . . Go to your husband's house. . . . Go! Go! Go die in his hands. You have AIDS!

As her lover shoves her away, Delta literally stumbles into the gutter.

The "AIDS" episode prominently featured women buying and using condoms, and the "Joke to Kill" episode initially seems to promote them as well. Delta believes that she has contracted HIV through Kaloua, who she presumes has refused to use the condoms that she had provided for him. (Interestingly, the show never suggests that Delta might have contracted the virus from her lover or that she could have transmitted it to Kaloua.) Although Delta had provided her husband with condoms, she had not used them with her lover, who believes that he also has been infected by Kaloua through Delta and that he has infected his other lover. But in the last scene, Delta's lover equates condoms, not AIDS, with suicide and death.[106] Her proposal that she and her lover use condoms triggers a more definitive rejection than her disclosure of her husband's HIV status did, a rejection that is a central goal of Kaloua's revenge strategy.

The episode mocks the dramatic threats underpinning the official AIDS prevention slogans—"AIDS is there. It kills" and "AIDS, don't die of ignorance."[107] It further defies the first 1989 government HIV prevention television campaign, which included repeated warnings not to take AIDS as a joke. Upending government prevention messages, the *How's it going?* "Joke to Kill" episode stages the widely circulating joke, including in *Ivoire Dimanche*'s Moussa's column, that the French acronym for AIDS, "the illness of the century," stands for "Imaginary Syndrome to Discourage Lovers" or "Invented Strategy to Discourage Lovers." However, the *How's it going?* "Joke to Kill" episode refers to the joke about AIDS as "invented strategy" but does not deny the existence of AIDS itself. Instead, the episode puns on the understanding of AIDS as nonexistent to reposition Delta as the target of the joke.

Sigmund Freud genders the teller of dirty or smutty jokes, which he describes as shared by men expressing sexual aggression toward a woman figured as passive and repressed.[108] "The Betrayed Husband" episode translates the structure of the smutty joke into viewers' complicity with the male elite at the expense of the woman, the dupe. In the episode, the viewer, along with Bagnon, is let in on the joke, while Delta remains oblivious. Delta's ignorance, unlike that depicted in HIV prevention campaigns and pedagogical television more broadly, is never rectified. Her ignorance is not about the fact of AIDS as Acquired Immunodeficiency Syndrome (as the HIV prevention message urges, "AIDS: Don't die of ignorance"), but about her jealous husband's performance, his pretending to suffer from AIDS-related illnesses. Put another way, the "Joke to Kill" is not that AIDS as a fatal disease is invented—a form of denialism—but that Kaloua uses AIDS and the real threat of death to control and punish Delta and her lover, the butts of the joke who remain unaware to

---

106. Perceptions that condoms cause AIDS have been documented as being widespread in South Africa. McNeill, "'Condoms Cause Aids,'" 360; Epstein, *The Invisible Cure*, 148. McNeill links the association of condoms and AIDS not to denialism but to attempts to create and maintain distance between individuals and those who suffered what was seen as an unnatural death. As he notes, female peer educators, particularly those who distribute condoms, have become "perceived as implicated in harboring and distributing a source of unnatural death" (367). A similar kind of association operates in the scene between Delta and her lover.

107. This slogan echoed a British government AIDS education campaign. Watney, "The Spectacle of AIDS," 72–73.

108. Freud, *Jokes and Their Relation*, 118.

the end that a joke is even being played. Kaloua's strategy is successful to the extent that fear of the virus circulates, that Delta and her lover actually fear the death that AIDS promises, and that they modify their behavior in response to their fears. At the same time, the joke can proceed as such only insofar as the show entirely forecloses the possibility that Kaloua, Delta, and her lover could actually have contracted HIV.

If AIDS as an "imaginary syndrome" serves as a pretext to extend control over and discipline sexual behavior, the unfaithful husband has adapted the tactic for his own ends. His invention of AIDS reproduces the very pedagogical efforts of state HIV education campaigns that it subverts. The show acknowledges the dangers of AIDS; in fact the narrative relies on acceptance of the message that "AIDS is there . . . It kills," but portrays prevention measures—especially the minimizing of sexual partners and condom usage—as deserved punishment of the sexually promiscuous woman who has promoted condom usage, whose punishment is effective only *because* of her awareness of HIV and of HIV prevention. If the joke about AIDS as an imaginary syndrome registers not only denial about the seriousness of the epidemic but also critique of how it has been deployed to control sexual behavior, "Joke to Kill" defuses and deflects the critique. Women, not state, medical, or foreign funder authorities, are the subjects and targets of heterosexual male aggression, which, like the previous episode demanding submission to prevention messages, reinforces a paternalistic and patriarchal economic, political, and sexual order.

WINTIN WINTIN AND OLD HEADSCARF

Wintin Wintin and Old Headscarf worked with the star Léonard Groguhet on *How's it going?* from 1980 to 1985 before breaking with him and creating their own weekly skits that aired beginning June 1, 1985, during what was originally a beloved Saturday afternoon children's program, "Call me Léo [Appelez-moi Léo]." They later featured in ten-minute skits on the weekly show "The Know-It-Alls [Les Incollables]" and, beginning in 1988, on the Saturday afternoon show *Tempo*. I was unable to find the exact date of broadcast of the *Wintin Wintin and Old Headscarf* skit "500 CFA If You Don't Come" in the RTI archives or in the state newspapers, and unfortunately the video of the show is undated. However, contextual clues situate its production around the early 1990s when condom campaigns were increasingly visible in the country.

Old Headscarf, or Léon N'Cho Assamoi, took his stage name from his father, Paul Atchié, a well-known musician who when he sang, would be covered by dancing women's headscarves. Atchié became known as "Chin doukou" or "the man with the headscarves" in Attié and, as he got older, "Old Headscarf," a name that his son adopted when he began work in the theatre.[109] Alain Djédjé Tiébé, or Mousso Dosso,[110] took the stage name Pierre Wintin Wintin because, as he put it during an *Ivoire Dimanche* interview, "wintin wintin," or *mosquito* in Baoulé and Attié, can never pass unnoticed: "I make noise and enliven sleepy places [Je fais du bruit et mets de l'ambiance dans les endroits endormis]."[111] Others have interpreted the name to refer to the mosquito's ability to bite and annoy everyone, regardless of social status[112]—though the word *wintin* in the urban slang nouchi also translates as "to have sex," or "to fuck."

Although Wintin Wintin insisted that he was merely playing a role, interviews represent him as resembling his character: "AIDS doesn't worry him at all. He finds that it's '*information merely to discourage lovers* [italics in original, *simple information pour décourager les amoureux*],'" which, like "'imaginary syndrome to discourage lovers,'" puns on Sida, the French for AIDS.[113] The "500 CFA If You Don't Come" episode depicts Wintin Wintin's resistance to HIV prevention as a hilarious example of his uncontrollable appetites, his failure to obey prevention messages, which signals a broader failure to practice self-discipline and rigor as urged by a woman who demands safer sex. As in the *How's it going?* episodes, the potentially subversive effects of refusals to comply with prevention directives and to practice austerity are managed through the rendering of the conflict in terms of gender struggle as Wintin Wintin defies the terms of sexual exchange set by a woman acting as the primary agent of HIV prevention.

The skit is set in what is clearly a poor neighborhood in Abidjan, where Wintin Wintin runs into a friend as he is heading to "a little visit" with a female friend. Wintin Wintin's friend warns him: "If you are going over there, you have to wear condoms [chaussettes, or *socks*]!" Wintin Wintin strides away,

---

109. Am Atta, "Vieux-Foulard, le bouffon raisonneur," *Ivoire Dimanche*, August 25, 1985, 8.

110. Thanks to Konan Amani who confirmed Wintin Wintin's names with Magnéto, a former colleague of Wintin Wintin. Magnéto said that Mousso Dosso was born of a Bété mother and a Dioula father and changed his name to Alain Djédjé Tiébé before he took the stage name Wintin Wintin. Personal correspondence with Konan Amani, May 8, 2015.

111. Am Atta, "Wintin-Wintin, le moustique tapageur," *Ivoire Dimanche*, August 25, 1985, 9.

112. A fellow performer on the show, Magnéto, offered this interpretation of Wintin Wintin. Personal correspondence with Konan Amani, May 8, 2015.

113. Moussa Zio, "Wintin Wintin Pierre et Vieux Foulard: Les Maîtres du gros rire," *Ivoir'soir*, April 1–4, 1988, 3. Evidently, Wintin Wintin experienced a change of heart, and in *Debauchery* [*La Débauche*], directed by Michel Didier Bro (2006), he narrativized his character's realization about the gravity of HIV/AIDS as part of a process of Christian conversion. The videocassette is dated 2006, but Wintin Wintin died in July 2005, so the production was shot before then.

reassuring him, "That, I'm up on that! I'm up on that! [Je suis au courant!]." To be "au courant" implies being informed, aware, in the know. The show educates by highlighting, mocking, and attempting to close the gap between Wintin Wintin's claims to knowledge and his actual ignorance. "500 CFA If You Don't Come" initially centers on Wintin Wintin's misunderstanding of the term *socks* [chaussettes] as a slang term for *condoms*. Over the course of the skit, Wintin Wintin reverses the joke: while he initially refuses to use condoms but agrees to practice safer sex and to pay a lower price by not ejaculating, he comes anyway.[114] Anthropologist Sasha Newell notes that in exchanges of money or gifts for sex, "money is not the antithesis of sentiment, but an integral part of it, and therefore, it would be a projection of Euro-American values to describe 'transactional sex' in urban Africa as the result of a process of commodification."[115] The skit parodies expressions of sentiment as pretext and expresses intense ambivalence around sexual economic exchanges, especially around women who attempt to set the terms of the exchanges, including by negotiating condom usage.

When Wintin Wintin finds out that the woman he has planned to visit has gone to the market, he unsubtly approaches the neighbor seated next-door (figure 2.7): "Do you know [au courant] that I love you?" The scene cuts quickly to a patas monkey (figure 2.8)[116] and then back to Wintin Wintin, who dismisses the woman's reservations about potential conflicts with her neighbor: "Neighbor! Neighbor! Is that marriage? That's not marriage! We can do a little something something! [On peut faire un peu un peu!]. Didn't you come here to earn a little money?" The shot of the monkey, who featured regularly in the show, has multiple valences, metaphorically linking Wintin Wintin to the figure of the monkey as a too-clever mischief-maker and trickster.[117] The shot also establishes metonymic correlation between Wintin Wintin and the woman's encounter and HIV. The quick shot of the monkey seeming to turn its head toward Wintin Wintin and the woman signals the threat of HIV and

---

114. France (through ORSTOM, *Office de la Recherche Scientifique et Technique d'Outre-Mer* [Office of Scientific and Technical Research Overseas] and UNESCO funded an HIV prevention campaign that incorporated research about young people's perceptions of condoms. They commissioned a musical cassette that included the Ivorian performer RAP-MC's "Young People, Put on a Condom [Jeunesse, Chaussez Capote]" that was incorporated into a cassette distributed for free in August 1992 and again at subsidized prices in December 1993. Reed, "C'est le wake up!," 182. The song also played on Ivorian radio and television. Deniaud, "'Chaussette De Vie,'" 123–24. Deniaud and Touré, "Présentahon de documents audiovisuels," 123–25.

115. Newell, *The Modernity Bluff*, 78.

116. Paleoanthropologist and physician Noel T. Boaz identified the monkey as probably "*Erythrocebus patas,* most likely a female"; primate researcher Darby Proctor similarly identified the monkey as probably a patas. Personal correspondence, March 5, 2015, and March 7, 2015.

117. Paulme, "Typologie des contes africains," 577.

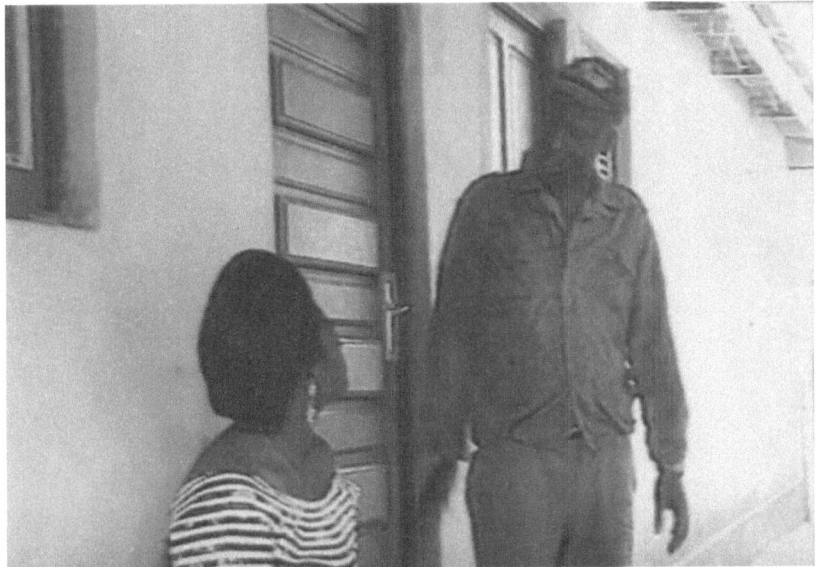

FIGURE 2.7. Wintin Wintin to woman: "Do you know that I love you?"

debates about its African origins. But in its playfulness, the image mocks the seriousness of AIDS and of HIV prevention. Wintin Wintin's comment that the woman is not married to the neighbor, and so can accommodate him, further travesties HIV prevention efforts that insist on fidelity and marriage as protection against HIV. It simultaneously acknowledges but disavows homosexuality and its link to the spread of the virus—naming marriage between women through Wintin Wintin's dismissal of such a possibility as impossible.

The woman agrees to take Wintin Wintin at the usual rates: "500 if you don't come [500 versé pas], and 1000 francs if you come [versé]." She refuses to accept Wintin Wintin's promise of later payment, and after he pays the 500 francs to just "have fun [s'amuser]" at the lower rate, they enter her room. The show continues to pun on Wintin Wintin's incomprehension of the directive to "put on a condom [chaussez capote]"—put on [chaussez] a condom in the sense of put on socks or shoes. As Wintin Wintin goes into the house, he politely asks the woman if he can wear his shoes: "I can enter with my shoes on [entrer avec mes chaussures-là]?"

After the woman leaves the room, Wintin Wintin strips down to his underpants and pulls up his red socks (figure 2.9), which ironically reiterate the red of the first HIV prevention posters from 1988, as well as the ribbon of solidarity in the fight against HIV/AIDS (beginning in 1991), and the name of

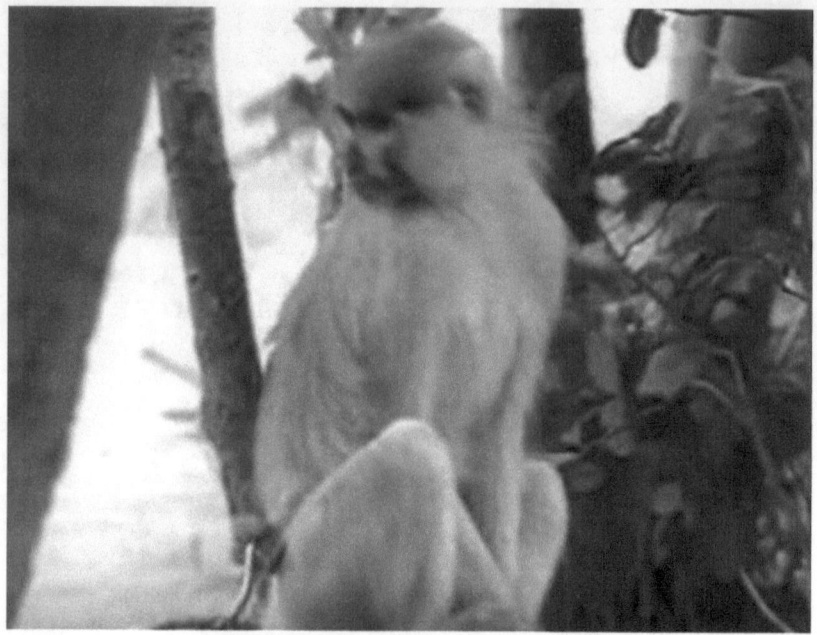

FIGURE 2.8. Patas monkey looks on skeptically.

one of the major AIDS organizations in Côte d'Ivoire (Red Ribbon, or Rouban Rouge, founded in June 1994). When the woman returns, she demands, referring to his socks, "What is that? What is that?" Wintin Wintin responds, "You're not up on this? [Tu n'es pas au courant?]. . . . My friend Bazo told me it's death [il y a la mort] without that. If you haven't put that on, death's going to get you [Si tu n'as pas mis ça, la mort va te guetter]." Wintin Wintin mangles the prevention messages from the first state AIDS prevention campaign that AIDS kills, and from the state and foreign funders that condoms can reduce the likelihood of HIV infection. Eliding AIDS, the most important term in the message, he understands "chaussettes" to literally mean socks, and not condoms, as in themselves ensuring well-being and protecting against death. He again identifies himself as aware, savvy, "You're not up on this [au courant]? My friend there just told me if you want to be in good health, when you go to a woman, you have to wear socks [chaussettes]."[118] The woman corrects him, gesturing at his feet, "Not those socks there!" Wintin Wintin sits up, "Which socks, then, the short kind?"

---

118. The closest equivalent translation would be if Wintin Wintin wore rubber boots, or perhaps gloves, to bed because his friend warned him to put on "rubbers."

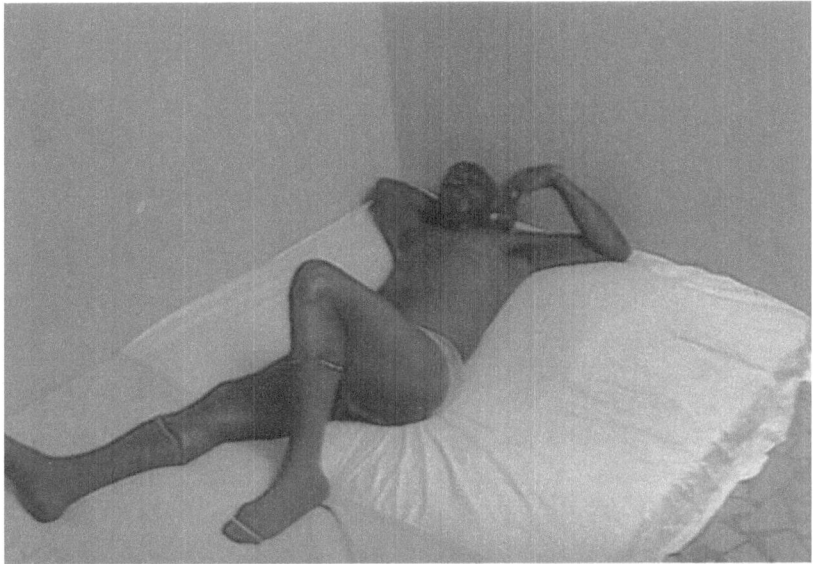

FIGURE 2.9. Wintin Wintin relaxing with his condom [chaussettes, or *socks*] on.

In his repeated insistence on being *au courant*, "in the know," Wintin Wintin only further underscores his lack of knowledge. As the woman points out, the protective "socks" are condoms, which in any event, Wintin Wintin won't need, since their agreement was that he would not come:

WOMAN: Not that [*gesturing to the socks*]! They're rubbers [préservatifs]!
WINTIN WINTIN: Rub-bers? What is that?
WOMAN: Condoms [capotes].
WINTIN WINTIN: You think that I'm going to put on a condom after all the money I gave you?
WOMAN: There are too many diseases now. So we have to protect ourselves [Donc on doit se préserver].
WINTIN WINTIN: Who told you I is sick [*sic*: que j'ai malade]? ... I'm going to give you money, and I'm going to put on a condom? You take me for a sucker [pour couillon] or what? You, young girls, you have no respect!
WOMAN: In any case, there's no problem. You're going to do it, but you're not coming.
WINTIN WINTIN: I said, to have fun [s'amuser] only, isn't that what I said?

Citing prevention and information messages urging the public to "protect yourself," the woman demonstrates that she has properly assimilated AIDS

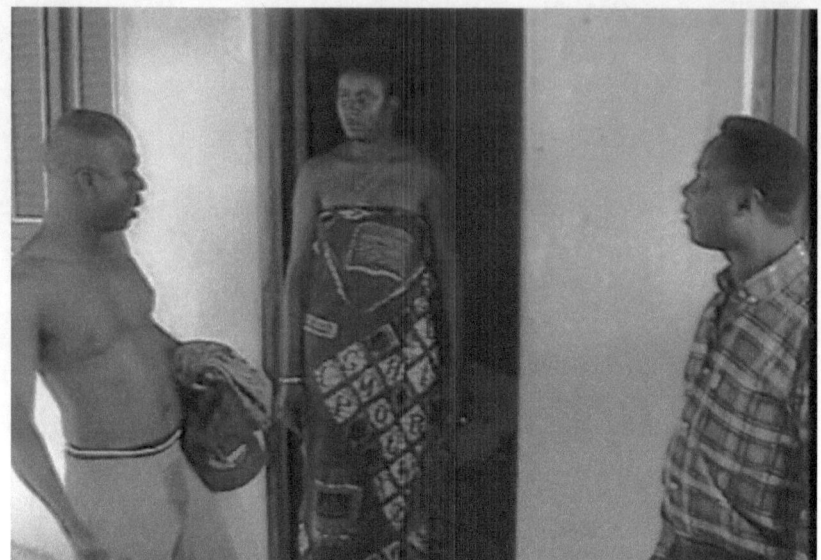

FIGURE 2.10. Wintin Wintin insisting that he did not come. Old Headscarf (on the right) looks on.

education directives. The initial transaction between the woman and Wintin Wintin implies a higher rate for unprotected sex—double the price—but the woman shifts the conditions so that both alternatives entail safer sex—no ejaculation or condom usage. Undercutting Wintin Wintin's contention that he would be a sucker for wearing a condom, the scene depicts him as a buffoon because initially, he does not grasp the import of his friend's and the woman's HIV prevention messages, or the terms of the sexual transaction with the woman, which have been transformed by the threat of HIV.

However, Wintin Wintin proves craftier than he seems. The second main character on the show, Old Headscarf, also looking for sex, knocks on the door of the absent neighbor who is still not home. The scene cuts to black. The woman with Wintin Wintin suddenly cries out into the dark: "You screwed [Tu as appuyé, vulgar slang for having sex]! For 500, you don't come!" The lights turn up to reveal Wintin Wintin scrambling out of bed and screaming that he has not come, as the woman counters, "You came! You came!" The two continue to argue as they get dressed and exit her house. As the woman furiously demands an extra 500 CFA, Wintin Wintin continues to insist "in the name of God" that he has not come—although his grey sweatpants are visibly soaked at his crotch (figure 2.10). At one point, standing in the entry of her room, the woman reaches inside the cloth wrapped around her body and extends her hand at Wintin Win-

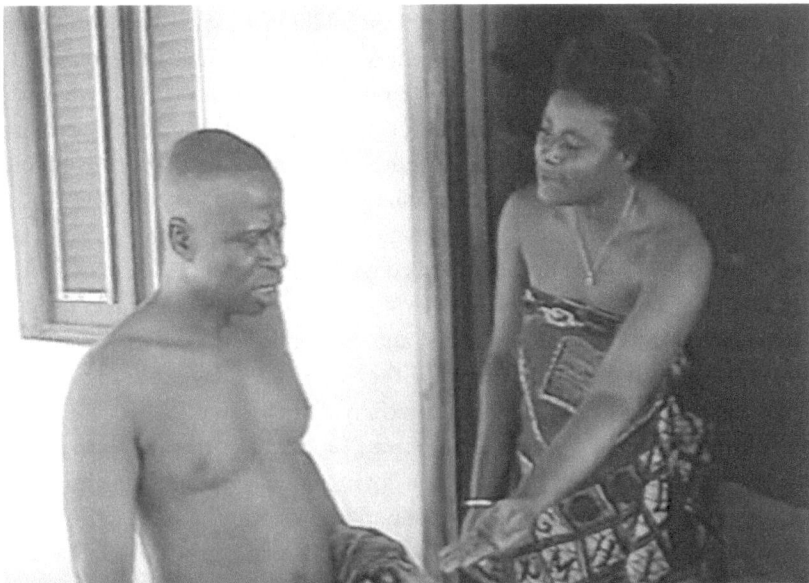

FIGURE 2.11. Woman to Wintin Wintin: "Isn't this your sperm in my hand?"

tin (figure 2.11): "You screwed me! Isn't this your sperm in my hand?" The scene finally resolves when the mediator, Old Headscarf, still standing at the neighbor's door and overhearing the argument, agrees to pay the difference.

Ultimately, the show reproduces the confusion about HIV prevention campaigns that it depicts. Despite repeated warnings from his friend and the woman about the threat of HIV, Wintin Wintin has unprotected sex. With his erratic grammar and bumbling, Wintin Wintin acts as a fool, a clown who does not understand HIV prevention messages, but also as a trickster who lives up to his name, both Mosquito and Have Sex. As a buffoon, he serves as a negative example about what not to do, his misinterpretations underscoring his ignorance and his ejaculation indicating loss of control over his body. But as a trickster, he ultimately prevails, having sex and coming—without a condom and for half price!

Although the woman and Wintin Wintin's friend had urged Wintin Wintin to use condoms, and the woman warns about the dangers of not doing so, the show depicts as humorous Wintin Wintin's failure to heed prevention messages. Even though ejaculation without a condom was not an option—the 1,000 CFA rate was for sex with a condom—the woman demands an additional 500 CFA as compensation from Wintin Wintin. The show never suggests that by coming without a condom, Wintin Wintin might have exposed her to HIV—or that he might have been exposed—and it depicts the woman as appeased once Old Headscarf offers her the additional 500 CFA. In correcting Wintin Wintin's misunderstandings, the woman had at first identified Wintin Wintin as the target of the show's humor, and at the same time, educated him and viewers about HIV prevention methods. In defying and deceiving her, Wintin Wintin effectively undermines the terms of sexual and economic exchange and of HIV prevention to situate her instead as the butt of the joke. As they exit the courtyard, Old Headscarf congratulates Wintin Wintin who has finally admitted that he did indeed come: "You are strong! [Toi, tu es fort!]."

Like the *How's it going?* episodes, *Wintin Wintin and Old Headscarf* depicts women dictating the terms of sexual and economic transactions and urging proper sexual self-discipline. But while the "AIDS" episode portrayed the male character who failed to comply as rightfully and swiftly punished, the "Joke to Kill" and "500 CFA If You Don't Come" episodes portray circumvention of HIV prevention as an effective strategy in comic gendered struggles. Misidentifying women as the cause of economic exploitation, and depicting them as mouthpieces for HIV prevention education demanding self-discipline and austerity, the later shows represent resistance to HIV prevention messages as the gleeful retaliation of the irrepressible heterosexual male. Sidestepping any challenges to or critiques of state or foreign funder policies, the satire directs its critical force at the women who demonstrate correct knowledge of HIV prevention methods. Regardless of how the shows depict the consequences of not using condoms, they all depict HIV prevention strategies as enabling the restoration of an upended social order—ironically, even if the strategies deployed do not align with measures identified as preventing the spread of HIV.

"TO CORRECT AND INSTRUCT THE PEOPLE"

A 1993 ceremony celebrating Groguhet underscores the role of satire in maintaining state authority. As the Grand Chancellor awarding Groguhet his medal underscores, the show serves as proof of the country's freedom of speech: "Thanks to your courage, these shows are the pride of Côte d'Ivoire, the subregion and beyond. They prove quite simply that freedom of expression is well and good in our country." In the speech's almost untranslatable, convoluted syntax, Groguhet's critical comedy [comédie critique] and comedy itself are figured as the basis of Ivorian culture:

> How not to accept that in West Africa, specifically, Côte d'Ivoire, where freedom of expression has never encountered any barriers [n'a jamais connu

d'entraves], at the risk even of becoming a license for expression [une licence d'expression] . . . how say I, not to accept, my dear Groguhet, that you inscribe your name on the base of Ivorian culture, especially on the record of laureates of critical comedy that makes of you today, tomorrow, and forever, another nationally distinguished person [personnage national] of the first order.

The Grand Chancellor describes Groguhet's satire as bridging the divides between elite/popular, French/African, and ruler/ruled. His speech locates Groguhet within a tradition of African humor from the popular Cameroonian Jean-Michel Kankan to the "critical comedy" of Ivorians: writer (and former Minister of Culture) Bernard Dadié's play *Monsieur Thôgô-gnini*[119] and popular comic actor Bamba Bakary.[120] During the awards ceremony, in the academic French of the formally educated, the Grand Chancellor also situates Groguhet within a tradition of European high art. He compares Groguhet to Victor Hugo, Voltaire, and Molière, satiric writers from France, "the country of our former ancestors," whom he extols as courageously critiquing their society. Like these writers, the Grand Chancellor continues, Groguhet and his show courageously serve society "to correct and instruct" "the people," both rulers and the ruled [gouvernants/gouvernés]. For the Grand Chancellor, the instruction and correction importantly provide further evidence: Groguhet and his show "prove quite simply that in our homeland [chez nous], liberty of expression is not an empty word [vain mot]."

The ceremony celebrating Groguhet as a national figure formally establishes *How's it going?* and popular humor as basis of "Ivorian culture" that is also rooted in France. It further situates as foundational to national culture "critical comedy," humorous critiques of society, or at least limited aspects of it. The ceremony celebrating Groguhet meant to highlight freedom of expression is not quite so simple. As exemplary national cultural product broadcast

---

119. A tradition of political satire in Ivorian theater has been dated to some of the first Ivorian theater productions, including Bernard Binlin Dadié's *Les Villes* performed in 1934 in the École Primaire de Bingerville. An early anticolonial and PDCI activist, Dadié was Director of Arts and Research and Inspector of Cultural Affairs in Abidjan, and from 1977 to 1986, Minister of Culture.

120. In response to a question about risks that Bakary took in his impersonations of Houphoüet-Boigny on his television show, Bakary insisted that he had never encountered any resistance from the government: "I don't believe so because in Côte d'Ivoire, democracy is real and effective. I respect the fundamental principles and ideals of the PDCI-RDA. I never asked for authorization before doing my sketches and I was never bothered by the authorities [je n'ai jamais été inquieté par les autorités], either directly or indirectly." D. Bailly, "En Couverture: Bamba." Bakary, *Ivoire Dimanche*, September 28, 1986, 4–9, 6.

on a state-run channel with the mandate to represent the interests of the ruling party, *How's it going?*, like *Wintin Wintin and Old Headscarf* skits, cannot and does not epitomize the freedom of expression as the state would claim. Rather it epitomizes a complicating of what even constitutes autonomous culture or cultural product, if defined as distinct from, much less in opposition to, the state or the official. It also challenges notions of critical comedy as counter-hegemonic if the state has deemed it foundational to national culture and to the media. As Howard Land notes, the annual cultural prizes were awarded only to those whose artistic work "exemplifies a positive image of the country."[121] As a final irony, the ceremony pays tribute to Groguhet as emblematic of Ivorian culture at a time when the elderly Houphouët-Boigny's power was waning (he died in December the same year) and when the show's popularity was declining.

The state, especially as embodied by Houphouët-Boigny, demonstrated characteristic resourcefulness in co-opting potential dissent through its control of the media. It aired shows framed as popular satire whose vulgar humor addressed pressing contemporary issues and offered instructions that mocked its own didactic mode but that served its interests and agendas. Although the programs represented a break from the formal pedagogical programming of PETV, they nevertheless supplemented and reinforced governmental campaigns underway. HIV proved no exception. In educating about HIV, the "AIDS" episode of *How's it going?* depicted AIDS as symptom of economic crisis that required the bolstering of austerity policies. In periods of intensifying economic and political instability, the later "Illness of the Century" and *Wintin Wintin and Old Headscarf* episodes questioned the efficacy of pedagogical television and of prior HIV prevention television campaigns. By targeting women as agents of HIV prevention as butts of the joke, the shows converted critique or resistance to austerity measures into the comedic triumph of the heterosexual male over his sexual partner.

---

121. Land, "Ivorien [sic] Television," 17.

CHAPTER 3

Regulating Female Reproductive Potential

Abortion and Family as HIV Prevention

EARLY EDUCATION around HIV/AIDS in the Ivorian media represented the solutions to HIV as self-discipline, self-denial, rigor, and maturity. By framing HIV prevention as a moral issue resolved primarily through sexual self-control, the state media promulgated neoliberal conceptions of free individuals who needed only to be educated to be induced to behave rationally and efficiently. The media represented health care, like other social services, as the responsibility of individuals and their families, of private corporations, and, later, of internationally funded nongovernmental organizations. However, directives to self-manage were not always consistent or coherent, and not surprisingly, for certain gendered bodies, injunctions to self-manage did not always suffice. The HIV-positive pregnant woman in particular provoked intense anxieties and fears around contamination, expressed in contradictory and shifting messages.

The previous chapters analyzed how during the first eight years after the first reported AIDS cases in 1985, the state press and television figured women as the mouthpieces of prevention efforts, especially condom usage, and depicted resistance to HIV prevention in satiric terms of gender struggle. Here, I focus on a selection of HIV prevention media and how it represents mother-to-child HIV transmission as instigating new forms of crisis and how, in response, women's reproductivity emerged as the site of intense interest and management. Over a period of ten years, from 1993 to 2003, HIV prevention media airing on state television in Côte d'Ivoire and throughout the region reversed their messages about abortion. The 1993 series *Gestures or Life* [*Les Gestes ou la vie*] by Ivorian director Kitia Touré was composed of four different segments. The four segments instructed women living with HIV to always use condoms with their male sexual partners and, if pregnant, to terminate their pregnancies. Although approved by the state, these astonishing officially unofficial (or unofficially official) messages directly contravened both state and religious prohibitions of abortion. The directives further implied acceptance, even endorsement, not only of legally banned procedures but also of female sexuality not securely oriented toward reproduction. The series contained such threats through insistent incorporation of HIV-positive women into the patriarchal family, a form of normalization that, like properly disciplined heterosexuality, was proposed as in itself a mode of HIV prevention. The series produced the heterosexual family as central line of defense and, alongside the private corporation, as the primary providers of care and support for people living with HIV. Women's submission to paternalistic medical and conjugal authority over their bodies and reproductive capacities figured as safety, solution, and reward. This self-reinforcing logic continued to frame HIV prevention television series even after drug regimens that decreased the likelihood of mother-to-child HIV transmission became more readily available in Côte d'Ivoire.

The telenovelas produced by Populations Services International (PSI), *AIDS in the City* 1 and 2, which were first broadcast on the state channel in 1995 and in 1996 to 1997, sidestep the issue of abortion. They instead depict the pregnant woman who refuses to test as a destroyer of families analogous to the unfaithful HIV-positive husband. While *AIDS in the City* 1 and 2 followed the story of the same group of characters, the 2003 *AIDS in the City* 3 was composed of four separate four-episode-long segments that each followed a different central character to explore a particular aspect of HIV prevention. The "Fatoumata: HIV-Positive Mother [Fatoumata: Mère séropositive]" segment of *AIDS in the City* 3 works as a corrective to prior HIV prevention messages directed at pregnant women. In this segment, pregnant women were urged to test and, if they tested positive, were admonished not to terminate their pregnancies but rather to obey the proscriptions of biomedical authorities. Women who submitted to medical and paternalistic authority, adhered to prophylactic regimens, and carried their pregnancies to term were redeemed and rewarded by the promise of their further subsumption into the patriarchal family. Those who did not suffered the expected punitive consequences. The segment insists that abortion, not HIV, threatens the fetus and the future of the community. It casts the homosexual, the drug user, and the "prostitute" as necessarily excluded to secure the future and the family—both of which are preserved through proper submission to biomedical authority and to the nongovernmental organization.

I focus on these examples of visual media because these productions, especially the *AIDS in the City* series, were repeatedly and widely broadcast and viewed. They particularly vividly elucidate how messages targeting pregnant women produced the family and control of female reproductivity as modes of HIV prevention. Almost twenty-five years ago, Simon Watney identified health education in response to HIV/AIDS as "the central site of hegemonic struggle" in which the family served as "the central term through which the world and the self are henceforth to be rendered intelligible." Watney was particularly concerned with the intensified marginalization and stigmatization of bodies in Britain marked as "homosexual," contaminated with AIDS, and against whom the heteronormative family served as defense—and against whom the family had to be defended.[1] In Côte d'Ivoire, the turn in prevention media to the heteronormative family as solution and protection against HIV served related, far-ranging ideological and political functions, functions that were, however, embedded in particular colonial and postcolonial histories and contexts.

The family has long been identified as a central organizing unit in Côte d'Ivoire. French colonial attempts to regulate sexuality were promoted as method of disease prevention and were explicitly linked to moralistic discourses on the family. For Christian missionaries in particular, combating diseases necessarily entailed promotion of Christianity and Christian morality and what Megan Vaughan describes as "a sanitized modernity and 'family life.'"[2] Lauren M. MacLean argues that the centralized and direct style of French colonial administration "encourage[d] the evolution of individual citizens living in smaller, nuclear families." French colonial authorities viewed the elimination of the extended family and the establishment of monogamous households through mutual consent as forms of emancipation for their colonial subjects. Under pressure from French missionaries and political groups, French colonial officials targeted family formations and bridewealth exchanges as oppressive to Ivorian women—a variation of what Gayatri Chakravorty Spivak in the context of colonial India has famously condensed as "white men are saving brown women from brown men."[3] In 1951, under French colonial law, monogamous marriages became the only family form acknowledged by

---

1. Watney, "The Spectacle of AIDS," 210.
2. Vaughan, *Curing Their Ills,* 57.
3. MacLean, *Informal Institutions and Citizenship,* 108, 125. Spivak, "Can the Subaltern Speak?" 50.

the state, and infractions were punished by imprisonment. However, under the dual colonial legal system, only a select few educated Africans, alongside French citizens, were subject to French law [statut civil français], while the majority of Africans were subject to customary law [statut coutumier]. Under the latter system, French colonial officials accepted customary polygamous marriages, which continued to be practiced, especially in rural areas.[4]

After independence, ironically, the Civil Code of 1964 no longer recognized customary law in regard to marriage. As the code declared, "Marriage creates the legitimate family."[5] Jeanne M. Toungara notes the central importance of the nuclear family to Houphouët-Boigny and his plans for economic, political, and social transformation after independence from the French: "President Houphouët used the state apparatus to make the conjugal family the only legitimate socio-economic unit and the only marital regime for Côte d'Ivoire."[6] As Toungara explains, the struggle for independence was in part instigated by an elite African planter class frustrated by their inability to access cheap agricultural labor and therefore compete with the French colonists who benefited from forced labor practices. Toungara suggests that the state's interest in enforcing monogamy was directly related to its interest in encouraging capitalist economic development and in maintaining a labor force that incorporated all adults assigned streamlined roles and responsibilities in male-headed single households.[7]

Defenders of the Civil Code certainly delineated its objectives in these terms. As Luzéni Coulibaly argued, the nuclear family was necessary to redress "all the economic servitude that is tied with the lineage family [famille lignagère]."[8] Houphouët-Boigny himself described laws enforcing monogamous marriage as necessary for the country's economic development, with the modern state essentially replacing polygamous marriage and the dowry payments exchanged within it: "Since it appears to us that the continuation [la survivance] of certain traditions constituted an obstacle or hindrance to the harmonious development [l'évolution harmonieuse] of our country, we have not hesitated to institute [imprimer] necessary changes. . . . A revised

---

4. Toungara, "Changing the Meaning of Marriage," 43–44, 55–57.
5. Code Civil, "Mariage." Loi 64-375 du 7 octobre 1964, article 50.
6. Toungara, "Changing the Meaning of Marriage," 57.
7. Toungara, "Changing," 57. In contrast, Eliette Abitbol maintains that laws prohibiting divorce on the grounds of sterility or impotence demonstrate the code's privileging of consent between individuals and the separating of sexual relations from reproduction. Abitbol, "La Famille conjugale," 149. See also Raulin, "Le Droit des personnes," 233.
8. Coulibaly, "Les Traits principaux," 80.

Civil Code [has been] devoted to the suppression of polygamy and reforms of bridewealth [la dot]; a modern civil state is put in place."[9]

The government further explained the need for the Civil Code for marriage in terms of gender equity, in other words, as the state's response to women dissatisfied with customary marriage laws. Closely modeled on French laws, the Civil Code required consent and mandated minimum ages (twenty for men, eighteen for women) for marriage. It formalized the primacy of monogamy through the prohibition of an additional marriage without the dissolution of the first. However, the appeal to gender equity was secondary to the rationale of state economic interests: The status of women in customary marriages hindered "the work of national construction [édification]" and served as "an obstacle to economic, social, political and cultural progress of the country."[10] Despite its claims to promote gender equity, the code further institutionalized new forms of gender subordination. It established "the husband" as "the chief of the family" established through a formalized union.[11] While the code declared that spouses owed each other "mutual fidelity, aid, and assistance," it held men responsible for their children born out of wedlock and thereby implicitly encoded expectations of male extramarital heterosexual relations.[12] In addition, the code, for the first time, authorized the husband's appropriation of the profits from his wife's labor after household expenses and denied women any of the proceeds from wealth or property inherited from their families.[13]

In 1983, the Association of Ivorian Women [Association des Femmes Ivoiriennes], an organization of mostly upper- and middle-class, professional, formally educated women, successfully advocated for changes in the law to enable women to retain control of their own earnings and inheritances and to exert more financial autonomy. However, the primacy of the conjugal monogamous unit remained unchallenged in this new iteration of what Toungara describes as the "invention of the 'legal family'" that served the interests of male elites.[14] The legal invention of the conjugal family enforced reproductive

---

9. Houphouët-Boigny, *Anthologie des discours*, 1.
10. D. Vangah, "Statut de la femme," 97.
11. Code Civil, "Mariage." Loi 64-375 du 7 octobre 1964, article 58.
12. Code Civil, "Mariage." Loi 64-375 du 7 octobre 1964, article 51. As Ivorian jurist Luzéni Coulibaly explained in a defense of the article, "Man, insofar as he is man, cannot stop himself [s'empêcher] from being an adulterer." Vangah, 102–3.
13. Code Civil, "Mariage." Loi 64-375 du 7 octobre 1964, article 74.
14. Toungara, "Inventing the African Family," 46–49; Code Civil, "Mariage." Loi 64-375 du 7 octobre 1964, article 50; Code Civil, "Mariage." Loi 64-375 du 7 octobre 1964 modifiée par la loi no. 83-800 du 2 août 1983, article 50.

heteronormativity as central to a national project of economic development. The upper classes conformed to the laws that already mirrored their practices, while the lower classes were unaware of the laws or ignored them, and customary polygamous marriages involving exchanges of bridewealth continued. The attempts to code heterosexual monogamy as essential to nation-building—and the gap between official discourses and lived realities—might be read instructively alongside efforts by more contemporary campaigns to reshape sexual behavior and families and to promote the monogamous family as modes of HIV prevention.

The insistence in HIV prevention media on the role of the family in properly containing female sexuality and reproductivity—and therefore the spread of HIV—echoed many of the prior attempts to legislate monogamous families as the foundational unit of the nation. During a period of state retrenchment, the turn to the family rationalized reductions in state services and facilitated the ascendance of the foreign-funded nongovernmental organization as primary source of testing, treatment, and care. Further, in HIV prevention videos in Côte d'Ivoire, the definition of certain bodies and behaviors as inassimilable into the patriarchal family contributed to intensifying debates about national identity and belonging, especially as they were invoked in conflicts around land ownership, political candidacy, and voting rights. By producing some categories of people as redeemable and others as necessarily expendable or excluded from the patriarchal family—and, by extension, community and nation—HIV prevention media reinforced the exclusionary logic of prevailing ethnic nationalism and expanded its terms to encompass sexual identities and behavior.

TERMINATION OF PREGNANCY AS HIV PREVENTION: *GESTURES OR LIFE*

In 1992, seroprevalence among pregnant women in Abidjan, the largest city and the economic capital of Côte d'Ivoire and of the region, was estimated at 15%. The effectiveness of the drug zidovudine (or azidothymidine, AZT) in lowering perinatal, or mother-to-child, HIV transmission was not established until results from the AIDS Clinical Trial Group 076 were published two years later, in 1994.[15] Produced in 1993, the *Gestures or Life* series attempts

---

15. The trial showed that AZT administered orally during pregnancy, intravenously during labor and delivery, and orally to a newborn in the six weeks after birth lowered perinatal HIV transmission by two-thirds, that is, from transmission rates between 15% and 40% in the absence of any AZT treatment down to about 8% when AZT was administered to the mother

to address the potential of perinatal transmission of HIV during the period when reported HIV prevalence rates among pregnant women were alarmingly high, but no protocols had yet been established to decrease the possibility of HIV transmission from mother to child. At the same time, the state, undergoing major cutbacks following the imposition of structural adjustment policies, continued to reduce health-care spending despite the increasing needs generated by the growing epidemic. President since independence from the French in 1960, the ailing Félix Houphouët-Boigny died at the end of 1993 after a thirty-three-year dictatorship. Coping with a weakening state on the verge of major struggles for political succession, *Gestures or Life* proposes as solution to perinatal transmission that all pregnant women who test HIV-positive end their pregnancies.

The four-segment *Gestures or Life* series was scripted and directed by Ivorian writer and filmmaker Kitia Touré, with funding from the European Union, the United Nations, the World Health Organization, the French government, and the Ivorian Ministry of Culture, with the support of state television and the National Committee for the Fight against AIDS [Comité national de lutte contre le Sida (CNLS)]. The series broadcast on state television and also screened at film festivals, where it won a number of awards.[16] Each of the four segments that each follow individual unrelated storylines urges HIV testing, explains various prevention methods, and attempts to combat stigmatization of people living with HIV.

One of the twenty-six-minute-long segments titled "Reasons for Fear [Raisons de la peur]" focuses on convincing pregnant women to test and on preventing mother-to-child transmission of HIV. According to the World Health Organization, in the absence of prophylactic regimens, a child born to an HIV-positive woman has about a 15% to 40% chance of becoming infected with HIV in utero, during delivery, or via breastfeeding.[17] A pregnancy is also by definition the product of shared bodily fluids, more specifically, in the absence of reproductive technologies generally unavailable in Côte d'Ivoire, of unprotected penile-vaginal heterosexual sex. According to the terms of HIV education media centering on inculcating individual responsibility for prevention, the HIV-positive pregnant woman therefore embodies a failure

---

and to the newborn. After the efficacy of the treatment was established, the trial was suspended and results released. Connor et al., "Reduction of Maternal-Infant Transmission," 1173–80.

16. *Gestures or Life* won the Promaco Prize for the Struggle against AIDS, the Telcripro Prize for Technical Quality at the Panafrican Film and Television Festival in Ouagadougou [Le Festival panafricain du cinéma et de la télévision de Ouagadougou (FESPACO)], and the special jury prize at the Festival of Scientific Film in Paris-Eiffel Tower.

17. WHO, *HIV/AIDS: Mother-to-Child Transmission of HIV*.

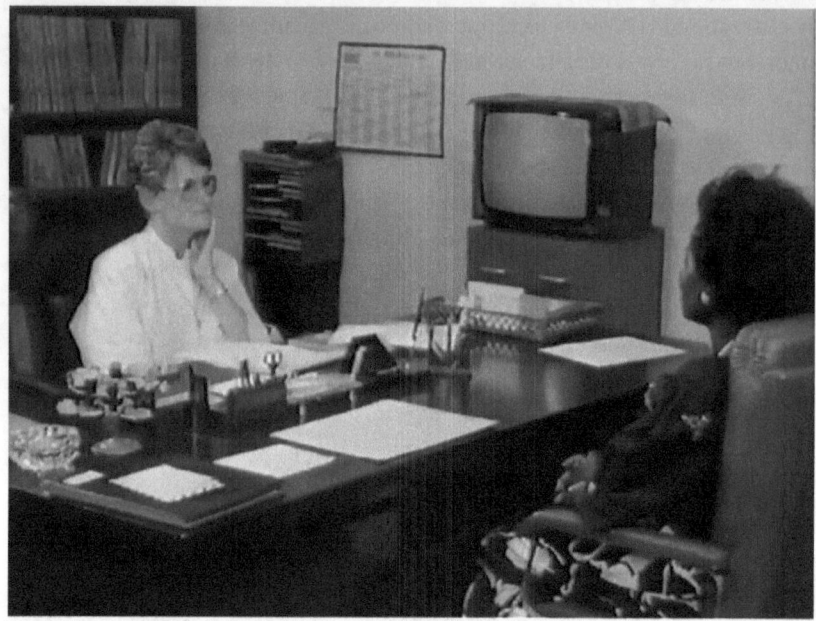

FIGURE 3.1. Jeanne (on right) and Sister Catherine (on left).

of HIV education and poses a double, even triple, threat to the health and well-being of individuals and of the community, to the future itself as symbolized by the child. "Reasons for Fear" attempts to counter and contain this threat.

Contrasting Muslim/Christian and rural/urban, the segment opens with the series theme song in Dioula, "Men and women, AIDS is not good. Allah help us," playing as establishing shots show a ferry landing in the country's economic and political capital city, Abidjan, followed by a woman entering an office. The camera then cuts to Kouako, a physician from the interior of the country, telephoning a white nun, identified in the credits only as "Sister Catherine." Sister Catherine runs an AIDS information hotline, AIDS Direct [SIDA Direct], in Abidjan, and the segment depicts her wearing a white habit and a crucifix in an office where she is seated next to a television and telephone. The film marks her as a central figure of white Christian religious, technological, and medical authority from whom others solicit advice. The nun's habit and crucifix symbolize her religious authority; the prominently displayed television, like the telephone, signals the modern technology and authoritative knowledge of HIV prevention information (figure 3.1). The woman who has come to consult with Sister Catherine in her office listens alongside viewers of the series as Kouako recounts his predicament to Sister Catherine, and the scenes that he narrates play out onscreen.

During a prenatal visit, Kouako tells his patient, Sita, that he will conduct routine screening but does not tell her that he has added HIV to the list of tests. When she tests HIV-positive, he feels conflicted about being unable to disclose the results to her because, as he explains to his own wife, they will "shatter her entire life." After Kouako's wife suggests that he wait until after Sita delivers to inform her, or her partner, about the test, Kouako counters, "No, she cannot keep this pregnancy [garder cette grossesse]. The child will have every likelihood of having the AIDS virus [L'enfant va avoir toute la chance d'avoir le virus de sida], not to mention that she can contaminate her partner if it hasn't already happened." His wife encourages him to tell Sita's partner and reminds him, "You are a doctor. Your work requires that you tell your patient what they're suffering from."

In the next scene, Sita's partner, Touré, comes to the clinic room where Sita lies recovering from what is clearly an abortion. Kouako takes Touré aside and confesses that he had lied: "There was no risk with Sita's pregnancy.... The truth, unfortunately, is that I did a test for the AIDS virus on your girlfriend. It is done with all pregnant women. She is seropositive.... I did not have the courage to tell her this truth." Kouako urges Touré to test but still does not inform Sita about her own test results. As Kouako later explains his actions to his supervisor [doyen], also a physician, he requested the HIV test and confirmed the positive result but could not tell Sita. Instead, he used the pretext [prétexter] of unspecified "serious complications, a pathological pregnancy, in order to advise a termination of the pregnancy [lui conseiller une interruption de grossesse]." For him, it was paramount "to avoid the birth of a child who could be born with the AIDS virus," since the child and Sita will confront "the anguish, the stress, the fear of the gazes of others [des regards des autres]" that could accelerate their decline and death, especially since they live in a rural area.

In 1985, the United States Centers for Disease Control recommendations stated that "infected women should be advised to consider delaying pregnancy until more is known about perinatal transmission of the virus."[18] As Ronald Bayer notes, in the context of the United States, "Only timidity and the bitter ideological politics of abortion precluded an open discussion" about whether the recommendations required that HIV-positive pregnant women be urged to terminate their pregnancies.[19] The *Gestures or Life* video displays no such

---

18. Centers for Disease Control and Prevention, "Current Trends Recommendations," 725.
19. Bayer, "Perinatal Transmission of HIV Infection," 502.

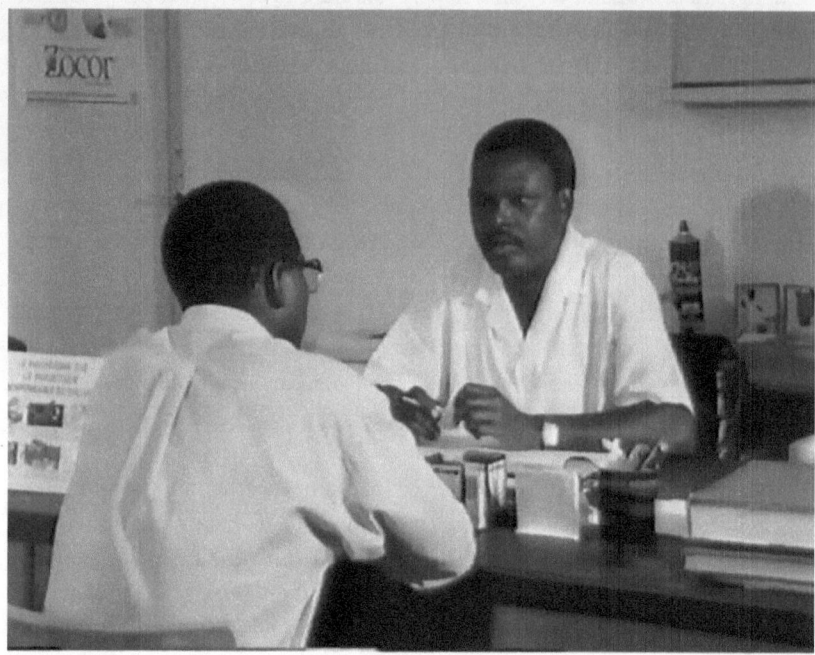

FIGURE 3.2. Supervisor with Kouako (in foreground).

timidity. In "Reasons for Fear," Kouako recounts that he has explicitly urged Sita to terminate her pregnancy and that she heeded his advice. Kouako's supervisor chastises Kouako for taking the risk of performing the procedure; Sita might have consulted another doctor for a second opinion. Nevertheless, the supervisor eases Kouako's faltering conscience and lingering doubts. The supervisor characterizes AIDS as instigating devastating social and medical disruptions that authorize physicians to act in violation of all previous norms and laws in order to save individuals and the community. His white coat signaling medical authority visually echoes the nun's white habit, and photographs of young children in the background further identify him as a father (figure 3.2). As the supervisor says to Kouako, "Listen my friend, AIDS is a new illness that comes to turn all customs and our morphology upside down [bouleverser toutes les moeurs et notre morphologie]. Know only that you have a duty [un devoir] to your patient and to society. We must avoid contamination on a grand scale."

As Kouako explains to Sister Catherine on the hotline telephone, his predicament centers on informing Sita about her HIV status, especially since Sita's partner, Touré, later also tested HIV-positive, and although Touré is full of self-recrimination about his many sexual affairs, he still has not told Sita. In contrast to Kouako's supervisor, the nun advises Kouako to inform Sita of her test results and to refer her to an HIV specialist. Significantly, however, the nun does not interrogate the assumption that pregnant women who test HIV-positive must not carry their pregnancies to term. The pregnant woman, Jeanne, who had come to consult Sister Catherine, tells the sister that she fears that she is HIV-positive but her doctor was hiding her results from her, just as Kouako did with Sita. Recounting the story of a young man who was convinced that he was HIV-positive, when he actually was not, the nun convinces Jeanne to test first: "Do the test and have your boyfriend do it." As Jeanne departs, she thanks the nun: "I will do it because of my baby. I am expecting a child, and I wanted to abort it. That's why I came to see you and to talk with you a little." While the nun and Jeanne both agree on the importance of testing for the sake of the child, neither one expresses any doubt that if Jeanne's results are HIV-positive, she will "abort [avorter]" the pregnancy.

The segment insistently frames HIV prevention as the responsibilization of pregnant women who must take initiative and decide to test for HIV and convince their partners to do so as well. However, the representation of HIV/AIDS as inaugurating a state of exception works to reinforce both existing legal prohibitions on abortion and to rationalize further assertions of paternalistic medical and conjugal authority over women, their bodies, and their reproductive capacity. In his influential theorizing of the state of exception, Giorgio Agamben considers how states of emergency that provoke and justify suspension of the law thereby strip certain bodies of human status, placing them outside the law's purview. For Agamben, the juridico-political decisions about whose lives are not worth living, and who as "bare life," or *homo sacer,* can be killed with impunity, define national sovereignty as the "politicization" of biopolitics.[20] As Penelope Deutscher argues, abortion law, and women's reproductivity more generally, represent symptomatic omissions in Agamben's analyses. Deutscher notes that abortion law inverts the states of exception that Agamben examines and that he reads as epitomized by the Nazi death camps. In contrast to these examples, recent abortion laws in the Global North have not decriminalized the practice of abortion, thereby expanding techniques of state sovereignty, so much as they have granted certain exceptions to preexisting regulations: "The state of exception is not the state, not the nation or a country's suspended legal system; rather, it is abortion 'itself' that has frequently existed in a state of suspension or exception to its own illegality."[21]

---

20. Agamben, *Homo Sacer,* 71–72, 142; Foucault, *The History of Sexuality,* vol. 1, 138; Foucault, "Society Must Be Defended," 250.

21. Deutscher, "The Inversion of Exceptionality," 55–70, 60.

Insofar as Côte d'Ivoire's abortion laws were modeled on French legislation, they too reproduce the inverted form of the state of exception—of abortion as the exception to its own illegal status. In France, the conflation of religious and legal doctrine made abortion punishable by death beginning in 1556.[22] The Penal Code of 1791 granted immunity to women who procured abortion but punished those who performed them with a twenty-year imprisonment. Article 317 of the Napoleonic Penal Code of 1810 eliminated the granting of immunity to pregnant women who procured an abortion. It imposed imprisonment on them as well as on anyone who administered or advised the administration of an abortion that took place. At the same time, the penal code did permit abortions performed to save the "gravely threatened" life of a pregnant woman. This law has become the basis for the most restrictive antiabortion laws persisting throughout Francophone sub-Saharan Africa.[23]

A 1920 French pro-natalist law that applied to Algeria and to French colonies, including Côte d'Ivoire, prohibited abortion and sterilization—as well as contraception and "propaganda" about contraception. In 1923, abortion became a civil rather than criminal offense, but penalties were expanded to encompass even attempted abortion and, in 1939, to women who procured or attempted to procure an abortion, regardless of whether they were even pregnant or actually succeeded in their attempts. In 1939, an important exception was also carved out for "therapeutic abortions" performed to save the life of a pregnant woman, although two additional physicians had to be consulted and attest that the procedure was necessary to save the life of the mother and that no other procedure could do so, a provision that was reiterated in 1955 law.[24] Significantly, while in 1975 France amended its laws to permit voluntary termination of pregnancies within the first ten weeks of pregnancy, the law was explicitly framed as a state of exception to the existing prohibitions on abortions, and article 317 of the Penal Code of 1810 still applied to cases outside the permitted exceptions.[25]

Both Agamben and Deutscher are particularly concerned with the United States and Western Europe, and Deutscher refers to these contexts

---

22. For a useful historical overview on abortion laws in Francophone countries, with a focus on Western Europe and Canada, see Knoppers, Brault, and Sloss, "Abortion Law in Francophone Countries," 889–922. Much of the historical background that follows is based on this article and on Knoppers and Brault, *La Loi et l'avortement*.

23. Knoppers and Brault, *La Loi et l'avortement*, 34.

24. Knoppers and Brault, *La Loi et l'avortement*, 94.

25. French Minister of Health at the time, Simone Veil, insisted that "abortion must remain the exception, the last resort for situations with no way out [l'avortement doit rester l'exception, l'ultime recours pour des situations sans issue]." BFM TV, "Le Discours de Simone Veil."

when she argues that "the repeated creation of abortion as a state of permanent exceptionality has been one of the essential workings of twentieth- and early-twenty-first-century biopolitics concerning women's reproductivity."[26] Deutscher reads reproductive biopolitics as a "parallel subregime" to those states of exception analyzed by Agamben. For her, the special dispensations that characterize abortion law constitute a modality of sovereignty that through the state of exception ensures the maintenance of the harshest forms of the rule targeting women's bodies.

In the context of postcolonial Côte d'Ivoire, the "biopolitics concerning women's reproductivity" were principally animated by postcolonial nation-building. Revising French colonial legislation, Côte d'Ivoire's 1981 abortion laws reflected the single-party state's continuing emphasis on population growth as enabling economic development and as reflecting the nation's wealth.[27] The 1981 law (as of August 2017 still in effect in Côte d'Ivoire) rejects the French 1975 revisions and preserves the language from the earlier laws that punished not just the person who performed or tried to perform an abortion but also the woman who procured, tried to procure, or consented to using methods that would result in the termination of her pregnancy. The Ivorian penal code further prohibits any dissemination of information or publicity about abortion but, following the 1939 and 1955 French laws, does permit the procedure in tightly restricted cases where the mother's life is in "extreme danger," in which case the abortion has to be carried out with the consultation of two additional physicians who must certify that the women's life can be saved only through the performance of the procedure.[28] Although in 1981, the July 31, 1920, law prohibiting "provocation to abortion and contraception propaganda" was abolished, the penal code imposed the death penalty for

---

26. Deutscher, "The Inversion of Exceptionality," 64–65.

27. Structural adjustment policies implemented from 1991 to 1993 marked what Anoh, Fassassi, and Vimard describe as a neo-Malthusian shift to population control rather than growth. The focus on a limitation of international migration as a form of population control corresponded with the rise of the exclusionary rhetoric of *Ivoirité*. They attribute the pronatalist perspective of the country to cultural and religious factors as well. Anoh, Fassassi, and Vimard, *Politique de population*, 8–14.

28. According to Ivorian law, if only one physician resides in the place where the abortion is performed, that physician must certify the procedure. If no other physicians reside in the place where the abortion is performed, the physician "must certify on his or her honor that the life of the mother can only be saved by the surgical or therapeutic operation employed." Code Penal. Loi 81-640 du 31 juillet 1981. Titre 2, Chapitre 3, Section 3, Article 367. See also Ngwena, "Reforming African Abortion Laws," 166–86, 170; Center for Reproductive Rights, "The World's Abortion Laws Map 2013 Update."

sterilization, "the act of depriving a person of procreative potential [la faculté de procréer]."[29]

The 1981 Ivorian law prohibiting abortion falls under the chapter "Crimes and Offenses against Children [Enfants] and People Incapable of Protecting Themselves by Reason of Their Physical and Mental State" and follows the sections "Infanticide, Acts of Violence and Aggravated Assault [violences et voies de fait]" and "Abandonment of Child or Incapable Person [d'incapable]." The Ivorian law frames the banning of abortion as protecting the lives of "children" and "infants," and at the same time, of pregnant women deemed incapable of "protecting themselves."[30] This formulation conflates "fetus" with "infants/children [enfants]" (and pregnancy with physical and mental incapacitation) as a life that, if aborted, would be deemed outside the law and able to be killed with impunity, or Agamben's *homo sacer*. In their arguments in the state weekly, *Ivoire Dimanche*, opponents of abortion in Côte d'Ivoire invoked this legal framing of abortion. An article in the state daily, *Fraternité Matin*, described a 1989 meeting in which Episcopal bishops condemned the widespread practice of abortion as a "plague" and a sign of "a certain decadence" that "menaces the moral order." Although some bishops disagreed and framed the issue as one of individual choice, the newspaper column writer countered, "Must be we then permit [Faut-il alors se laisser aller] a certain license, a certain licentiousness and kill unwanted children [qu'on ne désire pas]?"[31]

Deutscher critiques such antiabortion rhetorical, legal, and political slippages as false and pernicious, casting pregnant women as merely reproductive life, a competing and threatening sovereign from whom the child must be protected.[32] In the context of postcolonial Côte d'Ivoire, these slippages enable the assertion of a form of biopolitical postcolonial state sovereignty extended through laws that target not only women's bodies but also French laws or, rather, that target the French suspension of laws that Côte d'Ivoire insistently retains to produce and protect the new nation. Jan Stepan describes as a "tragic irony" that Francophone sub-Saharan African countries compelled to adopt French colonial antiabortion laws did not continue along the path of "modern legal development" after formal independence and similarly adopt the 1975 French "Veil Law," which permitted more-expansive exceptions.[33] In Stepan's implied narrative of progress, suspension of abortion prohibitions constitutes modern legal advancement, and Francophone sub-Saharan African countries'

---

29. Code Penal. Loi 81-640 du 31 juillet 1981. Titre 2, Chapitre 1, Section 1, Article 343.
30. Code Penal. Loi 81-640 du 31 juillet 1981. Titre 2, Chapitre 3, Sections 1–3.
31. Jean-Pierre Ayé, "Avortement: L'église s'inquiète," *Fraternité Matin*, April 10, 1989, 26.
32. Deutscher, "The Inversion of Exceptionality," 66–67.
33. Stepan, "Preface," ii.

refusals to adopt similar measures signal their lingering backwardness and failure to attain modernity. Such a narrative fails to recognize the reproductive biopolitics of the postcolonial nation aimed at producing subjects of and workers for a new nation and glosses over the extent to which women's bodies served as critical sites for definition and assertion of postcolonial national identity.[34] The paradoxes of asserting postcolonial state sovereignty through the maintenance of prior colonial laws exemplify the paradoxes of both postcolonial sovereignty and the condition of postcoloniality more broadly.

A further paradox of abortion in Côte d'Ivoire is the extent to which, despite its illegality, it is performed in "open secret." A population control program was not instituted in Côte d'Ivoire until 1997, and limited family planning services meant that although illegal, the termination of pregnancies was a common practice as a form of birth control and as a resolution for unwanted pregnancies.[35] An Episcopal bishop in Côte d'Ivoire in 1989 praised the country's restrictions on abortion but sharply condemned the well-known permanent incorporation of associations offering abortions in state Centers for Maternal and Infant Protection [Centres de protection maternelle et infantile (PMI)].[36] A series of articles in the December 2–8, 1990, *Ivoire Dimanche* lamented the "calamity" of frequent abortions: According to the weekly, 97% of unmarried women have abortions "very often" as a form of birth control. Another article noted that to obtain an abortion at the public hospital, "it suffices to know the hours of aborters [avorteurs] and to have a recommendation. This confirms the rumors that our public hospitals [Centre hospitalier universaitaire (CHU)] are veritable nests of aborters." The article reminded readers about the laws against abortion—although it also observed that the laws were rarely enforced.[37] For women living with HIV, as researchers note,

---

34. Much has been written on the subject of how women's reproductivity became the sites for colonial and anticolonial struggles for authority and for the definition and assertion of postcolonial national identities. See Boddy, *Civilizing Women*; Hunt, *A Colonial Lexicon*; Mikell, *African Feminism*; Thomas, *The Politics of the Womb*; Thomas, "Gendered Reproduction."

35. Guillaume and Desgrées-Du-Loû, "Fertility Regulation," 159, 161. Desgrées-Du-Loû et al. "Contraceptive Use," 466.

36. "L'État protège l'enfant," *Fraternité Matin*, April 11, 1989, 9.

37. Awa Ehoura and Agnès Kraide Masoso, "Avortement: La calamité," *Ivoire Dimanche*, December 2–8, 1990, 4. The accompanying article offered different statistics: 18% of girls between ages fourteen to sixteen, 72% of those between eighteen and twenty-five, and 9% of those between twenty-five and thirty-five had had an abortion at least once as an illicit form of birth control. Agnès Kraide Masoso, "Avec une aiguille, sans anesthésie," *Ivoire Dimanche*, December 2–8, 1990, 5. See also Awa Ehoura, "Tous les moyens sont bons," *Ivoire Dimanche*, December 2–8, 1990, 6–7. An *Ivoir'Soir* article noted: "Despite its prohibition . . . abortion today is extremely commonplace [banal]." Venance Konan, "Faut-il légaliser l'avortement?" *Ivoir'Soir*, December 29, 1990, 4.

abortion likely "exacerbated a practice already common and admitted by this population."[38] These paradoxes about abortion were amplified in the representations of HIV/AIDS as inaugurating a state of emergency that rather than provoke state response justifies its further attrition.

HIV/AIDS AS STATE OF EMERGENCY: "REASONS FOR FEAR"

In the segment "Reasons for Fear," for Kouako's supervisor, AIDS provokes a state of emergency essentially empowering medical authorities to suspend the law and locate both physicians and women who test positive for HIV outside its purview. "Reasons for Fear" explicitly represents HIV/AIDS as *not* activating the existing legal exception that permits the termination of a pregnancy (with required confirmatory medical opinion, if applicable) if this procedure constitutes the only means to save the lives of the women. Kouako states that he has lied, that "there was no risk" about the pregnancy. Similarly, Jeanne, who also consults Sister Catherine, states that she will terminate her pregnancy if her test is HIV-positive, not because of any threat to her life but because she cannot deliver a child who might be HIV-positive. Kouako's supervisor essentially agrees that such abortions must be performed on HIV-positive pregnant women—as, presumably, did the state, which coproduced the series. The segment further depicts Sister Catherine, the embodiment of white Christian religious and medical authority, as aligned with the state in its sanctioning of the further suspension of the law in the cases of pregnant women who test HIV-positive. This suspension of abortion laws affirmed the fundamental prohibitions against abortion and rationalized expansion of medical authority over pregnant women, and, at the same time, the denial of state responsibility for responding to the epidemic or to conditions of increasing social precarity.

Deploying a zero-sum biopolitical calculus, the segment insists that although in the absence of any prophylactic treatment, perinatal HIV transmission rates are estimated to be from 15% to 40%, an HIV-positive woman must avoid all risk of even the possibility of infecting her child. The segment implies that individuals and society would be best served if pregnant women were routinely—and mandatorily—tested for HIV and insists that if the results are positive, they must terminate their pregnancies. According to "Reasons for Fear," preventing *all* women who test HIV-positive from reproducing constitutes a necessary strategy to "avoid contamination on a grand scale."

---

38. Desgrées-Du-Loû et al., "Contraceptive Use," 466.

The segment relies on and reproduces what Linda Singer identifies as "epidemic logic," one that produces HIV as a threat in order to propose the solutions to contain it.[39] In its representation of HIV as inaugurating a state of emergency, the segment exempts pregnant women living with HIV and their physicians from the punishments outlined in state antiabortion law. The segment thereby produces HIV as the sole, or at least the most extraordinary, threat to the fetus, the overdetermined symbol for the future community in whose name pregnant women in particular must test. The series justifies the prohibition against reproduction for women who test HIV-positive through the establishment of maternal and child negative serostatus as guarantor of the safety, health, and vitality of the future and of the community. However, as UN statistics bear out, even when reported AIDS cases were relatively low, the health of the child and of the community were far from secure. Estimated mortality rates for children under five in Côte d'Ivoire, even before identification of the first AIDS cases in 1985, were about 154 out of 1,000 live births, a rate that remained consistent throughout the 1990s.[40]

In its figuring of HIV as extraordinary peril justifying extraordinary interventions, "Reasons for Fear" does not address the everyday perils resulting in high infant and child mortality *regardless of HIV status*. It does not only elide but also naturalizes as "safe" or acceptable how many infants and young children die from preterm or intrapartum complications and from other infectious diseases, like pneumonia, diarrhea, and malaria. The high rates of childhood mortality—which not incidentally are about equivalent to the likelihood of mother-to-child HIV transmission in the absence of prophylactic regimens—index poverty, a term that in turn indexes an array of conditions: lack of clean water, shelter, sewage, and nutrition, as well as health care, education, and other services. These conditions, which have come to serve as overdetermined and racist signs of "Africa," are not natural or inevitable but the results of specific local, as well as global, histories and economic policies, including structural adjustment.[41] The film further normalizes as acceptable

---

39. Singer, *Erotic Welfare*, 29–32.
40. For mortality rates among children under five per 1,0000 live births, see UNICEF, "Child Mortality Estimates: Côte d'Ivoire Under-Five Mortality Rate," 2016. http://www.child-mortality.org/index.php?r=site/graph#ID=CIV_Cote d Ivoire. For 2017 mortality rates among children under five per 1,000 live births, see the UN Inter-agency Group for Child Mortality Estimation, *Levels and Trends in Child Mortality*, 24.
41. Useche and Cabezas, "The Vicious Cycle," 25. A United Nations report titled "Globalization and Women's Vulnerabilities to HIV and AIDS," citing Colleen O'Manique's *Neoliberalism and AIDS Crisis*, among others, has acknowledged that structural adjustment programs have undermined health-care provision and negatively affected states' abilities to respond to HIV/AIDS (2). On the increase of infant and child mortality rates from the 1980s through the 1990s due to inadequate health resources, see Pégatiénan and Blibolo, "Impact

the high rates of maternal mortality, estimated in 1990 at around 20% of all deaths of women from ages fifteen to forty-nine, with rates tripling between 1978 and 1990.[42] It also does not acknowledge that illegal abortions were the major cause of maternal deaths—80% according to one study of maternal deaths in Abidjan hospitals from 1989 to 1992.[43] More broadly, the film produces the conditions in which all people with a negative serostatus live as a state to be defended against the threat of HIV, especially as embodied by HIV-positive pregnant women. It works in the service of preservation rather than transformation of the status quo.

While "Reasons for Fear" represents HIV as activating a state of emergency that impels direct interventions on pregnant women, the segment does not address the health of the women themselves, except insofar as it could potentially affect their children. In other words, while the threat of HIV prompts the tacit suspension of the state and Christian religious law, significantly, the terms and targets of that suspension are selective. While the segment sanctions the performance of technically illegal medical procedures on HIV-positive pregnant women, the international laws protecting pharmaceutical companies' patents, for example, remained fully enforced. In March 1987, the United States Food and Drug Administration approved AZT to treat HIV infection. However, limited provision of subsidized antiretroviral treatment in Côte d'Ivoire did not begin until more than ten years later—in Abidjan in August 1998.[44] The high costs of patented drugs in large part accounted for the long delay of treatment access for most people living with HIV/AIDS in Côte d'Ivoire and almost all of the Global South.[45] I will not here rehearse the

---

socio-économique," 46. See also Schoepf, Schoepf, and Millen, "Theoretical Therapies"; Poku, "Poverty, Debt and Africa's HIV/AIDS Crisis."

42. For maternal mortality rates, see WHO et al., *Maternal Mortality in 1990–2015*, 68.

43. Thonneau et al., "The Persistence of a High Maternal Mortality Rate," 1478–79.

44. As part of a UNAIDS Drug Access Initiative, six "'referral centers'" in Abidjan distributed antiretrovirals (ARVs) to "selected patients." Women who had participated in clinical trials for prevention of mother-to-child HIV transmission and active members of associations of people living with AIDS received the maximum possible subsidy for ARVs, 95%. Those identified as "low income" received subsidies of 50% to 75%. The plan to distribute ARVs was announced in November 1997, but distribution did not begin until August the following year. In 1996, highly active antiretroviral therapy (HAART) was identified as a significant improvement in treatment of HIV infections, but HAART distribution did not begin in Côte d'Ivoire until October 1999. Philippe Msellati et al., "Socio-economic and Health Characteristics," S64. See also Delaunay et al., "Prémices et déroulement de l'Initiative (1996–2000)," 38–40.

45. For more on the World Trade Organization's (WTO) Trade-Related Aspects of International Property Rights (TRIPS) and the Doha agreement of 2001, see UNAIDS, WHO, and UNDP, *Policy Brief: Using TRIPS Flexibilities*. The "Paragraph 6 solution" in 2003 (formalized as an amendment in 2005) finally permitted countries that did not have the capacity to manu-

heated debates about the safety and efficacy of AZT and the ethics of the clinical trials that led to provision of cheaper, shorter—but less effective—courses of treatment to prevent perinatal HIV transmission in the Global South. Nor will I detail the activism around treatment access that eventually led to the carving out of certain limited exceptions to international property laws so that cheaper generics could be dispensed in low-income countries. "Reasons for Fear" does not address treatment access at all. It produces not only the "reasons for fear" that it names—the threat of children becoming infected by HIV through their mothers—but also the protection against this danger: further interventions on women and their reproductive capacities.

"Reasons for Fear" identifies HIV-positive pregnant women as the most significant hazard to the fetus and proposes as safeguard the termination of their pregnancies. The series represents medical, religious, state, and family authority as aligned in approving procedures performed with impunity on pregnant women, especially pregnant women who test positive for HIV. The exemption of HIV-positive pregnant women and of medical personnel from laws restricting abortions affirms the necessity of the regulation of female reproductive capacity and frames such interventions as a critical mode of defense for the future of the community. At the same time, HIV prevention media effectively silences the state, which does not provide services or enforce—or officially suspend—its own antiabortion law. HIV prevention media that is financed by foreign funders themselves constitutes important demonstrations of international organizations' authority over that of the postcolonial state in crisis. The foreign-funded prevention media represents a consequence of state retrenchment—the state cannot fund its own prevention campaigns—even as it provides important legitimizing discourse for the cutbacks. Women's bodies and reproductive capacity serve as the familiar terrain for these struggles.[46]

---

facture antiretroviral drugs to import generics from developing countries granted compulsory licenses by the WTO. On paragraph 6, see WTO, "Implementation of Paragraph 6." See also Hanefeld, "Patent Rights vs. Patient Rights," 84–92; Beall and Kuhn, "Trends in Compulsory Licensing," 6; Abbott and Reichman, "The Doha Round's Public Health Legacy," 755–88. For necessary warnings about the embrace of biomedicine and medical intervention as a quick-fix solution to the HIV epidemic, see Wendland, "Research, Therapy, and Bioethical Hegemony," 1–23. For a critique of biomedical interventions as likely exacerbating the spread of HIV in Abidjan, see Nguyen, "Therapeutic Modernism."

46. McClintock, *Imperial Leather,* 354–55.

HETERONORMATIVE ROMANCE, FAMILY, AND THE "HEALTHY CARRIER": "IN THE NAME OF LOVE"

The "Reasons for Fear" segment seeks to persuade viewers that pregnant women, and, by extension, all women who test positive for HIV, must avoid even the possibility of transmitting HIV to fetuses. Women of reproductive capacity who test positive for HIV are therefore in a bind. If they defy prevention messages, they threaten the child, the family, and society. However, if they comply with medical directives and terminate their pregnancies and never reproduce, they cannot conform to heteronormative, reproductively oriented gender roles. Further, the insistence on abortion as the solution for mother-to-child transmission for all pregnant women who test positive for HIV implies that even the possibility of a life with HIV must be eliminated because such a life is not worth living. The prevention messages in "Reasons for Fear" thereby risk exacerbating the stigma that the series purports to combat. Two other segments in *Gestures or Life* attempt to resolve the impasses established by the series. "In the Name of Love" and "That Happens Only to Others" insist that HIV-positive women can be incorporated into the family constituted as what Linda Singer describes as itself a "strategic and prudential safe sex practice."[47] The series segments establish equivalences between family and corporation as responsible for the care of people living with HIV and as providing essential protection and support. In the segments, both family and corporation mobilize to take responsibility for the care of people living with HIV who have been defined as "healthy carriers."

In attempting to combat stigmatization of people living with HIV, the aptly titled segment "In the Name of Love" in effect delineates and enforces the terms of HIV-positive persons' reincorporation into family and workplace. "In the Name of Love" proposes that if HIV-positive women never reproduce and always use condoms, then they can be redeemed by heterosexual romance—and the corporation. In this segment, the central character, a middle-class office worker, Angeline, is set up by a friend with Serge. Angeline insists on being tested for HIV before having sex and then using condoms when they have sex before they have received their results. A poster on her bedroom door reminds viewers of the ongoing campaign urging usage of Prudence-branded condoms: "Trust okay. Prudence first. Prudence Condoms" (figure 3.3). As Angeline tells the friend who tries to dissuade her from testing, "I love him, so prefer to lose him than contaminate him if I am seropositive." After Angeline tests HIV-positive, she worries that Serge will abandon her

---

47. Singer, *Erotic Welfare*, 85.

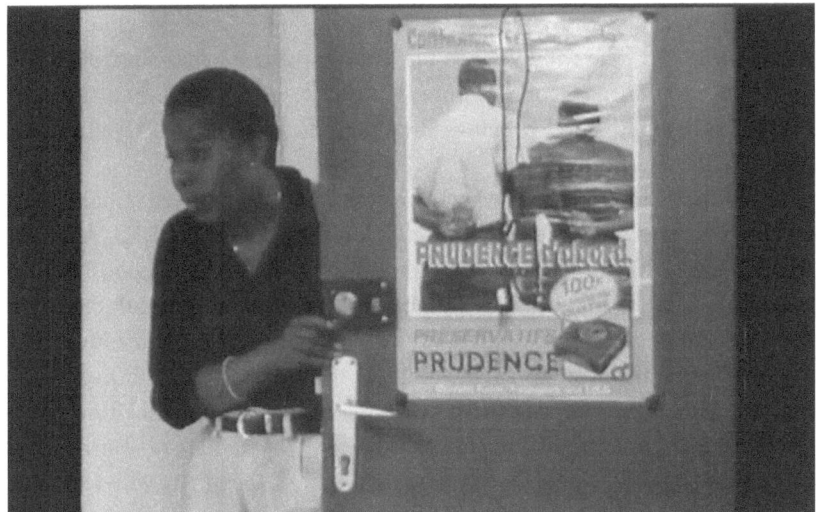

FIGURE 3.3. "Trust okay. Prudence first. Prudence Condoms," a campaign that the segment represents as effective.

but tells her friend that she "wishes him great happiness [je lui souhaite un grand bonheur] if he leaves me." Instead, Serge recognizes that "she spared me [m'a épargné] in demanding a test. She saved me.... Angeline needs care and help"—and marries her. As Serge's friend, Alain, a doctor, explains the sudden marriage plans to Serge's baffled mother, Angeline is HIV-positive, and the family serves as critical defense for Angeline: "Angeline is not sick. She is a carrier of the virus.... She needs love, the family's total support to help her fight."

On their way to a medical consultation with an HIV specialist, Angeline, Serge, and Alain pass by emaciated patients surrounded by doctors in the infectious disease clinic. Revising the stigmatizing script of the "AIDS carrier," Angeline's doctor in the next scene defines Angeline as HIV-positive, a "carrier of HIV," but "far from being sick." The editing of the images starkly contrasts Angeline with those suffering in the hospital and implies that Angeline's conformity to the doctor's directives will enable her to avoid their suffering and deaths. Angeline must have medical checkups every two months and never have sex without condoms. She must avoid reinfection, as well as alcohol, drugs, and stress. Nevertheless, Angeline "must lead a normal family life and continue to go to work." The doctor promotes "normal family life" and "work" as analogous to condoms, as themselves modes of protection, and at the same time challenges assumptions that "family life" by definition entails reproduction. In the next breath, the doctor warns, "No pregnancy, as you risk contaminating your spouse [votre conjoint] and the child." Serge agrees, insisting, "She will live with me. Everything will be watched over [On va veiller à tout]." Incorporation into the reconstituted family then serves as defense and support and provides necessary surveillance for Angeline, the family, and the community.

As ordered by the doctor, Angeline continues her job. When colleagues leave an anonymous note on her desk, "NO AIDS AT WORK," Angeline informs her boss and offers to quit: "I know that I am not contagious, but if I pose a problem for my colleagues' peace of mind [tranquilité], and for that of the department [le service], I am ready to leave." Having heard an educational radio program, the boss has been convinced that stigmatization of people living with HIV would impede the functioning of the corporation: "I heard on the radio that one in six in urban areas are [sic] contaminated [with HIV]. If all these HIV-positive people [séropositifs] are fired, then there will be no one at work." Although he recognizes the pragmatic reasons not to exclude HIV-positive people from the workplace, the boss further accepts the care of HIV-positive people as the financial responsibility of the company and promises to organize an information session for the department. As he tells Angeline, "It is terrible to carry the virus, but you need money and support. If I fire you, how will you live?"

The series depicts women living with HIV as necessarily dependent on the benevolence and compassion—what Angeline's husband describes as the "love and support"—of the family, as well as dependent on what Angeline's boss affirms as the "money and support" of the private corporation. Angeline will continue to supply her necessary labor to the workplace, where her colleagues, taught tolerance, shamefacedly apologize to Angeline and contribute to a collection for her care. Those unnamed and unrepresented who are excluded from sustaining love, support, and money include the pregnant woman who tests HIV-positive and the woman who is HIV-positive and becomes pregnant, who do not terminate their pregnancies. Similarly, the HIV-positive woman who contributes neither unpaid reproductive nor paid labor and who cannot be incorporated into heteronormative romance and the corporation as a "healthy carrier" and as worthy beneficiary of charity—humble, grateful, self-sacrificing—is cast aside. Like the woman who resists assimilation into heteronormative "family life," with the significant exception of the nun, they are the constitutive exclusions enabling the production of the heterosexual family and the corporation as primary sources of support and care and, at the same time, a method of protection against the danger of HIV.

THE GOOD WIFE AND THE CORPORATION AS SOLUTIONS: "THAT HAPPENS ONLY TO OTHERS"

The four segments of *Gestures or Life* attempt to counter stigmatization by carefully differentiating "healthy carriers" or "carriers of HIV" from those manifesting symptoms of AIDS-related illnesses. In an interview, director Kitia Touré stated that he had sought through the series to show that "being seropositive, doesn't mean being sick [quand on est séropositif, on n'est pas malade]." In particular, he wanted to film inside "a big corporation to show how you can be seropositive and work [on peut être séropositif et travailler]."[48] In attempting to challenge stigma surrounding HIV/AIDS, the series affirms the bodies able to work as worthy of reintegration—they demonstrate their worth through that reintegration into family and workplace—in contrast to those suffering from illness and who in the logic of the narrative, are abandoned and left to die.

Another segment, "That Happens Only to Others," casts the polygamous Muslim family and the corporation as protection for people living with HIV. In the segment, Mariam, a young pregnant third wife agrees to test for HIV during a prenatal visit. After she tests positive, her two cowives, Djereba and Assiata, avoid any contact with her and then abandon the household. After their husband, Abdul Diallo, also tests positive through his employer and is fired, he tries to commit suicide with Mariam and their child. The destruction of the family is narrowly averted when Djereba and her daughter return to the house and discover Abdul, Mariam, and their child unconscious on the sofa near a discharging cooking gas tank. The segment depicts Djereba's return as literally saving not only Abdul, Mariam, their child, and the family but also the community. As Djereba explains to Abdul, she has come back because she recognizes that leaving the family can spread the virus, just as returning can contain it: "Abdul, I was wrong to have left. I have come back with your daughter. It was stupid on my part to leave. Maybe I am already contaminated. It's not worth transmitting this virus to others."

In the next scene, a doctor announces to Djereba and Miriam that Djereba and the children have tested HIV-negative. Nevertheless, Djereba has agreed to stay with the household, and, as the doctor approvingly declares, she must provide "moral support" to her husband and cowife [sa rivale]. The doctor details the precautions necessary: If Adul or Mariam cut themselves, they

---

48. In "Sida et liberté" (86–87), Touré goes on to explain that because of the intense fear and stigma of HIV/AIDS, no private (including foreign-owned corporations operating in Côte d'Ivoire) or public company would permit him to film in their workplaces.

must clean up the blood themselves and use bleach as disinfectant. As for the "biggest problem, sex," the doctor instructs the two cowives that Abdul must always use condoms. Dismayed, Djereba asks the doctor, "So, I cannot have any more children? [Je ne peux plus faire d'enfants, alors?]." Without referring to Mariam's pregnancy—which is never directly addressed again after Mariam tests HIV-positive—the doctor responds to Djereba that he advises against her reproducing: she can be contaminated by Abdul, and "the child who will be born has a strong chance of being seropositive."

The segment seamlessly redirects Djereba's unpaid reproductive labor into maintenance of the HIV-positive household. As a self-described "good Muslim wife," the HIV-negative Djereba will remain in the household, accept condom usage, and perhaps most importantly provide her HIV-positive husband and her cowife with necessary care and support. In other words, the HIV-negative wife who cannot reproduce and who does not directly participate in the formal economy nevertheless must continue to play a central sustaining role as unpaid laborer in the polygamous household. She not only saves but also preserves the family and protects it by remaining—and enabling her husband and cowives to remain—firmly enclosed within it.

As in "In the Name of Love," the private corporation in "That Happens Only to Others" demonstrates its enlightened benevolence by also shouldering responsibility for people living with HIV. The scene with Diallo's two wives at the doctor's office cuts to Diallo entering his boss's office. The editing highlights and simultaneously renders mutually sustaining the divisions between the family and workplace and between gendered female and male labor. Having undergone HIV education exemplified by the series itself, Diallo's supervisor recognizes that HIV "does not happen only to others. We can all be victim of it." The boss informs Diallo that the company will rehire him to perform modified office duties for as long as he remains a "healthy carrier." The boss figures the corporation administration's response as a demonstration of their participation in "the fight against AIDS": "This tact is the workplace's support of people who are seropositive from this new plague [Ce tact c'est le soutien du monde du travail aux séropositifs de ce nouveau fléau]." Reincorporation into the company and sexual self-restraint serve as principal modes of prevention and are constituted as analogous individual and corporate responsibilities. The substitution of the private corporation for the state in public health provision constitutes a neoliberal solution, one that also draws from prior colonial enterprises, which were compelled to provide their workers with the health care that the state could not.[49] As the boss reminds Diallo, he should

---

49. Bekelynck, "Le Rôle des entreprises," 132.

not take advantage of the company's generosity to take a fourth wife or additional mistresses [d'autres bureaux en ville]. Diallo assures him that he will not, and the segment concludes with Assiata's return and the family's joyful reunification under the restored patriarchal order. The segment reinforces and naturalizes a gendered economic and social order as, paradoxically, under threat yet safe, desirable, in need of protection, and ensuring safety.

In the longest, most original, and frankly strange segment of *Gestures or Life*, "My Name Is 'Life' [Mon nom est 'La Vie']," an albino girl in a robe and glowing white veil thwarts HIV, depicted in a panting voiceover as an invisible ravening beast gleefully searching for victims. The girl, who calls herself "Life," appears magically at a dinner party and then beckons partygoers to the television where she stages interventions in a sequence of scenes that screen in close succession. In the only segment of an HIV-prevention video in Côte d'Ivoire that I have found directed at men and boys who have anal sex with each other, "Life" informs a startled group: "The anal mucous membrane is more fragile than the vaginal mucous membrane. Each penetration can create lesions [crée des lesions] in both partners. Thus, you are 100% exposed to the AIDS virus" (figure 3.4). She repeats this advice to a man and a woman in bed about to engage in anal sex. She also offers similar matter-of-fact counsel to sex workers on the street, a man and a menstruating woman about to have sex, a dentist cleaning teeth, a male circumciser, women performing a scarification ceremony, and so forth. In each scene, HIV howls in frustration as the girl advises different methods of protection: condom usage, sterilized blades, bleach as disinfectant, storing of blood for transfusions, and use of rubber gloves. The girl repeatedly refers to the advice she dispenses as saving the lives of the people in the scenes, including those of the partygoers depicted as in a trance in front of the television.

The director, Touré, described "My Name Is Life" as "in the register of religious syncretism,"[50] and the segment amalgamates the Gospel and the trance, the angel and the albino, to represent televised HIV education as initiating a successful process of conversion that ensures salvation. After the guests are jolted from their trance, the girl's final words echo those of Christ instructing doubting disciples after his resurrection: "Now that you have been informed, go tell your relatives, your family. Respond boldly without shame [sans gêne ni fausse pudeur] to the good news. I will always be among you."[51] The segment's self-referential framing of televised HIV prevention education lends author-

---

50. Déniaud and Touré, "Présentation de documents audiovisuels," 126.
51. "I am with you always, to the end of the age" [Je suis toujours avec vous jusqu'à la fin du monde] (Matt. 28:20). The albino girl as Christ might be productively read alongside "black Jesus" of Touré's novel, *Destins Parallèles*.

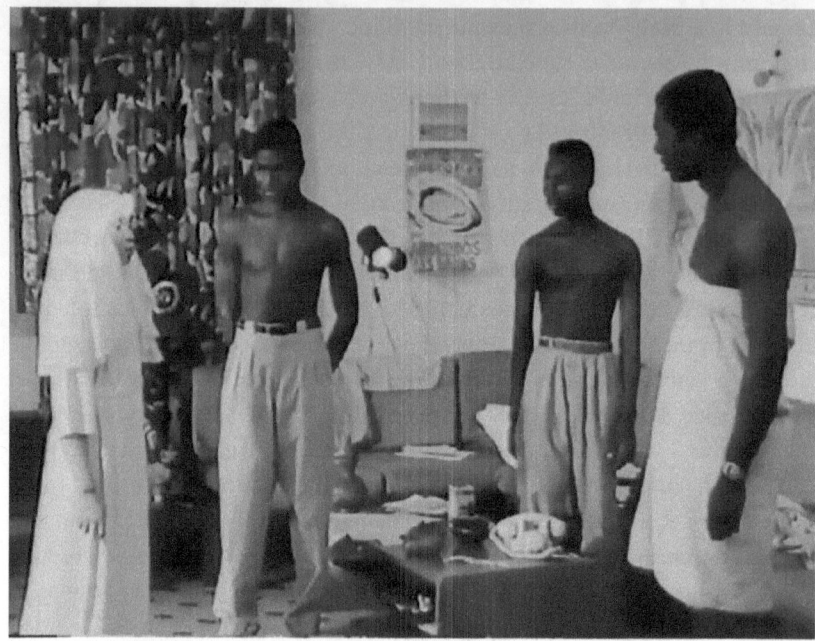

FIGURE 3.4. "Life" advises the group that "the anal mucous membrane is more fragile than the vaginal mucous membrane."

ity to its own messages and further detaches the series from the conditions and contexts of its production. In the series, HIV prevention education, and HIV itself, are not sites of ongoing negotiations and struggle but supernatural revelations with the categories of danger and safety—and HIV prevention media, such as *Gestures or Life*—constituting divine truths, with prevention a form of redemption.

THE PREGNANT WOMAN AS DESTROYER OF FAMILIES: *AIDS IN THE CITY* 1 AND 2

While *Gestures or Life* relied on European and United Nations financing, the telenovela *Sida dans la cité,* or *AIDS in the City,* was produced with funding from the United States Agency for International Development (USAID), both directly and through the United States–based Population Services International (PSI), which receives significant support from USAID. An eleven-episode version of *AIDS in the City* 1 was first broadcast weekly on the state-owned Channel 1 in Côte d'Ivoire Tuesday evenings, beginning February

1, 1995.⁵² Another twenty-episode-version, *AIDS in the City* 2, aired Thursday evenings between October 1996 and February 1997, and another sixteen-episode version (divided into four separate segments), *AIDS in the City* 3, in 2003.⁵³ The award-winning series screened widely throughout West and Central Africa, and cassettes of the series were also given and sold to organizations serving people living with HIV.⁵⁴

The first two versions of *AIDS in the City* center on Jacky and her husband, Sérapo, who had tested HIV-positive and tried to commit suicide when the first series begins. The series' plots are much too involved to detail, and in the next chapter, I will discuss how segments from the 2003 series draw on the melodramatic mode of the telenovela to socially market HIV prevention. Most relevant for this discussion is one of *AIDS in the City* 1's and 2's plot strands involving Mado, Jacky's pregnant best friend. Unbeknownst to Jacky, Mado is lovers with Sérapo (which is a pun on *seropositive*). Mado is also married to Kafongo, who during the entire first series is absent, working in Burkina Faso. The earlier *Gestures or Life* segments take for granted that a pregnant woman who tests HIV-positive will terminate her pregnancy, and they promote the heterosexual family as a form of social prophylaxis. In contrast, *AIDS in the City* 1 and 2 sidestep the question of abortion and instead promote fidelity, condom usage, and HIV testing.

The different approaches can in part be accounted for by producers' mandates. The 1973 Helms Amendment prevented any national government or nongovernmental organization from using U.S. government foreign assistance funding to provide abortions, or even information about abortions. On his first day in office, in January 22, 2001, George W. Bush had reinstated the

---

52. *Jeune Afrique* described the first *AIDS in the City* as entirely financed by USAID. Morand, "'Sida dans la cité,'" 44. Each episode was fifteen minutes long and was followed by fifteen minutes of publicity for Prudence condoms and discussion. Total budget for the first episode was about $50,000. Deutsche Gesellschaft für Internationale Zusammenarbeit, *Les Séries télévisées dans l'éducation sur le VIH*, 28–29.

53. Each episode of the second series was twenty-six minutes long, and the budget was about $100,000. GIZ and KfW, "Les Séries télévisées," 29. The series broadcast on state television Channel 1. On Wednesdays at 3:00 p.m., prior episodes were repeated, and Thursdays at 8:30 p.m., new episodes aired. Guenou, *Impact d'une campagne*, 19–20.

54. The *AIDS in the City* 1 series won the first prize for the best fiction film at the 1996 FESPACO Film Festival in Burkina Faso [le Festival panafricain du cinéma et de la télévision de Ouagadougou]. According to research funded by two of the series producers, USAID and the KfW, 80% of the people surveyed were familiar with *AIDS in the City* 2. Zoungrana et al., *La Prévention*, xi; According to additional research funded by PSI, 69% of people sampled in electrified regions knew about *AIDS in the City*, and 65% had seen at least one episode. Shapiro and Meekers, "Target Audience," 21–30, 28. About 40% of households were electrified at the time of the surveys. Shapiro, Meekers, and Tambashe, "Exposure," 304.

Global Gag Rule, suspended under Bill Clinton. First announced in Mexico City by Ronald Reagan in 1984, the so-called Mexico City Policy, or the Global Gag Rule, prohibited foreign NGOs receiving U.S. government funding for family planning from "perform[ing] or actively promot[ing] abortion as a method of family planning," even with non-U.S. funds. As a major recipient of USAID funding, PSI could not suggest, much less promote, terminations of pregnancies as a solution for perinatal HIV transmission. Further, by the time of the first two series' production, clinical trials (some conducted in Côte d'Ivoire) had established effective prophylactic regimens to lower perinatal transmission. These regimens were not widely available in Côte d'Ivoire, and promotion of abortions as prevention strategy might have too starkly highlighted the global racialized disparities and inequities in the conducting of clinical trials, implementation of prevention strategies, and access to treatment. The implications of urging HIV-positive women to terminate their pregnancies to prevent HIV transmission had already provoked comment. In 1998, a publication by the World Health Organization and the United Nations attempted to reframe abortion as an "option" for "individual women," rather than "public health intervention" to prevent perinatal transmission, an option that they noted was not exercised by most women: "Access to termination of pregnancy for HIV-positive women can also reduce the burden of paediatric AIDS cases, but should be viewed as an option for individual women, rather than a public health intervention for the prevention of transmission. Most women living with HIV will decide to continue with pregnancy, even where termination is offered."[55] In any event, the series neither mentions abortion as an alternative nor suggests family as protection. The series instead focuses on the depiction of the consequences of the failure to submit to HIV prevention messages as the destruction of the family—a scenario that was playing out on the political stage.

After the death of Houphouët-Boigny, commonly referred to as the "father of the nation," in December 1993, struggles for succession immediately ensued between the president of the National Assembly, Henri Konan Bedié, and the Prime Minister, Alassane Ouattara. The devaluation of the CFA in January 1994 precipitated further drops in prices for export crops, thereby increasing poverty. After Bedié claimed the presidency, Ouattara, the former Africa Director of the International Monetary Fund (IMF), who had been responsible for the implementation of many major structural adjustment policies in Côte d'Ivoire, resigned and left the country to return to work at the IMF. To ensure his succession and the continued dominance of the Democratic Party

---

55. WHO and UNAIDS, "HIV in Pregnancy," 16.

of Côte d'Ivoire-African Democratic Rally [Parti democratique de la Côte d'Ivoire-Rassemblement démocratique africain (PDCI)], Bedié deployed the concept of *Ivoirité*, a form of ethnonationalism, to disenfranchise particular groups—especially immigrants and Muslim Northerners—as outsiders and foreigners.

In 1995, the year the first *AIDS in the City* series broadcast, Bedié amended electoral laws to require presidential candidates to prove that both of their parents were of Ivorian birth and that the candidates had lived continuously in Côte d'Ivoire for at least five years before the elections. The laws were widely interpreted as intended to disqualify Bedié's primary political opponent, Ouattara, who was born in the North to a Muslim family. Ouattara's father—and, alternatively, his mother—were said to be from what was then Upper Volta, now Burkina Faso. Ouattara had been educated and had traveled regularly outside the country. While working for the IMF and the Central Bank of West African States, he had held a diplomatic passport released from Burkina Faso. In October 1995, Bedié won elections boycotted by the main opposition parties, including Ouattara's Rally of the Republicans [Rassemblement des Républicains (RDR)].[56] Karine Delaunay notes how Bedié differentiated himself from his predecessor, Houphouët-Boigny, and the latter's rhetoric of unity and inclusion through his invocation of the ideology of Ivoirité and its attendant stigmatization of foreigners and immigrants, whom he blamed for Côte d'Ivoire's high HIV/AIDS rates.[57] As national conflicts over citizenship, voting rights, and land ownership were deepening, *AIDS in the City* 2 depicted the family in crisis, eventually destroyed by unruly sexualities and illegitimate births.

In *AIDS in the City* 1, Mado refuses her lover's, Sérapo's, suggestions to use condoms because they indicate a lack of trust and imply that she is a "whore [une pute]." Mado later learns about Sérapo's HIV-positive status from her best friend, Jacky, who does not know about Mado and Sérapo's affair. Mado confronts Sérapo and castigates him for not informing her of his status: "You knew . . . I so needed a baby. And you condemned it to death even before its birth." Sérapo agrees that the child is "certainly" HIV-positive, but despite his pleas, Mado refuses to test. Underscoring a central, irresolvable conflict around HIV testing without available treatment, Mado argues with Jacky, who wants Sérapo to notify his sexual partners so that they too can test: "What

---

56. For more on the production of the Muslim Northerner as "foreigner" and on the discourse of Ivoirité, see Cutolo, "Modernity, Autochthony and the Ivorian Nation"; Dembélé, "La Construction économique"; Marshall-Fratani, "The War of 'Who Is Who.'"

57. Delaunay, "Réflexions sur les dynamiques socio-politiques, 115."

good is it to know that you had sex with a seropositive person [un séropositif] or not? Can a test treat [soigner]?"

The series does not refer to, much less promote, voluntary termination of pregnancy as an option for Mado. Nevertheless, it is the specter haunting Mado's pregnancy. Unaware of Mado's relationship with Sérapo, Sérapo's uncle argues with Mado that Sérapo should inform his sexual partners. The uncle addresses Mado: "But it's the test that lets you know if you're ill or not [qui permet de savoir si on est malade ou pas]. Let's take a concrete case. You are pregnant right now, my girl [ma fille]. Would you accept your pregnancy if it were of or from a seropositive person? [Est-ce que tu accepterais que ta grossesse soit celle d'un séropositif?]." The French ambiguously begs a series of questions. The uncle takes as given that Mado would not get pregnant with a partner who she knew was HIV-positive. He also implies that she would not "accept" the pregnancy, or carry it to term, if she learned that her partner was positive, and that she also would not deliver a child who could be HIV-positive. Mado later visits a friend, a nurse, who tells Mado about a woman who was unaware that she was HIV-positive until after the birth of a baby who became very sick: "The poor little child has AIDS! [Le pauvre petit a le Sida!]." The nurse underscores the importance of prenatal testing but also implies that if the mother had tested and learned her HIV-positive results, she would not have delivered the child who is suffering so terribly. Nevertheless, in a series of dramatic monologues, Mado resolutely continues to refuse to test, even as she laments that she is cursed and imagines that she sees signs of AIDS-related illness on her own body: swollen lymph nodes, fever, and rashes. When Sérapo proposes they continue their relationship but use condoms, Mado rejects him: "We are done. You are seropositive.... Get out! I do not want to see you again!"

The first series ends on a note of suspense, with Jacky having tested for HIV but not yet receiving her results, and then rushing to her home village where the chief's second wife, with whom Sérapo admits having also had an affair, has just died of what villagers suspect is an AIDS-related illness. The second *AIDS in the City* cuts between scenes in Abidjan, Jacky's home village (shot in Djibi), and Burkina Faso (shot in Ouagadougou and Saa), where Mado's husband, Kafongo, works as a UNICEF health educator.[58] The second series frames HIV prevention primarily in terms of gender struggle, with women demanding and promoting condom usage, and enlightened, self-described "traditional" and religious male authority—the village chief and the

---

58. Guenou, *Impact d'une campagne*, 17.

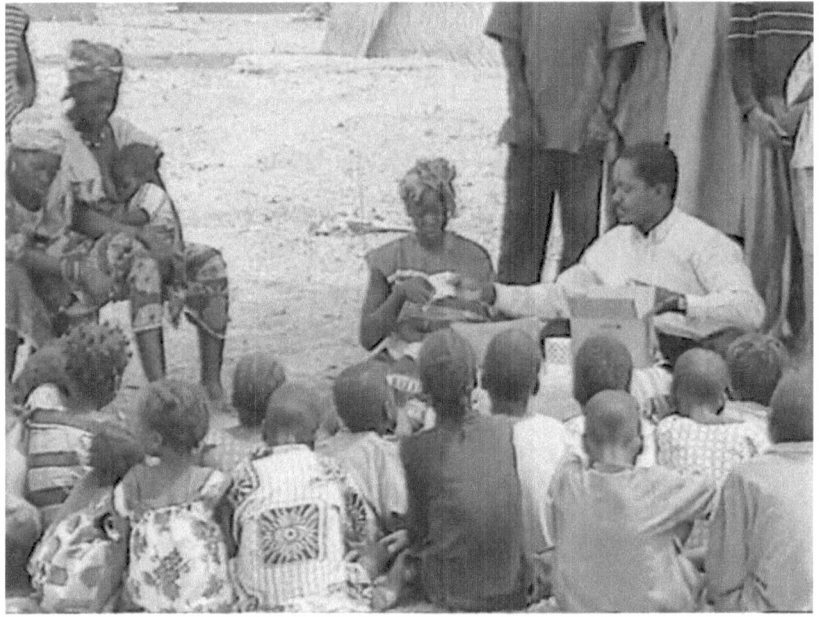

FIGURE 3.5. Agent of progress Kafongo (in white shirt).

imam—eventually publicly supporting their efforts. As representative of the authority of Western science and of the international development agency (as well as of the series' funders), Kafongo instructs the women in dusty villages in Burkina Faso, as well as viewers, to vaccinate their children and to administer oral rehydration salts in case of dehydration from diarrhea (figure 3.5). The series juxtaposes Kafongo as an agent of progress, and his accounts of disease prevention with representations of HIV as both curse and punishment.

Mado eventually leaves Sérapo in Abidjan to travel to Ouagadougou, Burkina Faso, with Kafongo, who presumes that the baby she carries is his. A fortuneteller mysteriously appears in front of Mado's house in Ouagadougou. Warning that Mado's attempt to flee her past will not be successful, the fortuneteller offers herbal treatments as protection: "The little one in the womb [Le petit dans le ventre], that's a lot of problems. I have good medication [bon médicament] for him. Otherwise, the future of the baby will cause a lot of problems. Be careful, woman [femme]! Baby misfortune! [Bébé malheur!]" (figure 3.6). Just as Mado has refused the interventions of "science," she rejects the fortuneteller as a charlatan. Sérapo similarly defies both medical directives to prevent the advancement of his illness and the spread of the virus, and

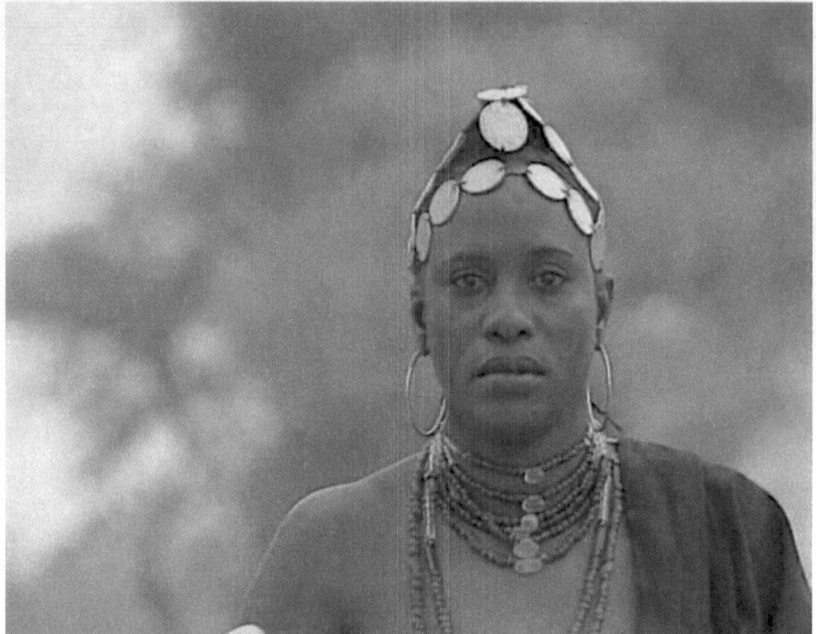

FIGURE 3.6. A mysterious fortuneteller whose warnings Mado ignores.

what the series refers to as "traditional" prohibitions against adultery with the chief's wives. As a result, Mado and Sérapo share what the series suggests are linked fates.[59]

The same fortuneteller who visited Mado's house in Ouagadougou ominously appears and disappears in the village where Mado has accompanied Kafongo. During a village dance under a full moon, Mado suddenly goes into labor. As she screams in agony on a mat on the floor, the fortuneteller enters the room and announces that Mado has hidden something and that she will not be able to deliver the child until she reveals the secret. Finally, writhing in pain, Mado begs Jacky and Sérapo for forgiveness: "I am cursed. Forgive me Sérapo. Forgive me Jacky. I destroyed your household [foyer]! I betrayed Jacky!" She confesses: "I slept with Sérapo! . . . No, leave the baby, you have AIDS! Sérapo, you have AIDS! Why did you do this to me? Why didn't you say anything to me? . . . Why? Why?" The scene dissolves to Sérapo rereading old letters and then dissolves back to Mado. The fortuneteller says that Kafongo must forgive [pardonner] Mado so that she can deliver the baby.

---

59. For contrasting ethnographic accounts of the status of secrets among women living with HIV in Northern Nigeria, see Rhine, *The Unseen Things*.

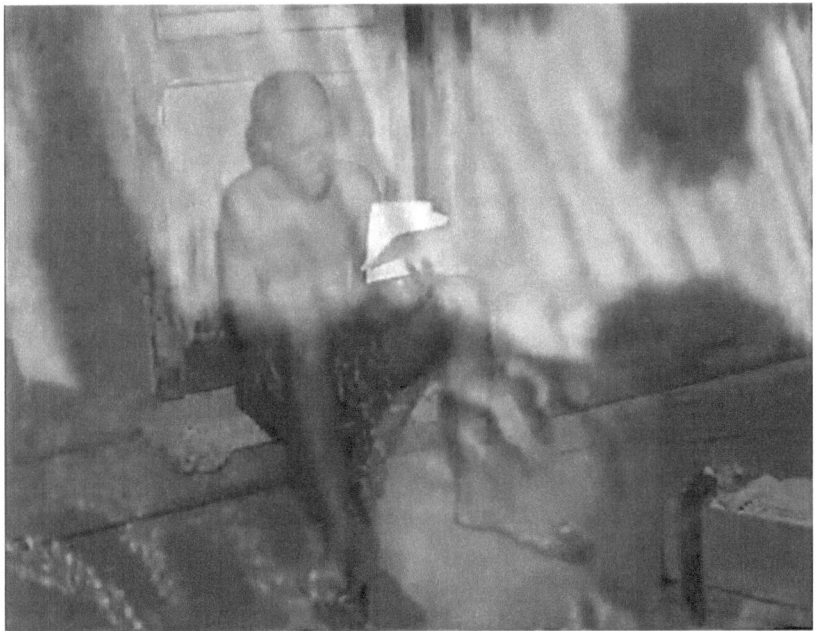

FIGURE 3.7. Slow dissolve of Mado screaming in labor to Sérapo reading letters.

As Kafongo shakes his head and clasps his hands, Jacky continues to chastise Sérapo: "I fled. I fled Abidjan. I fled Jacky. I fled AIDS." The camera dramatically undercuts her claims of escape. In a slow dissolve, the scene shifts to Sérapo collapsing and then returns to Mado's screaming, sweating face as she also collapses, while a baby's cries echo in the night (figure 3.7). The camera abruptly cuts back to Abidjan the next morning. In the concluding scene, a gathered crowd, including two of Sérapo's other lovers, have discovered Sérapo's body and sob outside his door, as concluding intertitles scroll: "As in a tragedy foretold [annoncée], Sérapo and Mado draw their last breath at the moment when their baby's cry reverberates [au moment où résonne le cri de leur bébé]."

The lyrics of the series' heavy-handed concluding song clarify the inevitable consequences of the failure to instigate the individual behavior changes that the series reminds are required to prevent the spread of HIV: "Hey, a lifetime of misery because I could not restrain myself [me retenir]. . . . An entire lifetime of suffering [Toute une vie de galère] because you wanted your freedom." In contrast to *Gestures or Life,* the first two *AIDS in the City* series avoid direct reference to the termination of pregnancies of women who test HIV-positive. Instead they focus on Mado as betrayer and home-wrecker who, like Sérapo, the unfaithful husband, suffers the terrible but deserved death of those who did not change their behavior and limit sexual partners, use condoms, and test for HIV.

In response to an interviewer's question about the decision to shoot segments of the second series in Burkina Faso, producer Hanny Brigitte Tchelley explained that PSI wanted to showcase their successful prevention efforts there and that she also saw an opportunity to expound on the role of the "foreigner [l'étranger]."[60] Although Tchelley does not further elaborate, her immediate association of Burkina Faso with the "foreigner" is suggestively symptomatic, underscoring the pervasiveness of the terms of ongoing political debates about definitions of foreigners and outsiders demarcated from autochthonous citizens. In depicting HIV/AIDS as a curse for sexual betrayals, the series invokes and reproduces potent circulating tropes collapsing political and reproductive legitimacy. The series closes on an ambiguous but portentous note, with the birth of a child of ambiguous parentage and unknown but likely HIV-positive status that will result in a "lifetime of misery" and "a lifetime of suffering."

HIV-POSITIVE PREGNANT WOMAN AS BEARER OF THE FUTURE: "FATOUMATA, HIV-POSITIVE MOTHER"

After prophylactic treatment began to be more widely distributed in Côte d'Ivoire in late 1998, the messages about perinatal HIV prevention and termination of pregnancies became much more sharply focused. In 1998, UNAIDS and the Office of the United Nations High Commissioner for Human Rights stated that pressure on HIV-positive pregnant women to undergo abortion constitutes a violation of human rights, and United States–funded media explicitly challenged prior state television representations of abortion.[61] In *Accidental Pregnancy,* a 1999 PSI (the funder of *AIDS in the City*) video broadcast in Côte d'Ivoire, a high school student, Behi, becomes pregnant with a classmate who refuses to acknowledge the pregnancy. In desperation, Behi turns to a nurse in a clinic to terminate the pregnancy. As Behi's friends look on in horror, the nurse exits from the clinic room, his apron soaked in blood, and bloody sheets and cloths wadded on the floor behind him. Behi almost dies, and as a doctor informs the families gathered around her coma-

---

60. Tapsoba, "Sida dans la cité II," 90.
61. Office of the United Nations High Commissioner for Human Rights and the Joint United Nations Programme on HIV/AIDS, *International Guidelines on HIV/AIDS and Human Rights*.

tose body in the hospital, she has been rendered permanently sterile from the procedure.⁶²

One of the four segments (each four episodes long) comprising the 2003 *AIDS in the City 3* series also produced by PSI, "Fatoumata, HIV-Positive Mother," reiterates the representation of abortion and sterility as threats to rather than solutions for pregnant women. However, it shifts away from techniques that by 2001 the World Health Organization described as centered on "fear arousal," deemed "rarely successful as a long-term campaign strategy," to focus instead on "emphasi[zing] positive behavior change."⁶³ Broadcast in 2003, the year after the country erupted in its first civil war, "Fatoumata, HIV-Positive Mother" insistently represents implementation of correct HIV prevention methods as enabling reconciliation, future, and family.⁶⁴

"Fatoumata: HIV-Positive Mother" centers on a minor character from the previous *AIDS in the City* series, a former neighbor of Jacky and Sérapo, Fatou, and on her conflicts after she learns that she has tested HIV-positive during a prenatal visit. Before she tells her husband, Joseph, that she has tested positive, Fatou poses as an abandoned, poor woman and begs a medical doctor to perform an abortion, but he refuses, interestingly, not because the procedure would be illegal but because, he says, her pregnancy at four months is too far advanced for him to risk performing the procedure. Fatou then obtains herbs from a market woman who instructs her how to prepare and administer them to induce an abortion. On her way home from the market, Fatou gazes longingly at young children playing in a schoolyard (figure 3.8); the bars of the fence literally block her access to the children and shadow both their play and her face (figure 3.9). Later that evening, while Fatou crushes the herbs in the courtyard, Joseph arrives home and, unaware of her HIV status or her plans to try to terminate the pregnancy, presents her with cloth [pagne] and a stuffed

---

62. In an article on illegal abortions, the state weekly reminded readers: "Abortion leads to sterility [L'avortement rend stérile]." Agnès Kraide Masoso, "Avec une aiguille, sans anesthésie," *Ivoire Dimanche,* December 2–8, 1990, 5.

63. Clift, *Information, Education and Communication,* 6.

64. Bédié was later overthrown in a 1999 military coup and replaced by a military general, Robert Guéï, who formalized the exclusionary tactics of his predecessor and oversaw the incorporation of a constitutional requirement that all presidential candidates be of Ivorian origin and born of parents of Ivorian origin. Bédié and Ouattara were disqualified from participating in 2000 elections. Former Houphouët-Boigny opponent Laurent Gbagbo claimed victory and then refused to hold new elections with a full ballot. Frustration and discontent at the structural exclusions of Ivoirité eventually culminated both in an unsuccessful military coup in 2002 during which Guéï was killed and in the first civil war. For more in-depth analysis of the civil war and the events leading to it, see McGovern, *Making War in Côte d'Ivoire.*

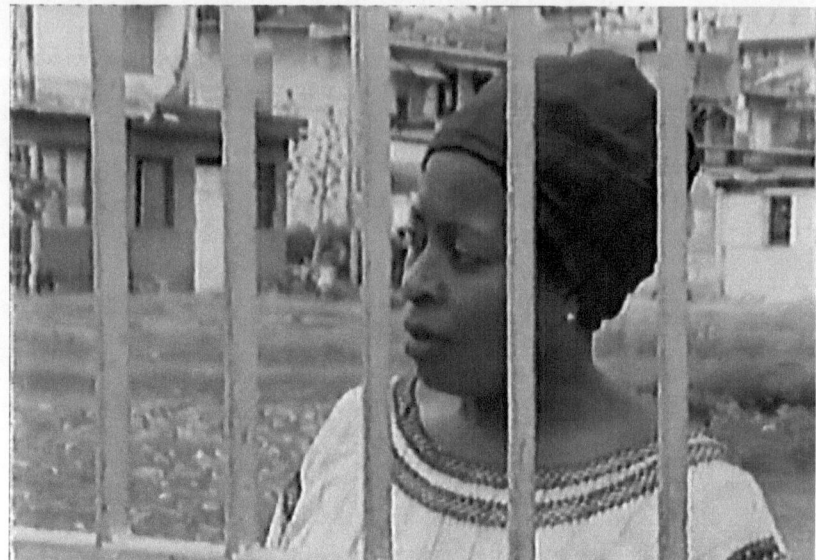

FIGURE 3.8. Fatou believing that she is barred from producing children.

animal for the baby. The music cues after Joseph enters the house, and a weeping Fatou cuddles the stuffed animal and then rises to throw out the herbs.

The scene cuts to a meeting of Fatou and Jacky, who has become an HIV counselor at a nongovernmental organization. Jacky chastises Fatou for trying to terminate the pregnancy: "You are seropositive. This is not a reason to kill your baby. With the development [l'évolution] of medicine, you can have [faire] a seronegative baby without any problems." Directly countering the messages from "Reasons for Fear"—and from the earlier series—the *AIDS in the City* 3 segment insists that women living with HIV can conform to normative gender roles centering on a heterosexual reproductive mandate. As "Fatoumata: HIV-Positive Mother" underscores, Fatou has not recognized the true barriers blocking her from children; the series recasts the bars that shadow her as not HIV, but her own attempts to terminate her pregnancy. The segment represents the suffering of the innocent, the child, as under threat from the mother, not because she might transmit HIV but because she might deliberately end her pregnancy. Through identification of the mother who seeks an abortion as the killer of babies, the segment figures the mother living with HIV who responsibly takes measures to avoid mother-to-child transmission of HIV as source of renewed life rather than of infection and death.

The segment emphasizes that locating the source of infection and attributing blame is useless. As a woman in Fatou's support group reminds another,

REGULATING FEMALE REPRODUCTIVE POTENTIAL • 131

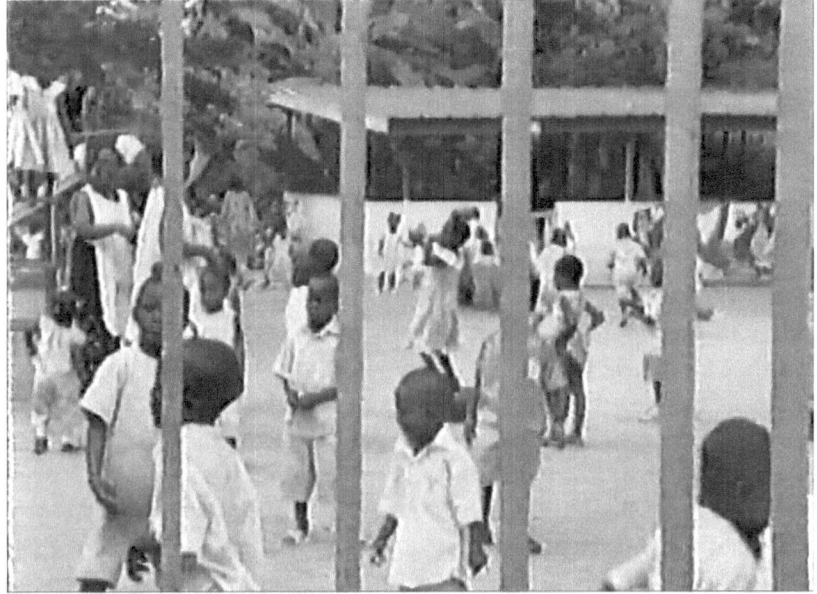

FIGURE 3.9. Reverse shot of the children playing in the schoolyard.

"What does it matter who infected whom?" But the segment simultaneously persistently represents Fatou as virtuous mother and wife and therefore, unlike Mado from the previous series, as blameless victim. After Fatou finally informs Joseph of her test, he throws her out of the house, and she returns to her parents' house. When she discloses her HIV-positive status to her mother, she carefully underscores her own fidelity: "I don't know if I got this from my ex-husband, or even from Joseph. I tried to explain [to Joseph], but he doesn't want to understand anything." After her return home, Fatou prepares Joseph's favorite meal and nervously tries to make conversation with him. When he ignores her, she follows him into the bedroom and again emphasizes her faithfulness:

> FATOU: Joseph, you're angry [tu m'en veux] because you believe that I am guilty [fautive], that I am unfaithful. The infection can be caused by things besides sex [L'infection peut avoir une source autre que les rapports sexuels]. [*She looks down at him*].
> JOSEPH: Listen, this won't change my mind. I know how you got that [Ce n'est pas pour me distraire. Je sais de quelle manière tu as eu ça].
> FATOU: Maybe I used a contaminated razor blade, or needle. You never know. And then what does it serve, trying to figure out who infected whom?

[Et puis, à quoi ça sert chercher à savoir qui a infecté qui?]. [*Sits on bed*]. Joseph, I am seropositive. We can't change that. We can at least think about our baby [*Joseph gets up and puts his shirt back on to storm out*].

Jacky reassures Joseph of Fatoumata's fidelity: "Because she had a positive test does not mean that she was unfaithful! Maybe she got the virus from her first husband before meeting you, or maybe you yourself were infected by another woman before meeting Fatou. Who knows?"

The show depicts Fatou not as sexually promiscuous and therefore culpable, like Mado and Sérapo of *AIDS in the City* 1 and 2, but as faithful and therefore blameless. As innocent victim, Fatou can be enlisted as mother into what Karen M. Booth, revising Lee Edelman, terms neo-imperial reproductive futurism, the project of protecting and caring for the fetus as the epitome of the possibility of a future in whose name parents must change their behavior.[65] The recoding of guilt and innocence casts Fatou as virtuous mother; a carrier and reproducer not of AIDS but of the child, an overdetermined, gendered, heteronormative trope for the future and life itself. The 1993 *Gestures or Life* had urged women who tested positive not to reproduce and, if pregnant, to terminate their pregnancies. *AIDS in the City* 1 and 2 portrayed those who reject HIV prevention mandates and who destroy families and the future as justifiably punished by death. Contesting the stigma and fear provoked by the portrayal of AIDS as curse, "Fatoumata: HIV-Positive Mother" represents ignorance and abortion, not HIV, as threats to the future child and family.

"Fatoumata: HIV-Positive Mother" shores up the normative heterosexual couple and family in large part through exclusion of the homosexual, the intravenous drug user, and the prostitute. Many scholars have critiqued how colonial-era stereotypes of exotic, promiscuous, violent, and inherently diseased African sexuality have been reproduced in mass media as well as in academic accounts of the high rates of HIV in sub-Saharan Africa.[66] As Marc Epprecht notes, in seeking to counter such racist representations, scholars have paradoxically reinforced another stereotype about so-called African sexuality: unsubstantiated claims that same-sex sexual relations are nonexistent or alien to Africa and that HIV in Africa is transmitted entirely through heterosexual contact, mother-to-child transmission, and intravenous injection. The insistence on the heterosexuality of so-called African AIDS has facilitated struggles against homophobia, especially in the Global North since, as Epprecht argues, gay rights activists can "deflect prevalent blame for HIV/

---

65. Booth, "A Magic Bullet for the 'African' Mother?" 351.
66. Stillwaggon, *AIDS and the Ecology of Poverty*, 133–57; Treichler, *How to Have Theory*, 35; Vaughan, *Curing Their Ills*, 205; Patton, *Inventing AIDS*, 77–97.

AIDS away from the 'homosexual lifestyle,' a huge political achievement."[67] However, like its antecedents, in attempting to educate Francophone West African audiences about heterosexual HIV transmission, "Fatoumata: HIV-Positive Mother" risks reinforcing a stigmatizing logic in which the lives of those who do not submit to medical and patriarchal authority and to monogamous reproductive heteronormativity are deemed expendable.

"Fatoumata: HIV-Positive Mother" differentiates the lives it seeks to save from those its narrative implicitly discounts as not redeemable; in fact, HIV prevention as promoted in the segment names homosexuality, drug use, and sex work only through its phobic disavowal. Early in the first episode of the segment, Fatou's husband, Joseph, a bus mechanic at the Abidjan Transport Company [Société des Transports Abidjanais (SOTRA)], dismisses a coworker's efforts to organize around HIV at their workplace since HIV is "whores' and fags' business [une affaire de putes et de pédés]. How does that concern us?" His coworker chastises him that "AIDS concerns us all." Joseph waves him away: "In any case, not me." The scene then cuts back to his wife in a solidarity group for women living with HIV who close their meeting, chanting in English, "LOVE!" and then in French, "Love, solidarity, support!" What Joseph does not know (and what the viewer is well aware of since the first scene of the segment) is that AIDS is definitely his concern: In the very first scene of the segment episode, Fatou, who had agreed to take an HIV test during a prenatal appointment, has learned she has tested positive.

The segment generates tension around the ignorance that it seeks to ameliorate and that leads to Joseph's rejection of Fatou, his refusal to test, and the possibility that Fatou might end her pregnancy. Initially, Joseph refuses to test and associates HIV/AIDS with the stigmatized others from whom he vehemently disassociates himself. As he tells Jacky, who comes to the house to counsel him, "I don't need to test. I'm not a tramp [vagabonde]. I am not a fag [pédé]. I am a respectable man who works hard to support his household [gérer son foyer]!" Joseph's consent to test signals his enlightenment and his successful education about HIV. His realization reinforces the category of the virtuous "normal" defined against the stigmatized categories of the nonrespectable, the unemployed, the sexually "promiscuous," prostitutes, intravenous drug users, and "fags" or "homosexuals" from whom the series carefully differentiates Fatou and Joseph. When Joseph finally agrees to test, he reiterates to the counselor, "I never imagined that my wife and I could be affected [touchés] by this disease. . . . I always thought that AIDS was a disease of prostitutes, homosexuals [homosexuels], and drug addicts [des drogués]. Because

---

67. Epprecht, *Heterosexual Africa?* 3.

I wasn't part of this milieu, I thought I was sheltered [à l'abri]." The segment attempts to underscore what the nurse reminds Joseph: "Millions from all social levels live with this infection." However, in representing the "respectable" and hardworking head of the household, like Joseph, as also affected, the segment represents certain parts of the population as inherently at risk, as blameworthy, and, implicitly, as dispensable, whereas the innocent—the good mother and child incorporated into the heterosexual family—can and must be saved.

Initially, Joseph views his wife as carrier not of a child but of AIDS. As he says to Jacky in a burst of anger, "So I ask my wife to give me a child. What does she bring me? AIDS!" The series transforms Fatou from "AIDS carrier" to the carrier and bearer of the HIV-negative child as embodiment of the future. Finally, Joseph reunites with Fatou. He proposes terminating the pregnancy, but in her eighth month of pregnancy, Fatou refuses: "This child could be our only child. Give him a chance." Challenging the representation in the prior series of the birth of a potentially HIV-positive child as equivalent to and cause of death, the "Fatoumata: HIV-Positive Mother" segment vindicates Fatou's refusal. She carefully follows the nurse's instructions about taking a single dose of medication during pregnancy and, after she gives birth to a son, about taking a short-course treatment over the days following delivery (presumably, single-dose nevirapine followed by AZT or short-course AZT). She also follows the nurse's advice; she does not breastfeed or mix breastmilk and formula, and, instead, only bottlefeeds her baby. "Fatoumata: HIV-Positive Mother" elides ongoing struggles for HIV treatment access as well as debates about clinical trials of shorter courses of treatment to prevent perinatal HIV transmission in so-called developing countries at the time of the series production. In particular, it elides the ethics of provision of less effective but cheaper prophylactic regimens and the potential for future treatment failure for HIV-positive women and for their children who became infected with HIV despite the administration of prophylactic therapy.[68] Nor does it question the underlying assumptions governing directives that women living with HIV who cannot afford formula or fuel to sterilize water must accept increased risk of HIV transmission through breastfeeding. The segment entirely sidesteps addressing governmental or public responsibility for the provision of care and treatment of people living with HIV.

Like prior prevention media, "Fatoumata: HIV-Positive Mother" encourages dependence on the private sector for support and care. According to the Ivorian Minister of Health and Public Hygiene, the bus company where

---

68. Fowler, Mofenson, and McConnell, "Editorial," 308–11.

Joseph works, SOTRA, served as a model instance of private-sector engagement in the battle against HIV.[69] In the show, after Joseph also tests HIV-positive, the SOTRA doctor reassures Joseph that he can live a long time provided that he immediately alerts the doctor if he is feeling sick and quickly treats any opportunistic infections. The doctor further promises that he will try to find a program in a nongovernmental organization offering free antiretroviral treatment and that SOTRA will treat him "like any other sick person." Joseph then, like all people living with HIV, must rely for his care on the benevolence of the corporation and of nongovernmental organizations.

The segment reinforces the silences around provision of care for the woman living with HIV, for the person suffering from AIDS-related illness and unable to function as productive laborer, and for the child who despite prophylaxis (or in its absence) becomes infected with HIV.[70] While the SOTRA doctor reassures Joseph that he will receive medical care from SOTRA, neither the doctor nor the segment addresses what will happen to Joseph when he can no longer work. The segment does not represent Fatou as enjoying access to the corporation's private health care, and the medication that she receives from a Center for Maternal and Infant Protection (PMI) is focused exclusively on preventing mother-to-child HIV transmission. The segment elides questions of treatment or care for Fatou herself, just as it declines to address what it must exclude to offer a narrative of hope and redemption: the child who becomes infected with the virus despite prophylactic treatment.

Gliding over these omissions, the segment affirms the authority of biomedicine and of the nongovernmental organization depicted as displacing and superseding the authority of the parents who represent tradition. Fatou is never able to disclose to her father that she has tested HIV-positive, and Joseph avoids explaining to his uncle and to his father-in-law the real reason why he has thrown Fatou out. The segment associates insurmountable stigma with the older generation, who remain uninformed or, worse, urge administration of what the segments depicts as harmful traditional remedies. While

---

69. In 2001, SOTRA created a committee for the fight against AIDS which was charged with educating employees, providing "psycho-medico-social" care for people living with HIV, and protecting the rights of infected employees." Ministère de la Santé et de l'Hygiène Publique, PEPFAR, and Johns Hopkins University, "Stratégie Nationale," 20. SOTRA modeled its AIDS awareness campaign on the Ivorian Electricity Company's [La Compagnie ivoirienne d'électricité (CIE)] earlier efforts. UNDP, UN-HABITAT, and Urban Management Program, Regional Office for Africa, *HIV/AIDS and Local Governance in Sub-Saharan Africa*, 26; Bekelynck, "Le Rôle des entreprises privées," 136.

70. According to WHO estimations, adult prevalence in Côte d'Ivoire was 7% at the end of 2003: 570,000 people (from 0–49 years) were living with HIV/AIDS in Côte d'Ivoire, but in 2005, only 17,600 of 110,000 who needed antiretroviral treatment were receiving it. WHO, *Côte d'Ivoire: Estimated Number of People*, 1–2.

the prior *AIDS in the City* narrative suggests that Mado should have heeded the fortuneteller's warnings and accepted offers of herbal treatments, "Fatoumata: HIV-Positive Mother" urges firm rejection of such advice. Following the instructions she has received from the hospital, Fatou administers AZT to her son to decrease the risk of his HIV infection, and she steadfastly resists her mother's insistence on adding herbal treatments, even when her mother storms away, crying in disgust, "You are not going to respect any tradition?"

"Fatoumata: HIV-Positive Mother" depicts the rewards of proper conformity to biomedical and nongovernmental organizational authority. It closes with Joseph and Fatou with their relatives and friends celebrating their son's fifteen-month "birthday" portrayed as his symbolic rebirth—the day Joseph and Fatou learn that he has seroconverted and tested HIV-negative. Rather than lead to the termination of pregnancies figured as the killing of babies, HIV testing and HIV-positive diagnosis enable reproduction within the patriarchal heterosexual conjugal family, continuation of paternal legacy, and the role of woman as wife and mother, all attained through individual education, decision making, and compliance with biomedical directives, including those conveyed through the segment. Through the representation of the termination of pregnancies and not HIV as threat to the child and to motherhood, the segment narrative insists that women living with HIV can conform to normative gender roles as wife and mother and that she can serve as carrier and reproducer of the child and the future. The challenge of "Fatoumata: HIV-Positive Mother" to stigmatization of women living with HIV essentially reinforces stigmatization against those who do not conform to reproductively oriented, heteronormative gendering.

CONCLUSION

Gestures or Life and the three versions of *AIDS in the City* were produced during periods of intense turmoil in the country. Broadcast on state television, all of the productions avoid any direct reference to ongoing electoral struggles and allude only elliptically to economic crises and conditions of increasing economic precarity. Through their persistent attempts to shape female reproductivity, they nevertheless actively reflected, participated in, and deflected debates about economic retrenchment. According to all of the series, the central obstacles to the prevention of perinatal HIV transmission were not structural adjustment policies mandating decreases in public services and intensifying poverty, or the global inequities limiting life chances—in part through the restriction of access to treatment or prophylaxis for HIV—or the ongoing political crises.

Rather, inadequate surveillance of women's bodies and reproductivity was the central obstacle. *Gestures or Life* suggests that mother-to-child transmission of HIV instigates a state of emergency to be addressed by the suspension of state laws prohibiting abortion. Confronting a state in crisis, the series proposes abortion and family as forms of prevention, and the patriarchal family in tandem with the corporation as the primary providers of care and support.

The promotion of the patriarchal family and of the policing of female reproductivity as HIV prevention strategies dovetailed with disputes about definitions of citizenship and intensifying attempts to marginalize those categorized as foreigners and outsiders. During conflicts over political succession after the death of Houphouët-Boigny, *AIDS in the City* 1 and 2 represent HIV/AIDS as centrally implicated in questions around reproductive and political legitimacy. Both series associate ambiguous parentage with HIV-positive status which leads to ruination of the family and future, a cursed legacy as retribution for improper sexual behavior. After increasing conflicts culminated in a civil war and the division of the country, *AIDS in the City* 3 offers a narrative of redemption, with submission to biomedical and nongovernmental organizations' authority enabling the reunification and restoration of the family and the safeguarding of the child as emblem of the future.

Attempts to redefine heteronormative gendering to combat stigma and prevent the spread of HIV reiterated and reinforced the exclusionary logic underpinning debates about legitimacy and national belonging. The challenge to the stigmatization of women living with HIV relied on an affirmation of their procreative function that bolstered not only heteronormative gendering but also the exclusion of the homo/fag, the prostitute, and the intravenous drug user, as well as the HIV-positive child and the person with AIDS-related illnesses as inassimilable to the family, the community, and the future. Women's reproductive capacity—appropriately monitored by biomedical and patriarchal authority—constituted the conditions of possibility of incorporation and redemption.

CHAPTER 4

The Melodrama and the Social Marketing of HIV Prevention

THE FIRST two *AIDS in the City* series (1995 and 1996–97), produced by the United States Agency for International Development (USAID), represent the death and destruction of individuals and the family as the inevitable consequence of the failure to comply with HIV prevention messages. They portray HIV as a terrible, fatal biomedical condition and also as a curse and punishment for those who did not properly manage and contain their sexualities within heterosexual monogamous marriage. The later *AIDS in the City* 3 (2003) series, produced by Population Services International (PSI), shifts away from these punitive approaches to affirm what it portrays as positive behavior and choices and their happy consequences. *AIDS in the City* 3 nevertheless continued to presume and promote individual responsibilization as public health solution to the HIV epidemic. The series centers on heterosexual romantic love and family as prophylactic and on the nongovernmental organization as the primary source of information and support. Shot while the country was divided by civil war, the series portrays marriage and reproductive futurity as particularly potent tropes for the hope of future national union.

Producer Hanny Brigitte Tchelley has stated that *AIDS in the City* was created to "raise awareness" and was initially conceived as a "dramatic comedy,"

This chapter significantly revises and expands Cynn, "*AIDS in the City*: Melodrama and the Social Marketing of HIV Prevention in Francophone West Africa," originally published in *Camera Obscura*.

emphasizing drama and comedy equally "in order to win people's trust."[1] However, *AIDS in the City* centers less on dissemination of education and information and more on instigating behavior change, a shift in prevention strategy and focus that corresponds with a generic one. The series relies primarily on what Peter Brooks, in his important study of nineteenth-century European and American literature, has termed the *melodramatic mode*, its intense moral claims around contemporary issues and social problems, its "heightened dramatization" of guilt/innocence, and its linear progression of cause and effect climaxing in the triumph of virtue and truth.[2] As Brooks notes, when social orders were upended in a process of "desacralization" which culminated in the French Revolution, the melodramatic mode staged not merely punishment for the guilty but "the promise of a morally legible universe."[3] The *AIDS in the City* 3 series, in particular, simultaneously depicts and seeks to instigate the restoration of moral legibility in the social order. According to its circular logic, this restoration of moral legibility both results from and effects the prevention of HIV. The series conflates narrative resolution with policy solution. Drawing on social marketing and its consumerist ethos, it depicts desired behavior change as acceptance of personal responsibility and produces and promotes neoliberal conceptions of rational and free individuals, whom Aiwha Ong characterizes as "induced to self-manage according to market conceptions of efficiency, discipline and consumerism."[4] In *AIDS in the City* 3, the melodramatic mode provides the basis for the social marketing of HIV prevention and the production of HIV as an issue of individual responsibility and self-care.

Through *AIDS in the City* 3, PSI sought to transform behaviors of specific groups that range across different ethnic groups and economic classes. According to PSI, the four segments in the 2003 series, each individually comprised of four episodes, highlights a different "risk behavior" associated with the epidemic: "Adams the Driver [Adams le routier]" "informs the public of the unsafe behaviors surrounding mobile populations"; "The Story of the Fiancés [L'Histoire des Fiancés]" underscores "the importance of pre-nuptial testing and accepting one's HIV status"; "Amoin Séry" (which I will discuss in the next chapter) "addresses the consequences of risky behaviors such as multiple partners and polygamy"; and "Fatoumata: HIV-Positive Mother [Fatoumata: Mère seropositive]" (which I discussed in the previous chapter) "profiles the problem of mother-to-child transmission." The identification of

---

1. Tapsoba, "*SIDA dans la cité* II," 88, 90.
2. Brooks, *The Melodramatic Imagination*, xiii.
3. Brooks, *The Melodramatic Imagination*, 201.
4. Ong, *Neoliberalism as Exception*, 4. See also Harvey, *Brief History of Neoliberalism*; Povinelli, *Economies of Abandonment*.

risk behaviors as opposed to risk groups circumvents the problematic stigmatization and stereotyping of certain identities cordoned off as threats to the "general population"—for example, "gay/bisexual men" and "intravenous drug user"—to focus on behaviors.[5] However, while *AIDS in the City* clearly delineates the transformations that it represents as required—condom usage, monogamy, HIV testing, increased sympathy, acceptance of medical authority, and so on—the series encourages these measures to secure not only the health of the individual but also companionate marriage and the heteronormative, reproductively oriented family. As underscored by the *AIDS in the City* 3 segments "Adams the Driver" and "The Story of the Fiancés," heterosexual marriage and patriarchal family serve as both the rationale and the reward for proper self-management. Broadcast shortly after the country's first civil war divided the country, *AIDS in the City* 3 never refers to ongoing conflicts. Nevertheless, the series allegorizes monogamous marriage as symbol for and condition of national reunification.

MELODRAMA AND THE TELENOVELA

The melodramatic mode has provoked intense debate among Anglo-American feminist film critics, much of it centering on the affective responses Hollywood melodrama provokes and the masochistic identifications it is seen as eliciting from female spectators.[6] This scholarship also seeks to reclaim melodrama from its degraded status as feminized popular mass art form. Tanya Modeleski identifies the "unique pleasures" soap operas offer to women in the home and argues that they "may be in the vanguard not just of T.V. art but of all popular narrative art."[7] Linda Williams goes further and contends that rather than exemplifying an archaic mode of popular entertainment superseded by more realist and modern narratives, or a degraded feminized genre of entertainment epitomized by the soap opera or the "women's film," melodrama "typifies popular American narrative in literature, stage, film, and

---

5. As Nina Glick Schiller, Stephen Crystal, and Denver Lewellen note in the U.S. context about "subgroups" at risk for AIDS education and the accompanying "hierarchy of exposure," "The use of these categories to characterize who was 'at risk'—and therefore who was *not* at risk—diverted attention from the vital distinction that individuals were at risk for HIV infection not only because of what they did but also because the person they did it with was already infected." Schiller, Crystal, and Lewellen, "Risky Business," 1338. Seidel and Vidal further argue that the "epidemiological discourse of 'risk groups' is reductionist in that it proposes a single explanation for what is a complex social phenomenon." Seidel and Vidal, "Implications of 'Medical,'" 51.

6. Doane, *The Desire to Desire*; Kaplan, "Theories of Melodrama."

7. Modleski, *Loving with a Vengeance*, 80.

television when it seeks to engage with moral questions."[8] She argues that the melodramatic mode is quintessentially U.S. American in its generation of racialized spectacles of pathos and action, scenes that continue to inform conceptions of race and animate ongoing claims to rights and redress in the United States. Williams quotes Henry James's description of *Uncle Tom's Cabin* as a "'wonderful leaping fish'" that easily shimmied through a number of adaptations, a metaphor that for Williams characterizes the melodramatic mode and its prevalence across multiple media in the United States.[9]

Hiram Pérez has argued for an expanded understanding of the melodrama, what he describes as "a hemispheric—regional, transnational, extranational—mode or symbolic structure that in the excesses and peregrinations of its performances may indeed reinforce nation-state racial formations but also subverts, or at least recodes, those formations."[10] Consideration of how the melodramatic mode has not so much leapt back and forth but been adapted and readapted in HIV prevention media across the Atlantic enriches feminist scholarship on melodrama, as well as on HIV/AIDS prevention, fields that have not in the past been in dialogue. Although West African media scholars have argued for a reconceptualization of melodrama that considers the particular conditions and contexts of its production, dissemination, and reception, I am not aware of any who have considered the melodramatic mode in the HIV prevention videos marketing behavior change that circulate widely in the region.[11] Similarly, critics of HIV prevention media have not considered how social marketing, which has become increasingly popular among governments and donors as a form of health education in the Global South, has enlisted melodrama in its efforts to prompt behavior change in viewers.[12] Analysis of how and to what effects social marketing, HIV prevention efforts, and the melodramatic mode converge in "Adams the Driver" and "The Story of the Fiancés" segments of *AIDS in the City* 3 offer particularly useful contributions to feminist challenges to behavioral approaches to HIV prevention and to various neoliberal technologies of domination. To the extent that *AIDS in the City* draws from the techniques and tropes of Hollywood melodrama, Anglo-American feminist film criticism can provide useful critical frame-

---

8. Williams, *Playing the Race Card*, 17.
9. Williams, *Playing the Race Card*, 44.
10. Pérez, "*Alma Latina*," 2.
11. In *Signal and Noise*, Brian Larkin argues for the importance of a redefinition of melodrama through his analyses of Nollywood videos. See Katrien Pype's *The Making of the Pentecostal Melodrama* for more on Pentecostalism and the melodrama in television productions in Kinshasa. See Green-Simms's "Occult Melodramas" (25–59) for more on the "occult melodrama." See also Meyer, "'Praise the Lord.'"
12. Pfeiffer, "Condom Social Marketing."

works to read the series, even as such readings necessitate a broadening of the terms of aesthetic and political debates about melodrama and African media and complicate Anglo-American feminist attempts to recuperate the melodrama as a quintessentially American mode. Christine Gledhill maintains that melodrama in soap operas and its conversion of "topical social, economic, or political reference into personal, family dramas" provide generative sites to consider female desire, pleasure, and spectatorship.[13] In the Francophone West African context, this conversion has produced additional, different ideological and political effects.

SOAP OPERA AS EDUCATION

The term *soap opera* emerged in the 1930s United States to refer to daytime dramatic serial radio programs developed to pitch products—initially, literally soap—to women presumed to be listening as they did housework. Later, the term *soap opera* came to refer to television serials, which dominated U.S. daytime television from the 1950s onward.[14] The Latin American telenovela shares not just formal but also commercial origins with U.S. soap operas. The same corporations that sponsored the first soap operas in the United States—Procter and Gamble, Lever Brothers, and Colgate-Palmolive—also sponsored the first telenovelas in 1940s Latin America. While the soap opera, like the melodramatic narrative film, was not developed for pedagogical purposes, its form and its origins as advertising vehicle for its producers rendered it particularly suitable for such uses.[15]

Writer-producer-director Miguel Sabido first created telenovelas intended to impart social messages to audiences after he witnessed the tremendous success of *Simply Maria* [*Simplemente Maria*], a Peruvian soap opera broadcast in Mexico in 1971. *Simply Maria* portrayed the forty-year struggles and eventual triumph of a rural-to-urban female migrant who toils as a maid and seamstress before marrying her literacy teacher and becoming a world-famous, wealthy fashion designer. Produced by Panamericana de Televisión (PAN-TEL), 448 hour-long episodes of the telenovela screened from 1969 to 1971 in Peru, where enrollment in literacy classes skyrocketed after the series began broadcasting. Inspired by intense audience response to *Simply Maria*, Sabido developed seven educational soap operas in Mexico between 1975 and 1982, all

---

13. Gledhill, "Speculations," 122.
14. R. Allen's book remains the most comprehensive analysis of U.S. soap operas. R. Allen, *Speaking of Soaps*, 4. For a history of the U.S. soap opera, see 96–129.
15. R. Allen, *Speaking of Soaps*, 106, 116.

broadcast on Televisa, Mexico's largest TV station. These soap operas focused on imparting social messages around issues that Televisa glosses as "adult education and literacy," "responsible parenthood," "family planning," and "sexual responsibility among teenagers." Influenced by Sabido, Johns Hopkins University's Population Communication Services (JHU/PCS), which controls much of the communications funding from USAID, began launching educational television and radio soap operas in Kenya, Tanzania, and India.[16]

In the 1980s, *Dallas* and *Dynasty* were the first American serials to be distributed internationally (to fifty-seven countries). Dubbed into French, these shows enjoyed wide popularity in Côte d'Ivoire. More recently, televised half-hour soap operas, especially Brazilian and Mexican telenovelas, were dubbed into French, including *Catalina y Sebastián* [*Catalina and Sebastián*] (Azteca 13, 1999); *Laços de família* [*Family Secrets*] (Rede Globo, 2000–2001); and *Marimar* [*Marimar*] (Canal de las Estrellas, 1994). Domestically produced Ivorian shows like *Comment ça va?* [*How's it going?*] (RTI, 1975–94); *Qui fait ça?* [*Who's Doing That?*] (RTI, 1990–2002); and *Ma famille* [*My Family*] (RTI, 2002–7) were broadcast weekly in the evenings on one of the two national television stations in Côte d'Ivoire.[17] Likewise, *AIDS in the City* 3 aired primetime (after the 8:00 p.m. evening news in Côte d'Ivoire), and all the *AIDS and the City* 3 segments were eventually broadcast throughout Francophone West and Central Africa. In 2012, selected segments were posted on YouTube. As of early 2018, one segment, "The Story of the Fiancés," has been viewed over 905,000 times.[18]

With its relatively short individual storylines, *AIDS in the City* 3 might be better characterized as an abbreviated telenovela—which can run more than four hundred episodes—rather than as a soap opera. The 1995 and 1996–97 series featured a continuous storyline centering on Jacky and her husband, Sérapo. In contrast, the 2003 series was divided into four independent, four-episode segments, with Jacky featured as an HIV counselor for different central characters in each. While the U.S. soap opera typically endlessly defers narrative resolution, the telenovela, in contrast, consists of a limited number of episodes that build toward a climax and close with a predetermined resolution that Vitoria Barrera and Denise D. Bielby condense as follows: "Problems solved, lovers reunited, long lost family members found, villains getting what they deserved."[19] *AIDS in the City* 3 draws from the melodramatic mode of

---

16. Singhal and Rogers, *Entertainment-Education*, 48, 52.
17. Touré, "Telenovelas Reception," 43–44.
18. Shapiro, Meekers, and Tambashe, "Exposure to 'SIDA dans la cité,'" 304; Shapiro and Meekers, "Target Audience Reach," 21–30. https://www.youtube.com/watch?v=U63nl2TVokM.
19. Barrera and Bielby, "Places, Faces and Other Familiar Things," 2.

the public education film, the telenovela, and the soap opera to offer complex, crosscut plots incorporating flashbacks, family drama, wild coincidences, and heterosexual romance, with each episode closing on a note of suspense to encourage viewers to return for the next installment.

Relying on pathos, especially the spectacular suffering of its female protagonists, the telenovela represents social types or moral positions rather than psychologically complex characters. It also deploys melodrama's moralistic, Manichean framework of virtue/villainy that juxtaposes the ignorance of certain characters with the spectators' superior knowledge. The educational telenovela thereby reinforces moralistic frameworks to distinguish what it depicts as particular "good" or desirable behaviors from those which are "bad," to be eschewed or shunned. It also attempts to generate strong emotional responses so as to better impart those moral lessons to viewers and compel them to rethink and modify their own actions.

Brian Larkin argues that Nollywood videos produced in Nigeria and widely disseminated throughout sub-Saharan Africa "wage a political critique through the language of melodrama," an "aesthetics of outrage" that through representations of excess and the grotesque, and of extreme transgression, not only reveal the suffering, insecurities, and inequities of everyday life but also incite viewers' intense physical responses that serve as "moral commentary."[20] *AIDS in the City*'s melodramatic mode carefully avoids inciting outrage: As a form of sentimental politics, it compels audiences to empathize with people living with HIV/AIDS and to value and enact what the series depicts as necessary individual and personal—not political or economic—transformations. *AIDS in the City*'s melodramatic mode propels narrative action as well as resolution in the form of public health policy as the solution to the spread of HIV: behavior change as a moral imperative, instigated by individual identifications and sympathy rather than by any project of collective social transformation.

"Behavior change" and "Information, Education and Communication" (IEC) have become central goals and key terms of reference in global HIV prevention programs and health education. The definition of the terms and what they presume about the role of social and economic contexts in which "target audiences" live continue to be subject to debate. A 1997 study commissioned by the World Health Organization on twenty-five years of global IEC interventions defined IEC "as an approach which attempts to change or reinforce a set of behaviours in a 'target audience' regarding a specific problem in a predefined period of time." Ideally, such health communications transform individual and institutional practices and "contribute to sustainable change

---

20. Larkin, *Signal and Noise*, 183–94.

toward healthy behaviour."²¹ A World Bank report defines Behavior Change Communication (BCC) as an improvement on prior IEC's "unidirectional," top-down production and dissemination of educational information. The report identifies BCC as centering on more-collaborative approaches and concentrating on "outputs" rather than "inputs," in other words, on "effectiveness and outcome," or "behavior change results" as "the principal success criteria."²² In a 2003 report, USAID similarly endorsed BCC as "an interactive process with communities" that uses various modes of communication "to develop positive behaviors; promote and sustain individual, community and societal behavior change; and maintain appropriate behaviors." According to USAID, BCC is essential to the development of "a comprehensive HIV/AIDS prevention, care and support program."²³

In sub-Saharan Africa, the behavioral focus of HIV education, what Eileen Stillwaggon, among others, has termed the culture and behavior paradigm, risks trafficking in and reiterating colonial-era efforts centering on reforming or "modernizing" African "culture."²⁴ The focus on modifying behavior further highlights what Ezekiel Kalipeni, Susan Craddock, and Jayati Ghosh identify as one of the central paradoxes of HIV education itself: "[HIV] outreach campaigns are based implicitly on the notion of rational behavior, that is, that with new knowledge comes automatic adjustment in social or sexual practices. This approach elides the broader context of power relations, economic necessity, and resource limitations within which HIV transmission occurs."²⁵ Economic and political factors not only provide context for but also further exacerbate the spread of the HIV/AIDS epidemic, just as the epidemic intensifies economic and political crises.²⁶ HIV prevention telenovelas such as *AIDS in the City* ignores this more dynamic interplay and instead insistently focus on instigating individual behavior change and on socially marketing products and services. In a self-perpetuating, self-reflexive loop, the media represents social marketing campaigns as effective HIV prevention strategies. In other words, through portrayals of successful transformations that the series seeks to effect, *AIDS and the City* 3 promotes "behavior change"—and the series itself.

---

21. Clift, *Information, Education and Communication*, 3.
22. Elmendorf et al., "Behavior Change Communication," 2.
23. Family Health International, "Behavior Change Communication (BCC) for HIV/AIDS," 5.
24. Stillwaggon, *AIDS and the Ecology of Poverty*, 133–57.
25. Kalipeni, Craddock, and Ghosh, "Mapping the AIDS Pandemic," 65.
26. O'Manique, *Neoliberalism and AIDS Crisis*, 5.

SOCIAL MARKETING OF HIV PREVENTION

In *Marketing Social Change,* Alan Andreasen defines social marketing as "the application of commercial marketing technologies to the analysis, planning, execution and evaluation of programs designed to influence voluntary behavior of target audiences in order to improve their personal welfare and that of their society."[27] He describes the "domain of social marketing in the 21st century" as "*influencing* individual behavior [italics in original]" for the benefit of larger communities.[28] Until January 2018, PSI defined its mission as implementing the social marketing of family planning products and services in particular, a mandate that explicitly entails incorporation of the poor into neoliberal markets:

> The mission of PSI is to measurably improve the health of poor and vulnerable people in the developing world, principally through social marketing of family planning and health products and services, and health communications. Social marketing engages private sector resources and uses private sector techniques to encourage healthy behavior and make markets work for the poor.

PSI's website further claims that it is "the leading nonprofit social marketing organization in the world."[29] In the last twenty years, social marketing has become what James Pfeiffer describes as "the dominant approach to health education and communication in the developing world," with the social marketing of condoms the centerpiece of such campaigns in much of sub-Saharan Africa.[30] In contrast to French-funded, Francophone African cinema that necessarily engages in a dialogue with French conceptions of Africa and of African cultural identity, PSI actively seeks to produce "culturally sensitive" behavior change communication "tailored to specific groups to encourage health-seeking behaviors."[31] To advance PSI's mission of "build[ing] local capacity," *AIDS in the City* was scripted by Ivorian writers (with extensive oversight by PSI) and featured many established Ivorian actors.[32] The

---

27. Andreasen, *Marketing Social Change,* 23.
28. Andreasen, *Social Marketing in the 21st Century,* 10.
29. In January 2018, PSI changed its mission to: "PSI makes it easier for people in the developing world to lead healthier lives and plan families they desire by marketing affordable products and services." http://www.psi.org/about/at-a-glance/. Accessed Jan. 3, 2018.
30. Pfeiffer, "Condom Social Marketing," 77.
31. On "cultural sensitivity," see Patton, *Inventing AIDS,* 84–87.
32. Population Services International, "PSI at a Glance." In March 2018, PSI described its work on HIV/AIDS in Côte d'Ivoire: "We're a nonprofit, but we take a business approach to

first two series were produced by well-known Ivorian actor Hanny Tchelley. Filmed in Côte d'Ivoire, the third 2003 series was directed by a prominent Ivorian playwright and theater director, Alexis Don Zigré. Globally renowned Ivorian musician Alpha Blondy composed the single that served as the inspiration for the title of the entire series and as *AIDS in the City* 1's and 2's theme song.

Although *AIDS in the City* relied on Ivorian talent and was produced for Ivorian and African viewers, it was financed and its production administered exclusively by foreign funders, primarily from the United States. The series therefore represents a sort of inversion of French production of Francophone African cinema that has provoked sustained critiques for reinforcing dependence on French funding and for shaping an African cinema intended almost exclusively for French and European audiences.[33] The 2003 series was produced by the United States–based PSI, with the majority of the $175,000 budget (some of the budget was used to purchase studio equipment) provided by the U.S. Centers for Disease Control (CDC), with additional subsidies from the German governmental development agency Gesellschaft für Technische Zusammenarbeit (GTZ), and the German government development bank Kreditanstalt für Wiederaufbau (KfW).[34] The 2003 series was produced in collaboration with AIMAS (Ivorian Agency of Social Marketing, founded by PSI); Radiodiffusion Télévision Ivoirienne (RTI); UNAIDS Intercountry Team for West and Central Africa; Family Health and AIDS Prevention (SFPS); Projet Rétrovirus de Côte d' Ivoire (RETROCI); and the Ministry for AIDS Control in Côte d'Ivoire (MLS) and the Ministry of Health (MOH). The Coca-Cola Africa Foundation underwrote broadcasting costs.

Social marketing campaigns explicitly cultivate these convergences of public, private, and commercial sectors and the enlistment of local talent to promote products, services, and behavior change as a form of commodity. The attempts to inculcate in target audiences the value of commercial markets replicate techniques of colonial health management. In particular, they recall colonial-era missionaries' practice of charging for treatments so as to intro-

---

saving lives. We break the traditional development model and tackle the toughest health problems by using proven business practices like marketing and franchising, by helping build strong health systems in the private and public sector, by tapping into the expertise of 8,000 local staff in more than 50 countries around the world, and by measuring our impact." Population Services International, "PSI: Approaches".

33. Diawara, *African Cinema*, 77; Genova, *Cinema and Development*, 130–31.

34. Jeff Barnes, personal interview, October 28, 2013. The first series had a total budget of $50,000; the second, $100,000 (though some of that budget was for studio equipment). Deutsche Gesellschaft für Internationale Zusammenarbeit, *TV Soap Operas in HIV Education*, 28–30.

duce colonial subjects to monetary exchanges. They also recall colonial efforts to produce thrifty, efficient consumers through health education that elided social and economic contexts, even as they compelled insertion into cash economies as a route to "civilization." Such campaigns set colonial subjects on the path of managing their own health in market and moralistic terms, as what Jean Comaroff has described as "moral achievements to be secured by hard labor, effective management, and rational consumption."[35]

While the *AIDS in the City* 3 series as a whole constitutes an HIV prevention social marketing campaign, individual segments also foreground such campaigns as central to their narratives. According to Neil Price, the commodities promoted through social marketing are usually subsidized and branded: "Social marketing's behavior change strategy seeks to promote access to and demand for goods and services by integrating health education with commercial brand advertising."[36] *AIDS in the City* 3 advertises and promotes a PSI-funded testing center, le Centre l'Éveil [The Awareness Center], in Abidjan, where all the main characters receive counseling and eventually test. PSI-brand condoms, Prudence, feature conspicuously in all the segments, as do social marketing campaigns themselves. In the song, for which the entire series is named, Alpha Blondy punningly reminds viewers to buy Prudence condoms:

> I went to the pharmacy
> To buy some condoms.
> I am going to explode!
> We are going to have some fun.
> Trust, okay.
> But Prudence first!
> There's panic on board! . . .
> There's AIDS, AIDS in the city.
> There's AIDS, AIDS in the city.
> AIDS in the city.
>
> [Je suis allé à la pharmacie
> Acheter des préservatifs.
> Je vais m'éclater!
> On va s'amuser.
> Confiance, d'accord
> Mais Prudence d'abord.

---

35. Jean Comaroff, "The Diseased Heart," 319.
36. Price, "The Performance of Social Marketing," 231.

Y'a la panique à bord.
Y'a le Sida, Sida dans la cité.]³⁷

Not incidentally, Prudence condoms are an actual product sold in Côte d'Ivoire. PSI began subsidizing the distribution of Prudence brand condoms in May 1991. By 1995, according to PSI, Prudence enjoyed the same brand recognition as Nescafé and Toyota, and by 1997 Prudence sales constituted 95% of the condom market in the country. By 2003, Prudence condoms were the centerpiece of the largest nongovernmental social marketing HIV prevention program in the country.³⁸ The Ivorian government viewed the promotion of Prudence condoms as conspicuous enough to warrant a demand for payment of 7 million CFA to screen the 1995 series; it argued that the short spots promoting Prudence condoms before each episode constituted advertisements.³⁹

HIV/AIDS AND INDIVIDUAL BEHAVIOR CHANGE

African ministries of health and international nongovernmental organizations have embraced social marketing of behavior change as central to HIV prevention. With its emphasis on the so-called free market and attendant retraction of government services, neoliberalism of the latter part of the twentieth and early twenty-first century radically shifted prior liberal ideological strains of Keynesian economics and their underpinning of the "welfare state."⁴⁰ Although neoliberalism rationalizes economic policy agendas, and neoliberal technologies manage and regulate through economic, political, or military processes and practices, neoliberalism also operates on the level of the social and the individual. HIV prevention media such as *AIDS in the City* promotes the central tenets of neoliberalism—privatization and individual responsibility—with regard to HIV prevention, thereby representing HIV as a problem to be resolved through proper self-management and regulation.⁴¹ Those characters practicing what it deems "unsafe" or improper sex subsequently suffer the

---

37. Blondy, "Sida dans la Cité," recorded 1991, track 5 on the album *SOS Guerre Tribale*. EMI France, compact disc.
38. Dodd, "AIDS Soap Opera," 16; Shapiro, Meekers, and Tambashe, "Exposure to the 'SIDA dans la cité,'" 304. PSI turned over sales and distribution of Prudence condoms to AIMAS (which was launched in 1991) around the time of the 2003 *AIDS in the City* production. Barnes, interview.
39. Morand, "TV passionne les Ivoiriens," 44.
40. Connell and Dados discuss neoliberalism as it has impacted the Global South, primarily in the arenas of global trade, state and military force, and land and agriculture. To this list, I would add health and health care. Connell and Dados, "The Market Agenda," 117–38.
41. Duggan, *Twilight of Equality*, 12.

consequence of HIV infection, represented as a form of sanction at the level of the individual person/body. But *AIDS in the City* also depicts such individual as culprits, a menace to others. Thus, the danger posed by people living with HIV and their "unsafe" behavior extend beyond contamination of other individuals to threaten the population and the species. Like the masturbating child, hysterical woman, Malthusian couple, and perverse adult identified by Michel Foucault, the person living with HIV or possibly living with HIV represents a "node" where body and population, and disciplinary and regulatory processes, are articulated, with the *AIDS in the City* series both representing and itself constituting medical and hygienic intervention.[42]

With its focus on individual behavior change and its attempt to bolster the production of individual consumers, social marketing suits the mandates of the World Bank and the International Monetary Fund (IMF), as well as those of major bilateral and multilateral donors such as USAID, a major funder of PSI.[43] However, as many have noted, the imposition of structural adjustment programs in sub-Saharan Africa and their mandated cuts in public spending, especially on health and education, have had particularly adverse effects on the poor and have in fact intensified the impoverishment of the poor, especially women.[44] The spread of HIV is exacerbated by the very policies that the IMF promotes. Economic instability in Côte d'Ivoire steadily increased after a number of political crises following the 1993 death of Houphouet-Boigny after a thirty-three-year dictatorship. Mandated structural adjustment aggravated the country's shift to ethnonationalist politics and contributed to a series of political and economic crises that culminated in Côte d'Ivoire's first military coup in 1999 and to a political and military division of the country from September 2002 to May 2011.[45]

---

42. Foucault, "*Society Must Be Defended*," 252. Foucault, *History of Sexuality, Volume 1*, 105.

43. Pfeiffer, "Condom Social Marketing," 78.

44. A UNESCO publication described the effects of structural adjustment on women as the "feminization of poverty," a term that circulates widely in UN literature. UNICEF critiqued Structural Adjustment Policies as early as 1987. Moghadam, "The 'Feminization of Poverty'"; Afshar and Dennis, *Women and Adjustment Policies*; Harrison, *Neoliberal Africa*, 39–41; Kalipeni, Craddock, and Ghosh, "Mapping the AIDS Pandemic," 67–68; Oppong et al., *Sex and Gender in an Era of AIDS*, 8–9; Poku, "Poverty, Debt and Africa's HIV/AIDS Crisis," 538; Schoepf, "Assessing AIDS Research in Africa," 134–35.

45. Akindès, "La Côte d'Ivoire depuis 1993"; Akindès, *The Roots of the Military-Political Crisis*; Dembélé, "La Construction économique," 123–72; B. Campbell, "Defining New Development Options," 36; McGovern, *Making War*, 157; Klaas, "From Miracle to Nightmare," 113–15; Charbonneau, *France and the New Imperialism*, 154. In "Africa's New Territorial Politics" (59–81), Catherine Boone describes the shift to neoliberal policies in slightly different terms, as undermining national integration and instituting new forms of territorial politics, and state control and management. Boone, "Africa's New Territorial Politics." See also Boone and Kriger, "Multiparty Elections and Land Patronage."

Although the need for vigilance about statistics, especially when they reinforce stereotypes of "Africa" as a region of dire poverty, should not be understated, the IMF itself notes that poverty rates in Côte d'Ivoire rose from 10% in 1985, to 36.8% in 1995, to 48.9% in 2008 (with poverty defined as living on CFA 661, or $1.35/day). The ensuing military deployment and increased sex work and impoverishment; the widespread displacement and migration; and the destruction of health-care facilities following the failures of structural adjustment and the division of Côte d'Ivoire have been well documented as contributing to the spread of HIV.[46] While the World Bank and the IMF coerced compliance with neoliberal policies, including structural adjustment programs, the General Agreement on Tariffs and Trade and the World Trade Organization (GATT/WTO) initiated the first comprehensive protection of intellectual property rights through the trade-related aspects of intellectual property rights, or the TRIPS agreement, which prohibited governments from purchasing or manufacturing low-cost generic antiretroviral treatments.[47]

Social marketing as HIV prevention in *AIDS in the City* ignores and obscures these larger structural constraints. The 2003 series in particular elides the widely acknowledged failure of the insertion of Côte d'Ivoire into the "free market" to "make markets work for the poor" and instead insistently centers on individual characters represented as deciding to make rational decisions to care for the self and the family. The series codes HIV testing and prevention as the only obviously moral choice: Education and enlightenment effect what are depicted as necessary, healthy, and ethical, transformations in behavior. (Significantly, in 2007, the cost of a package of three Prudence condoms was 200 CFA, about a third of what a person living in poverty—close to 50% of the population, according to the IMF definition of poverty—would live on in a day.) The *AIDS in the City* 3 series ignores global inequities, which were reinforced by the WTO through the TRIPS agreement and which rendered antiretroviral treatments prohibitively expensive for almost all people living with HIV in the Global South.[48] Instead, it turns to the mode of melodrama to reinforce its identification of HIV as a problem of ignorance and denial.

---

46. For an overview of such research, see Parker et al., "Structural Barriers." See also Iliffe, *The African AIDS Epidemic*, 40, 55; Karim, "Heterosexual Transmission of HIV," 246–47. On the history of health-care facilities and the effects of the civil wars on health care, see Gaber and Patel, "Tracing Health System Challenges."

47. On TRIPS, the Doha agreement of 2001, and the "Paragraph 6 solution," see chapter 3, footnote 44.

48. In "Prémices et déroulement" (13–86) Karine Delaunay et al. offer an overview of the UNAIDS 1996 initiative (which did not begin until 1998) to provide limited antiretroviral treatment and efforts, especially efforts by organizations of people living with HIV/AIDS to obtain antiretroviral treatment.

According to the logic of the melodramatic narratives of the series, HIV transmission occurs because of improper control of individual sexual behavior, a failure that threatens the health and future of the individual, the family, and the community. Its promotion of HIV testing and prevention in the form of behavior change seeks to secure the heteronormative body for romantic love represented as enabling reproductive future and family.[49]

AIDS IN THE CITY
"You can't eat bananas with their skin!": "Adams the Driver"

A segment comprised of four episodes in the 2003 "Adams the Driver" represents the transformations that the video attempts to initiate as the culmination of a series of effective HIV prevention events and interventions.[50] The series opens at a roadside kiosk where an HIV prevention radio message from the *Drive Protected* [*Roulez Protégé*] campaign plays: "My girlfriend, the condom, of course! It's my travelling companion! [Mon amie, la capote, bien sûr! C'est mon compagnon de route!]." The message provokes a series of remarks by the server and the male clients at the kiosk, including Adams, who dismiss the message as an annoying interruption of the song. They comment that AIDS is an invention of the news [les brèves] designed to amuse and distract listeners [nous distraire]; that villagers say that anyone suffering from diarrhea and rashes has AIDS; that people are created in the image of God, so those with rashes must be the children of demons; that AIDS was created to discourage lovers; that people with HIV are skinny and sick at home or in the hospital; and doctors, nurses, and military must undergo HIV testing, but such testing offers no diploma.

The men's attempts to grapple with new forms of disease and suffering provide multiple alternative explanations for the spread of HIV, all framed as "local," or everyday. Mixing French with Dioula, or Malinké, their com-

---

49. In "Targeting the Empowered Individual" (67) Hansjörg Dilger traces a shift in HIV prevention media in Tanzania from what he terms an "approach of deterrence" ("AIDS kills") to one that focuses on a growing urban middle class and that centers on the promotion of condom usage as a sign of true love, trust, esteem, communication, and health.

50. As of 2018, the PSI website outlines the desired effects of social marketing as "program exposure" positively influencing "behavioral factors," "behavioral change," and "health outcomes" (Population Services International, "Social Marketing: Evidence Base"). In "Adams the Driver," social marketing instigates behavior changes, including condom usage, reduction in number of sexual partners, HIV testing and counseling, and treatment of HIV/sexually transmitted infections. This revises PSI's previous account of social marketing as "product distribution and communication," followed by "behavioral factors" ("opportunity," "ability," and "motivation") resulting in "behavior change."

ments further launch a critique of the media itself and its attempts to distract from the realities of the hardships of their everyday lives. Underscoring the central importance and role of educational media, the segment counters their interpretations. The men at the kiosk exemplify what the entire series consistently frames as the need for social marketing and education, a process that Adams successfully undergoes through the kind of sustained pedagogy which the series suggests that social marketing media, exemplified by the segments themselves, provides. After another man at the kiosk, Solo, announces his HIV-positive status, he disrupts the other men's presumptions: He is a friend in "good shape," not wasting or hospitalized, like the people with HIV whom the men have seen on television. Solo further prompts Adams to action. After Adams has heard the message about condoms on the radio, visited Solo to talk with him again, and seen the Prudence billboard by the side of the road, he demonstrates what social marketing identifies as the correct factors—opportunity, ability, and motivation—to institute behavior change. He breaks off his relations with another girlfriend on the road and purchases Prudence condoms to bring back to the house that he shares with his partner, Kadi.

While the segment alludes to prevention of unwanted pregnancy as a benefit of condom usage, its focus is clearly on condoms as method of HIV prevention. Through its insistence that condoms enable heterosexual reproduction within the monogamous nuclear family, the segment recognizes and seeks to resolve the contradiction between condom usage as a method of HIV prevention and what it represents and reinforces as the heterosexual reproductive mandate. The conflict is gendered and intergenerational, and centers on what the segment portrays as a clash between tradition and modernity; the conflict is also articulated as generic, between the comic and the melodramatic. Significantly, the series depicts condom usage as necessary for reproductive heterosexual normativity and portrays nonusage or incorrect usage as comic disruption to the seriousness of the melodramatic narrative—of HIV itself.

In reply to questions from the host at a Prudence condom event, a male spectator, another stand-in for the series audience, raises the issue of decreased male pleasure. To the laughter of the audience, he repeats a widely circulating metaphoric objection to the use of condoms: "I don't like condoms. You can't eat bananas with their skin! [On ne peut pas manger la banane avec sa peau!]." Adams, who has joined the audience of the Prudence event, volunteers to demonstrate proper condom use. The slapstick scene of the Prudence condom event positions the viewer alongside the audience of the event. In a series of medium shots, Adams is encouraged with vigorous thumbs up from Ladji, his buffoon assistant apprentice sidekick (the actor playing Ladji, Abass

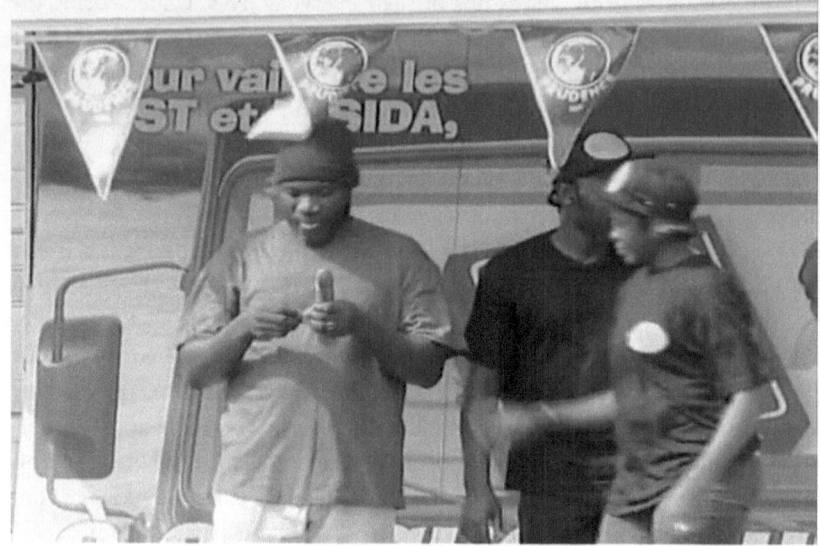

FIGURE 4.1. Adams as he attempts to put a condom on a prosthetic penis during a Prudence event.

Ibn, is a well-known comedian), to mount the stage. The scene abruptly cuts to Adams's mother grimly informing Kadi that they must have a woman-to-woman talk. The video then cuts back to the Prudence condom event where, in his attempts to slide the condom on a wooden prosthetic penis, Adams has shredded the condom (figure 4.1). As a woman displays how to correctly open the packet and pinch the air out of the tip of the condom, the video cuts back to a close-up of Adams's mother chastising Kadi for not having produced a child and threatening that if Kadi does not become pregnant in two months, she will give her son another wife (figure 4.2). After a close-up of Kadi looking downcast, the video cuts back to a medium two-shot of Adams insisting to a laughing and joking to Ladji that HIV/AIDS is a serious issue.

As the conflict between Kadi's mother-in-law's mandate to produce a child and Adams's insistence on condom usage intensifies, the telenovela narrative eventually assimilates the nonusage of condoms rendered as a comic, negative lesson into the properly serious melodramatic plot. In an intertextual reference to the prior *Drive Protected* HIV prevention social marketing campaign, Adama, the apprentice in the *Drive Protected* video, becomes Adams the master in "Adams the Driver" who begins to serve as a peer educator, trying to convince a driver friend to also stop having sexual relations on the road and giving his own apprentice, Ladji, Prudence condoms to use with one of the

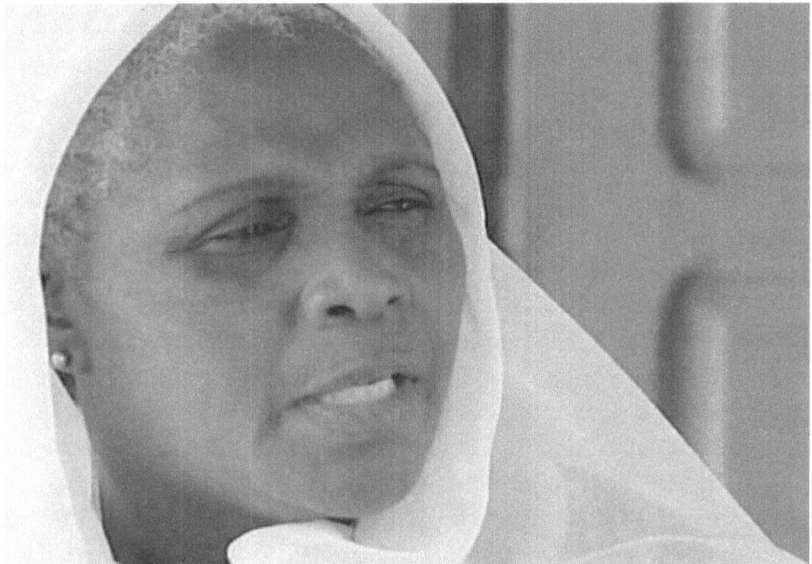

FIGURE 4.2. Adams's mother warning her daughter-in-law.

market girls, Sally. In the *Drive Protected* video, the apprentice refuses to use condoms; as a result, he is infected with a sexually transmitted disease and his girlfriend becomes pregnant. Similarly, in "Adams the Driver," Sally announces that she is pregnant, but testing reveals that Sally actually suffers from gonorrhea, which has prevented her from menstruating. Failure to use condoms, then, not their usage, results in gonorrhea, Sally's false pregnancy, and potential sterility. Clutching properly dispensed prescription medication (and not the black-market medication he had used in the past), Ladji vows that he will use condoms in all future sexual relationships. Appropriately subdued, finally serious [sérieux, an adjective that also connotes *maturity*], he and the comic plot disappear from the narrative of progress in which Adams fulfills his role as an exemplary subject of social marketing as a form of HIV prevention.

The HIV counselor, the peer educator, and social marketing media supersede the mother and the village as sites of authority and wisdom, just as the melodramatic supersedes the comic. Kadi tries to share her concerns about her conversation with Adams's mother, but after perfunctorily reassuring her, Adams brushes her aside to continue to watch a television program in which a central character from the prior series, Jacky Sérapo, reminds viewers that HIV is not transmitted by mosquitoes or witchcraft [sorcellerie] and that condoms are necessary for young people, for mobile populations, and for those who have multiple sexual partners. The scene cuts to Adams sharing the same bowl of food with Soro (another successfully internalized lesson: HIV is not transmitted through casual contact like sharing food) and declaring that he has decided to test.

Despite his mother's continuing opposition, Adams insists that he and Kadi use condoms until he has obtained his test results. Unlike Kitia Touré's 1993 *Gestures or Life* and unlike prior HIV prevention messages, the segment does not insist that women living with HIV never reproduce. "Adams the Driver" accepts what it depicts as a heterosexual reproductive mandate and foregrounds the stigmatization confronting "sterile" women. Initially, Kadi firmly rejects condom usage: "What about what I want? I want a child! I don't want others to think that I am sterile. Make a child with me!" When Adams receives his negative results but nevertheless complies with medical directives that he continue to use condoms until after the necessary three-month-window period, Kadi is furious: "I do all Adams asks and instead of making me a child, he gives me problems. If this continues, I will leave get my bags and leave. Two years without children! We are not sterile in my family." Through counseling with Jacky Sérapo, Kadi, too, eventually becomes convinced of the importance both of condom usage until Adams's test results can be confirmed and of HIV testing for herself and the health of her future child(ren). While Solo and Jacky code Adams's willingness to test as sign of his responsibility and his concern for her and their future child, Adams's mother represents "tradition" and the conditions of improper reproduction—polygamous (conflated with "Muslim"), compelled not by romantic love but by matriarchal dictate; and ignorant, undertaken without heeding HIV prevention messages about testing and condom usage. The social marketing of HIV prevention through radio, television, billboard, group spectacle, and the authority of biomedicine then literally displace the older generation as sources of correct information and as the model for future behavior.[51]

The segment concludes with what the segment depicts as the rewards of obeying HIV prevention messages. Adams and Kadi wait for her results outside the Awareness Center and affirm that they will have a child together, a son, whom they will name Adams, to whom his father will bequeath his truck. As in other segments of the series, "Adams the Driver" portrays characters undergoing the process of education and increased awareness followed by individual transformation and behavior changes that it seeks to reproduce in viewers. It represents proper behavior, in this instance, HIV testing, condom usage, and sexual fidelity, as facilitating the restoration of the moral

---

51. In *Visual Pedagogies* (181–87) Brian Goldfarb provides an account of cinematic representations of the transfer of pedagogical authority to the younger generation as challenging both precolonial and colonial, traditional and imperial, modes of authority in West Africa.

and social order conflated with a certain "modern" reproductive heteronormativity: monogamous, companionate, nuclear, patriarchal, and patrilineal. The segment cannot depict the actual test results that might threaten the very reproductive future that they are supposed to secure, so it closes instead with the promise of heteronormative romantic love undergirded by the nongovernmental organization. When Kadi worries about testing HIV-positive, Adams reassures her: "I am with you today. I will be with you tomorrow, whatever your [HIV test] results. You know why? Because I love you." In the closing shot, they walk hand-in-hand back into the testing center.

"Hope is allowed": "The Story of the Fiancés"

While "Adams the Driver" centers on a Muslim, Dioula, or Malinké working-class couple, a different segment of the *AIDS in the City* 3 series, "The Story of the Fiancés," takes up the issues confronting an HIV-discordant couple through the narrative of the familiar drama of heterosexual love between a couple from different social classes and ethnic groups. A young woman, Nathalie, the daughter of a wealthy Beté family, and Alex, an upwardly mobile young man from a more modest Baoulé family, want to marry. While Nathalie's mother is supportive, Nathalie's father opposes the match and prefers another suitor, since Alex is not of the same social class [milieu]. The telenovela narrative of class and generational conflict shifts when Nathalie's father eventually grants his approval, but Nathalie insists that she and her fiancé test for HIV before their marriage because they both have had lovers—though she is careful to note that although he has had multiple girlfriends, she has had a single affair [une aventure]. For the sake of their future children, Nathalie argues, they should test. As she tells Alex, it would be "cruel to have a child and learn that it is positive because we did not have the courage to test."

What Nathalie does not realize—but in that familiar melodramatic shuttling of ignorance and knowledge, what the viewer does—is that Alex has recently been contacted by a former girlfriend, Bintou, who informs him that she is HIV-positive. The segment establishes conventionally punitive melodramatic consequences of unregulated sex, with a single lapse in vigilance leading to disease and ruination. Bintou refers to a 1989 National Committee for the Fight against AIDS [Comité national de lutte contre le Sida (CNLS)] prevention clip featuring a seated, emaciated man in shadow who speaks over an ominous drumbeat: "Don't risk your life as I did, for one little moment of pleasure. Protect yourself. Protect your life. Be faithful . . . It's the advice of a sick man." Bintou echoes the clip, as does Mado, a character from the 1995 *AIDS in the City* 1, who lamented having an affair with her best friend's husband who learns that he is HIV-positive: "God, help me. To die for a few minutes of pleasure, by recklessness [l'inconscience], negligence."

Bintou acknowledges to Alex that she did not obey such directives: "I had never thought I could have AIDS. I went out with good, serious people. I thought I was sheltered [à l'abri] from all that. Alas, AIDS strikes everyone. Unprotected sex just once is enough [Il suffit d'un seul rapport nonprotégé]. One tiny little moment [un tout petit moment] of pleasure and everything collapses [tout bascule]. Life is ruined." The narrative further relies on the reversals familiar in melodrama to establish a rationale for the behavior change that it promotes, one that also governs "Adams the Driver": failure to properly regulate behavior as advised, failure to use condoms and to test, threaten heteronormative reproductive future. While Kitia Touré's 1993 *Gestures or Life* promoted abortion as the solution for mother-to-child transmission, an exchange between Nathalie and her HIV counselor identifies the termination of the pregnancy, not the unprotected sex leading to the pregnancy, as a potential source of contagion:

> NATHALIE: Before my fiancé, I had an affair [une aventure] so I want to know my serological status before my marriage.
> COUNSELOR: You think you took risks during this affair?
> NATHALIE: Yes, once. In high school, I had to have an abortion [J'étais obligée d'avoir un avortement] to continue my studies. I was marked by this experience, and I broke up with this boyfriend. But since then, I have always demanded condoms with my partner.
> COUNSELOR: Even with your fiancé?
> NATHALIE: Yes, always, each time.
> COUNSELOR: Let's go back to this termination of pregnancy. Did you test afterward?
> NATHALIE: No. This is the first time. It's because of that that I want to definitively know [avoir une idée nette] my status. I will marry soon, and I want children in complete safety [en toute sécurité].
> COUNSELOR: That's wise.
> NATHALIE: But tell me, Madame, because of this youthful love, can I be at risk [exposée] of AIDS now? Can just a fling [un simple flirt] ruin my life as a couple?
> COUNSELOR: To be frank with you, you took a risk with this abortion.

The counselor deflects the question about unprotected sex to instead identify abortion as the "risk" leading to potential HIV infection and concurs with Nathalie that marriage offers protection against HIV. But, more significantly, the counselor does so to promise, as does "Adams the Driver," that proper condom usage and HIV testing will ensure rather than threaten Nathalie's impending marriage and the safety of her future children. By identifying the termination of the pregnancy as a "risk," the series then challenges prevailing assumptions that women living with HIV should not reproduce.[52] The segment represents as ideal "companionate marriage," what anthropologists Holly Wardlow and Jennifer S. Hirsch usefully define as the "marital ideal in which emotional closeness is understood to be both one of the primary measures of success in marriage and a central practice through which the relationship is constituted and reinforced." As Wardlow and Hirsch argue, companionate marriage is not an inevitable signifier of modernity but a place where struggles to define and access it, and where conceptions of individuality, individual fulfillment, and happiness, are articulated and shaped. In "The Story of the Fiancés," the melodramatic visual vernacular of companionate marriage, the segment's "discursive intertwining of gender, marriage, and progress," links the conflict between generations and classes with the crisis and the drama around HIV testing.[53] The segment's melodramatic visual vernacular of companionate marriage further links the conflict between generations and classes over marriage with the crisis and the drama about HIV testing.

After Alex tests seropositive, and Nathalie negative, their counselor reiterates the theme of the segment, "Hope is allowed [L'espoir est permis]." The phrase revises the slogan of the Vancouver 1996 XI International AIDS Conference and of the UNAIDS World AIDS Day: "One World, One Hope [Tous Unis en Espoir]," later taken up as a slogan by people living with HIV in Côte d'Ivoire. The 1996 conference highlighted the importance of antiretroviral treatment, especially new three-drug regimens, to treat HIV, and during both the conference and World AIDS Day that year, the Ivorian government and representatives of groups of people living with HIV/AIDS in Côte d'Ivoire demanded access to the expensive but promisingly effective new therapies. Significantly, the segment revises the assertion of a shared hope for a future free of HIV, a future that, as activists and government officials repeatedly underscored, would be enabled in part through universal access to HIV treat-

---

52. A 1989 *Fraternité Matin* article noted the pervasiveness of "polemics about the possibility of forbidding especially women with HIV from reproducing [la possibilité d'interdire notamment à la mère séropositive de procréer]." Léon Francis Lebry, "Sida: Ordonner sa sexualité." *Fraternité Matin*, January 18, 1989, 2.

53. Hirsch and Wardlow, "Introduction," 4, 20.

ment.⁵⁴ The counselor invokes the slogan but only to affirm their future as a heterosexual, reproductive couple. Eliding any mention of treatment for HIV, the counselor reassures the couple about treatment for opportunistic infections and offers support services through nongovernmental organizations.

Despite the counselor's reassurance, after Alex and Nathalie return to Nathalie's house, Alex tries to end their engagement:

> ALEX: I am infected, Nathalie. I have the virus of AIDS in my body. That is what you want?
> NATHALIE: Alex, we can live with this illness [maladie].
> ALEX: What life are you talking about? Making love forever [en permanence] with a condom? To have a household [foyer] condemned to sterility? That is the life that you want to lead with me?
> NATHALIE: And love, Alex? We love each other, don't forget that. [*Hugs him*]. Listen, you had promised to stay with me no matter the result. Did you forget that?
> ALEX: Try to understand. This sickness is incurable. It is fatal [mortelle]. No, I cannot. I cannot marry you knowing I have AIDS. That will transmit death to you [Ce sera te transmettre la mort].

Descending the stairs of the family villa, Nathalie's mother overhears their argument and, although she had been supportive of the couple, immediately agrees with Alex when he asks her to convince Nathalie that they cannot marry. That the entire exchange takes place on the staircase is not incidental. In his important essay on Hollywood melodramatic cinema, Thomas Elsaesser notes the significance of the staircase's vertical axis in signaling dramatic downward narrative and emotional shift.⁵⁵ "The Story of the Fiancés" further uses the staircase both to shift and to analogize the conflict between Nathalie and her father to that between Nathalie and her mother. When Nathalie's father initially refuses to approve of the marriage between his daughter and Alex because of their different social status, Nathalie expresses her frustration to her friend, Juliette, on the staircase of her villa (figure 4.3). The long shot of Juliette walking up the stairs and of Nathalie descending cuts to Nathalie's confrontation with her parents, a scene in which Nathalie tries to assert her

---

54. The English slogan "One World, One Hope" asserts a global optimism; it effectively defines a global community through that shared optimism. The repetition of "one," emphasizing unity, is not translated into the French phrase, which might be translated more literally as "All United in Hope."

55. Elsaesser, "Tales of Sound and Fury," 83.

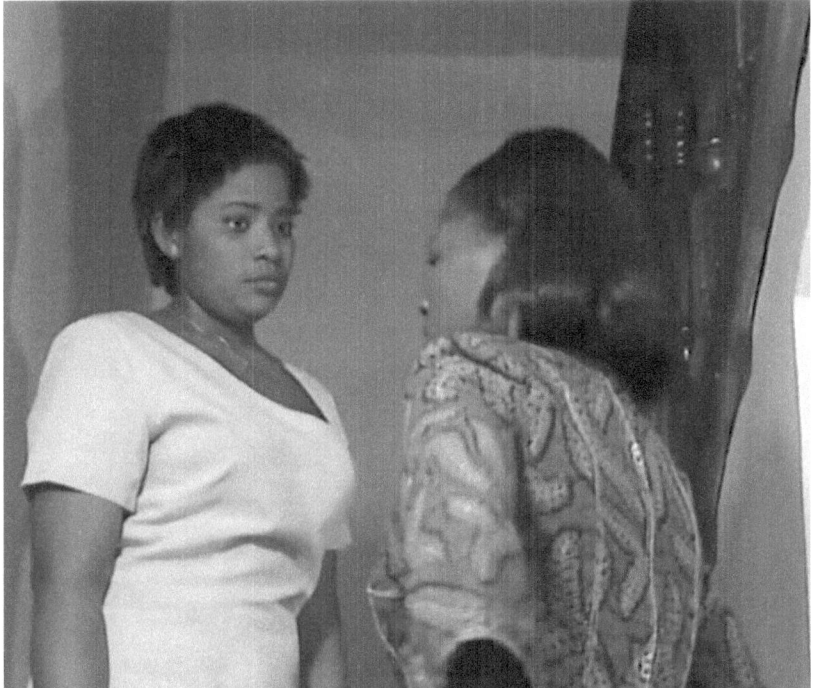

FIGURE 4.3. Juliette (left) urges Nathalie to calm down and listen to her parents.

independence and her desire to marry Alex despite her father's disapproval: "I am an adult [Je suis majeure] and work!" Later, after Alex tests HIV-positive, Nathalie's mother pauses and then descends the same staircase to dissuade Nathalie from marrying him (figure 4.4). Later, as they descend the staircase outside their workplace, Nathalie and Alex continue their argument about testing for HIV before their marriage (figure 4.5). The visual conventions of the melodrama render contiguous the conflict that it codes as between upper and lower classes, HIV-negative and HIV-positive partners, younger and older generations, HIV testing and refusal to test, traditional and modern, and family and individual.

The segment highlights another unresolvable contradiction: It must acknowledge the risk of HIV transmission both to Nathalie and to her child(ren) if she and Alex reproduce, what Alex calls the transmission of "death," even as the segment attempts to persuade that testing for HIV and potentially having an HIV-positive result can enable and affirm, rather than destroy, heteronormative love, marriage, and the continuity of the family.

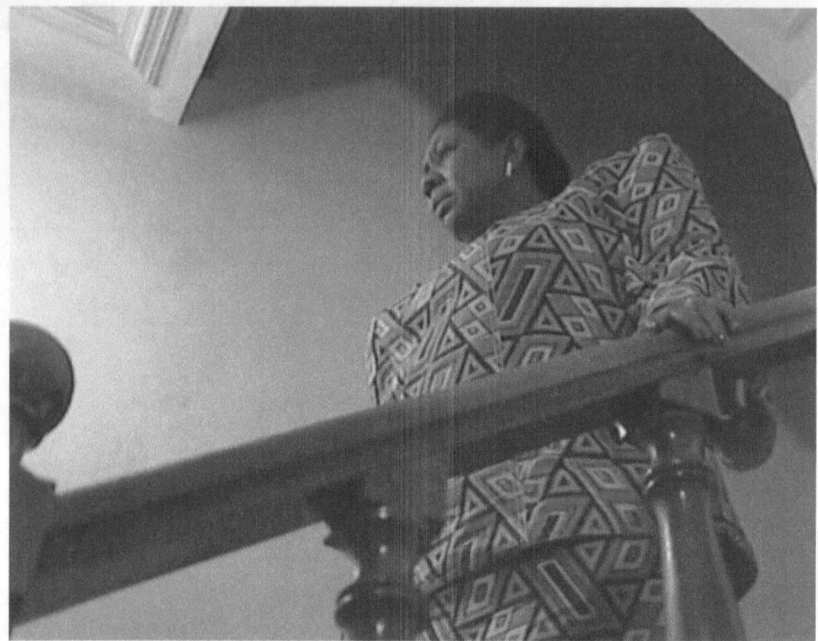

FIGURE 4.4. Nathalie's mother overhears Alex trying to end his engagement with Nathalie because he has tested HIV-positive.

To attempt to resolve the conflict, "The Story of the Fiancés" segment, like "Adams the Driver," insists on its own status as melodrama; it explicitly turns to a central trope of the melodrama: the overwhelming force of true love as an affirmation of the genre itself. Nathalie's confrontation with her mother about marrying Alex is figured as that between the individual and the family, the modern and the traditional. Nathalie argues, "Mom, it's not you or Dad who is marrying. It's about me, about my life [Il s'agit de moi, de ma vie]." Her mother responds, "But it's about your father, about me. It's about the family. You are not alone in the world. We are all concerned [Il s'agit de ton père, de moi. Il s'agit de la famille. Tu n'es pas seule au monde. Nous sommes tous concernés]." They continue to argue until Nathalie's mother extends her hand and pulls Nathalie toward her and says, "Come my daughter [ma fille], come into your mom's arms." As music swells, Nathalie's mother tenderly brushes back Nathalie's hair. At this moment of high-pitched melodrama, Nathalie's mother criticizes as patronizing the very terms of emotion that the video evokes and that its underscores are necessary to show toward people with HIV: "Tell me, this passion you have [for Alex]. Isn't it guided by pity, compassion?" Nathalie nestles onto the maternal bosom and replies that Alex requires precisely this

THE MELODRAMA AND THE SOCIAL MARKETING OF HIV PREVENTION • 163

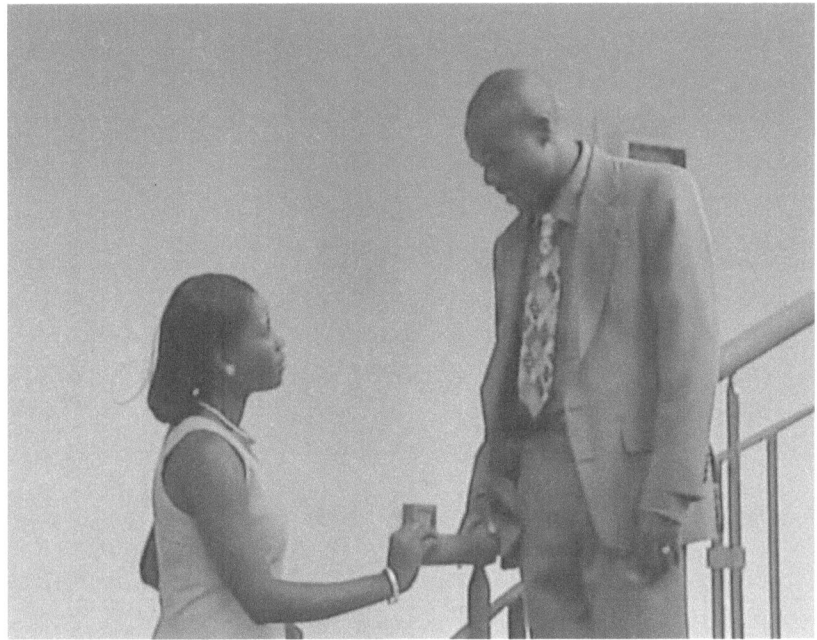

FIGURE 4.5. Nathalie and Alex argue about testing for HIV as they descend the staircase outside their workplace.

compassion: "I love Alex. I cannot abandon him. He needs affection, tenderness. Mom, it's not his fault that he is HIV-positive. I must support him, help him, be at his side. You know, living with the virus is not easy, and living with someone with the virus is even harder. For that I need you, Mom. I need your help [concours], your aid, your advice too. You cannot refuse me that" (figure 4.6). Finally, Nathalie's mother stands up and walks out of the frame and then to the other side of the room. She responds that the best support for Alex would be to provide material and financial aid—money to go to Europe to obtain treatment: "The boy, leave him, forget him."

The segment never explicitly states that antiretroviral treatment for people living with HIV/AIDS was widely available in the United States and Western Europe at the time of the video's production, but not for the vast majority in Côte d'Ivoire.[56] In typical melodramatic mode, "The Story of the Fiancés" con-

---

56. According to a 2005 World Health Organization report on HIV/AIDS treatment in Côte d'Ivoire, in 1998 UNAIDS, along with the CDC, began an initiative that provided subsidized two-drug treatment for some, but it was not well publicized and served only a fraction of those requiring it. In 2001, the Ivorian government announced that it would subsidize free antiretroviral treatment for children younger than fifteen; adults whose income did not exceed

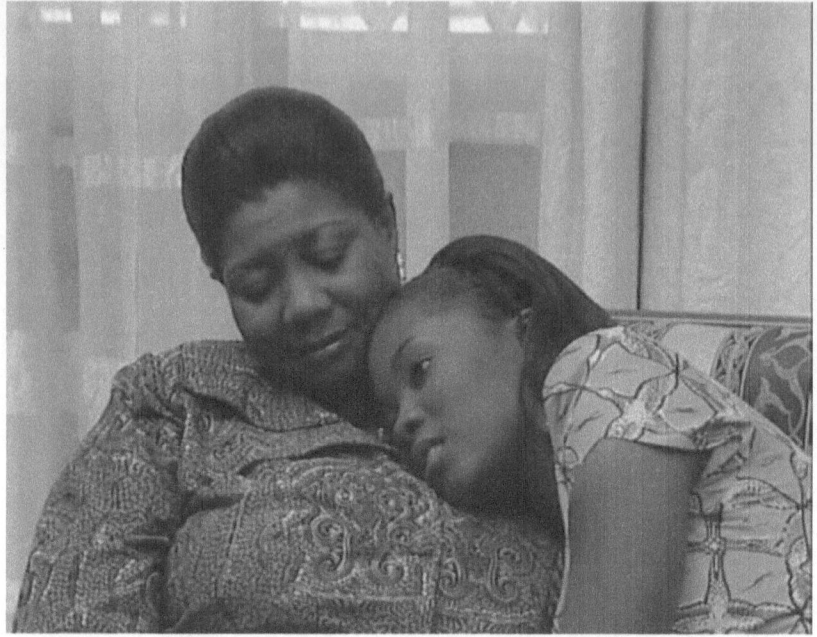

FIGURE 4.6. Nathalie and her mother.

verts the economics and politics about HIV treatment access into individual and family drama, a move reiterated by the cinematic vocabulary of the film. Nathalie's mother's assessment of Nathalie's emotion—the pity and compassion that she feels toward Alex and that the segment seeks to provoke in viewers—levels a critique of melodrama in a scene saturated with the cinematic techniques and conventions of the melodramatic mode: the domestic mise-en-scène, the dramatic gestures, silent close-ups of expressive female faces, surging music, and shot/reverse shot of scenes of extended dialogue. Nathalie's response to her mother suggests that the attempt to give Alex money to obtain treatment is unfeeling, at odds with the dramatic emotion of the scene itself. Reference to the economic or material is crassly insensitive since the issue is not the injustice of the inequities that make treatment accessible for those in the Global North and for the wealthy but not for most Ivorians, but that emotion, love, and individual, female sacrifice—the melodramatic mode itself— must prevail, as it literally does as the scene draws to a close.[57]

$830 monthly would pay a fixed annual rate of $17.00. However, in September 2004, only 4,536 were reported to be receiving antiretroviral treatment of an estimated 78,000 (in 2003) people needing it. WHO, *Côte d'Ivoire: Estimated Number of People*, 1–2.

57. In "Beyond Bare Life" (206), Jean Comaroff underscores how the focus on HIV treatment access has actually displaced or occluded other equally important struggles: "Why is it

Nathalie dismisses concern about lack of treatment access as a failure of empathy: "Mom, you have not yet understood anything. It's not about money. It's about love. I love Alex. I stand by him." In a close-up, Nathalie covers her face, then her throat, then walks back into a two-shot with her mother as she places her hand on her shoulder and demands, "Tell me, Mom, if Dad were infected with the HIV virus, would you leave him?" Her mother remains silent in a close-up shot/reverse shot, and music again surges as Nathalie presses: "Would you abandon the man you love?" Nathalie's mother sinks to a chair, and the women stare at each other in a dramatically silent final shot/reverse shot.

The structure of the melodramatic telenovela mandates an unambiguously happy ending or, at least, in Peter Brooks's terms, the restoration of moral legibility. Drawing from Brooks, Linda Williams analyzes how classic melodrama seeks a return to home as emblem of a "'space of innocence,'" a space that she argues in U.S. racial melodramas actually stood more for nostalgia for such a space than for an actual location.[58] The social marketing of public health film or soap opera and its melodramatic mode cannot fulfill its mandate of education and behavior change and still restore or mourn the loss of this "space of innocence," since innocence implies the ignorance that it seeks to remedy. The narrative therefore depicts the forest and the lagoon, nature and the rural village, the ancestral home, not as sites of innocence but of sexual contamination and secrets. When Bintou announces to Alex, "I am seropositive," the camera frames her face in a close-up, music swelling; then it cuts to Alex in a close-up in profile, and then to a black-and-white, slow-motion flashback, camera angle askew, of long shots of Alex and Bintou on the grass enjoying a picnic, laughing and chasing each other, and then embracing. In an unsubtle visual metaphor of their unprotected sex, the camera zooms quickly in and out as Bintou sits on Alex's lap. A disorienting pan of the treetops cuts back to Alex at the lagoon with Bintou. Significantly, Alex meets Bintou in Tiagba, a coastal community of the Ebrié, people considered the original inhabitants of Abidjan, and bucolic establishing shots—a boy on a pirogue skillfully tossing a fishing net into the lagoon, Alex riding in a pirogue, women preparing fermented, dried, steamed cassava [attiéké]—visually correspond to the forest of the flashback scene in which Alex and Bintou have unprotected sex.

In the face of HIV, neither rural nor urban space provides comfort, reassurance, or safety. "The Story of the Fiancés" instead offers as a narrative resolution a literal flight from the family, the country, and the frame—a flight not toward political transformation but toward affect, confidence, and hope.

---

that, in many places, access to medicine—rather than, say, jobs, clean air, or freedom from war—has come to epitomize citizenship, equity, and justice?"

58. Brooks, *The Melodramatic Imagination*, 29; Williams, *Playing the Race Card*, 188–89.

Nathalie talks with the recurring character, Jacky, the HIV counselor, who addresses Nathalie's fears that if she marries Alex, she will, as she echoes Alex, "be condemned to sterility." Jacky explains that medical treatment can reduce the likelihood of HIV transmission from mother to child, but she also stresses that Nathalie and her baby would still risk HIV infection. Jacky suggests adoption as an alternative and encourages hope of future medical advances that would further lower the risk of transmission. The segment does not allude to controversy about the provision of different drug regimens that reduce mother-to-child transmission in the Global South versus those in the Global North, and, like Alex and Nathalie's post-testing counselor, Jacky does not refer to intense, ongoing political struggles for broader access to existing HIV treatment.[59] Like the testing counselor, she offers hope instead.

In the final shots of the segment, Nathalie in a voiceover reads a letter that she has left for her parents. The image cuts back and forth from her mother reading the letter to slow-motion shots of Nathalie driving with Alex in a car. In her voiceover, Nathalie says that she and Alex have departed Abidjan: "Alex and I must leave [s'éloigner] Abidjan to think about our lives together [réfléchir sur notre union]. Should we [faut-il] marry legally? Should we [faut-il] stay forever abroad [a l'étranger]? Should we [faut-il] adopt a child? In all cases, I know that there is hope [l'espoir est permis]. We can live with AIDS and confidence." Responses to the questions that Nathalie poses about the possibility of reproductive heteronormative family and future, as in "Adams the Driver," necessarily remain suspended even as the segment attempts to impose a generically reassuring, heterosexual romantic resolution. At the close of the segment, Nathalie and Alex drive away as the series theme song affirms emotional closure both to the segment and to the issue of HIV: "I love you [Mi fè]. I love you. My love, I love you [Mon amour, mi fè]. I say, live your life. There is hope."

"The Story of the Fiancés" never explicitly addresses ethnic difference, but Alex's and Nathalie's surnames, Kouassi and Dobe, unambiguously identify the characters as Baoulé and Bété, groupings produced as "families," then as ethnicities during the French colonial period.[60] These differences increasingly

---

59. As Mark Hunter writes about "LoveLife," a campaign designed to reduce HIV prevalence among young people in South Africa, financing from foreign donors and government funders made advocating for treatment access (as did the Treatment Action Campaign [TAC]) difficult. Hunter, *Love in the Time of AIDS*, 206. Similarly, in an interview, director Don Zigré noted that his mandate was to educate about HIV prevention, not engage in political commentary. Don Zigré interview with the author, November 11, 2013.

60. See Chauveau's "La Part baule [sic]" (150) for more on historic French colonial production of the Baoulé as ethnic-territorial identity positioned in hierarchal relation to other groups

congealed under Houphouët-Boigny, who refigured colonial hierarchies to position the Akan-Baoulé, the group with which he identified, as inherently superior and predisposed to rule other groups. At the bottom of the hierarchies were the Bété and the Dioula. The director, who was also one of the writers of the earlier *AIDS in the City* series, notes that writers were careful to include a variety of ethnic groups, both to reflect a kind of realist aesthetic— historically in Cote d'Ivoire, people from what have been defined as different ethnic groups did intermarry—and to avoid seeming to attribute blame for the epidemic on a single group.[61] But the optimistically indeterminate terms of Nathalie and Alex's union could also be read as allegorizing the hope for a political union, especially as boundaries between those demarcated as "Ivorians" and those excluded as "outsiders/foreigners" congealed, and as those categorized as from different ethnic groups increasingly rallied behind opposing political parties: the Democratic Party of Côte d'Ivoire-African Democratic Rally [Parti Democratique de la Côte d'Ivoire-Rassemblement démocratique africain (PDCI)] of the Baoulé Houphouët-Boigny (and later Henri Konan Bédié) and the Ivorian Popular Front [Front Populaire Ivoirien (FPI)] of the Bété Laurent Gbagbo.

While Nathalie asserts her confidence about her future union with Alex, the story defers the promise of the fulfillment of her hopes: the story is of fiancés, a term that implies impending marriage, but the story does not close with nuptials. Similarly, the country remained divided at the time of the series' production, and the conflict ongoing at the time of shooting repeatedly interrupted the production of the series.[62] To the extent that the "Story of the Fiancés" allegorizes the hope for future union of the country, the *AIDS in the City* 3 series represents as a national project the possibility of reproductive heteronormativity for the serodiscordant couple. That union, significantly, ascribes impending death to the Baoulé, Alex, and entirely omits those cast as foreigners, often conflated with Muslim Northerners, or Dioula.[63] But it also excludes those whom the series depicts as inassimilable to the telenovela marriage plot—those for whom the series entirely forecloses the hope extended of a heteronormative future.

---

defined by "ethnic characteristics." See also Memel-Fotê, "Un Mythe politique"; Nguyen, *The Republic of Therapy*, 121–26.

61. Zigré, interview.

62. Barnes, interview.

63. For accounts of the production of Dioula, or Muslim Northerners, as foreigners and outsiders, see Akindès, *The Roots*; Cutolo, "Modernity, Autochthony and the Ivorian Nation"; Dembélé, "La Construction économique"; Dozon, "La Côte d'Ivoire entre démocratie, nationalisme et ethnonationalisme"; Marshall-Fratani, "The War of 'Who Is Who.'"

CONCLUSION

Robert C. Allen argues that while soap opera serials represent the concealment and revelation of dirty secrets or threaten to disseminate "dirt" about other characters, the commercials for cleaning products that interrupt and finance the serials reproduce the figuring of dirt—dirty laundry, dirty secrets, and dirty houses that require women to clean using the product being promoted: "According to the commercials' logic, it is [women's] inadequacy in controlling dirt that creates a problem, and it is their responsibility to eliminate the home's sources of filth."[64] HIV prevention media in the form of soap opera or telenovela integrates the commercial product into the serial itself; it reproduces the tropes of dirt, contagion, contamination, and secrets, as well as the logic of the soap commercials, to suggest that the control of the spread of dirt as HIV is the individual responsibility of characters in the series—especially of women—as well as of the viewers being targeted. The series promotes what it deems proper individual HIV behavior change, as well as commercial products and health services (e.g., condoms and HIV testing centers), through the techniques of social marketing.

Deploying the melodramatic mode, HIV prevention media oriented toward the social marketing of behavior change elides ongoing struggles and debates about HIV treatment access. The segments further avoid any explicit reference to ongoing political and military conflict in the country at the time of filming and initial broadcast. Explicitly framed as attempts to intervene in and change individual behavior, the segments promote integration into commercial markets and nongovernmental organizations as the solutions to the spread of HIV. The 2003 *AIDS in the City* series relies on tropes and techniques of the melodrama to appeal to affect, in particular, not the mobilization of political action but the creation of hope, love, and compassion for some (the properly monogamous and heterosexual) but not for others ("fags," injection drug users, and sex workers). The series therefore not only educates about HIV but also constitutes the communities whose lives it defines as worth saving, those who constitute community itself.

---

64. Allen, *Speaking of Soap Operas*, 4.

CHAPTER 5

"Stay away from unhealthy places"

Sex Work, Condoms, and the NGO

AFTER THE country's first reported HIV cases in 1985, the media in Côte d'Ivoire consistently associated prostitution with modernity and with the immorality and corruption of urban life. The state press urged men to avoid prostitutes identified as foreigners and outsiders, and as sources of dangerous contagion, with HIV rates as high as 90%.[1] As a February 1989 article in the state daily, *Fraternité Matin*, warned readers, "Stay away from unhealthy places, the milieu of prostitution. . . . Perhaps we have espoused [épousé] modernism too soon through our openness to the outside world [l'extérieur]."[2]

The most visible film and video productions promoting HIV prevention in "the milieu of prostitution" in Côte d'Ivoire—Henri Duparc's 1993 feature film *Princess Street* [*Rue Princesse*]; and Population Services International's (PSI) videos, the 2003 "Amoin Séry" segment from the *AIDS in the City* 3 series and the videos *Amah Djah-Foulé* 1 and 2 (2001, 2005)—counter such conflations of prostitution, immigration, and disease, even as they attempt to

---

1. See chapter 1 and Léon Francis Lébry, "L'Afrique alarmée par le fléau," *Fraternité Matin*, January 16, 1989, 25. A 1987 *Ivoire Dimanche* article warned that 40–80% of prostitutes would soon be infected. Venance Doudou, "Les Ivoiriens face au SIDA: Entre la capote et la fidélité," *Ivoire Dimanche*, March 15, 1987, 9. On April 4, 1986, the first television program devoted to prostitution, *Le Temps social*, aired. A January 1989 Radio Côte d'Ivoire program featured an interview with a man living with AIDS who warned listeners, "Avoid unhealthy places. Prostitutes. Homosexuals." "J'ai 26 ans et j'ai le SIDA." *Ivoir'soir*, January 17, 1989, 1.

2. Marcellin Abougnan, "Sida et . . . Valeurs Morales," *Fraternité Matin*, February 2, 1989, 2.

educate about the importance of condom usage among sex workers and their clients. The productions depict the sale of sex as a tactic deployed by women to cope with and challenge their economic marginalization in the city. They portray HIV and the sale of sex as the by-products of economic crises that intensified gendered precarity in Abidjan, the de facto capital of the country and a major migratory hub of the country and region.[3] At the same time, the productions depict the redemption of female protagonists from sex work, especially through marriage and reincorporation into a redefined heteronormative family, as resolution and as a key strategy both to combat the spread of the virus and to resolve the economic issues compelling them to engage in such transactions.

Like other HIV prevention media, in their emphasis on marriage and family as simultaneously narrative and policy resolutions, the productions either displace larger structural inequities or represent them as remedied through informal networks, entrepreneurialism, and romantic love. The productions thereby deflect state responsibility both for HIV prevention and for the support and care of people living with HIV/AIDS. By depicting the effects of such displacements as gendered empowerment, the film and videos rationalize state reductions in spending, including on health care, as the most effective response both to prevent the spread of HIV and to redress the gendered effects of economic crisis. The productions critically represent and at times even urge the casting aside of what they mark as "tradition" and traditional practices as harmful to women—witchcraft, fetishers [marabouts], hierarchal village leadership, and polygamy—in order to establish the reconstituted monogamous family as protection, and as a central prevention strategy and source of support.

The film and videos shift in their representations of sex work, more specifically, in their representations of the elimination of sex work as enabling HIV prevention and women's empowerment. *Princess Street, Amah Djah-Foulé* 1 and 2, and "Amoin Séry" were written and directed by Africans and featured African actors, but they relied almost exclusively on external funders, including United States Aid for International Development (USAID), which provided financing for all the productions, especially through the United States–based PSI (a recipient of USAID funding).[4] Shot over a period of twelve

---

3. Although the film *Princess Street* was actually shot in the coastal city of San Pedro, the references to Princess Street, which the mayor of the popular Abidjan neighborhood of Yopougon created as an entertainment district in 1990 (and which was mostly razed in 2011), situate the film in Abidjan.

4. Most of *Princess Street*'s 6.5-million-franc budget derived from French sources—Canal+, *Écrans du sud,* and the French Ministry and Development Agency—but Duparc received a

years, the productions reflect debates about sex work that in the context of the United States are intensely polarized, with certain radical feminists viewing what they term *prostitution* as the epitome of patriarchal oppression that dehumanizes and exploits women. In contrast, activists and sex workers challenging such views consider sex workers as agents rather than victims. Their preferred term, *sex work,* rather than *prostitution,* conveys their perspective on the sale of sex as a form of labor that under certain conditions proves more profitable and pleasurable and less arduous, dangerous, or inherently degrading than available alternatives. Related discussions have focused on the extent to which Anglo-American feminists have relied on the production of the "Third World sex worker"—often conflated with the trafficked woman or child—to bolster efforts to criminalize sex work globally.[5] My use of the term *sex work* rather than *prostitution* signals my own position in these debates. However, in this chapter, I am less interested in engaging with the extensive literature on sex work than I am in tracing how visual media promoting HIV prevention reproduces its terms and how these terms represent the devolution of HIV prevention onto the individual and the local, coded as community and as gendered empowerment.

Radical feminist perspectives on sex work have prevailed in U.S. government policies directed at HIV prevention globally, in part through alliances between radical feminists, evangelicals, and conservative politicians. In 2003, U.S. President George W. Bush's President's Emergency Plan for AIDS Relief (PEPFAR) promised billions of dollars in funding for HIV treatment and prevention in fifteen initially targeted countries, including Côte d'Ivoire. Directly invoking the rhetoric of radical feminist critiques of "prostitution" as victimizing and degrading, Republican Congress member Chris Smith revised PEPFAR legislation to affirm that "prostitution and other sexual victimization are degrading to women and children and it should be the policy of the United States to eradicate such practices." PEPFAR identified "eradicating prostitution" as a priority in prevention efforts focusing on "reduction of HIV/AIDS

$58,000 grant from the United States Agency for International Development (USAID), with additional funding through Family Health International (which receives funding from USAID). Barlet, *African Cinemas,* 227. Letter from USAID, May 12, 1992. Thanks to Henriette Duparc for making this letter available to me.

5. On "prostitution" as sexual slavery, see Barry, *Female Sexual Slavery.* For an overview of some of the literature that parses distinctions between trafficking and prostitution, but argues that prostitution is fundamentally exploitative, see MacKinnon, "Trafficking, Prostitution and Inequality." For a critique of the conflation of sex work and trafficking, of "prostitution" as sexual slavery, and of Western feminists' investment in liberating the "Third World Prostitute," see Doezema, *Sex Slaves and Discourse Masters*; Doezema, "Ouch! Western Feminists' 'Wounded Attachment.'"

behavioral risk" and, further, made funding contingent on compliance with the legislation's stance on prostitution:

> No funds made available to carry out this Act, or any amendment made by this Act, may be used to promote or advocate the legalization or practice of prostitution or sex trafficking....
>
> No funds made available to carry out this Act, or any amendment made by this Act, may be used to provide assistance to any group or organization that does not have a policy explicitly opposing prostitution and sex trafficking.[6]

The requirement that all organizations receiving PEPFAR funding declare their explicit opposition to "prostitution and sex trafficking" extended to those based in the United States beginning in 2005, but this provision was successfully challenged in the Supreme Court in 2013. As of early 2018, the stipulations were still in effect for non-United States–based organizations. The "antiprostitution pledge" has generated intense controversy for deploying the pejorative term *prostitution*, rather than *sex work*; rendering sex trafficking and "prostitution" as equivalent; and hindering HIV prevention efforts among sex workers.[7] As Jennifer Chan further argues, following the passage of PEPFAR, the implementers of PEPFAR funding—USAID, the National Institutes of Health, and the Centers for Disease Control and Prevention—have become the "anti-vice police" of international development aid.[8]

In Côte d'Ivoire, exchanges of sex for money are legal, although soliciting, pandering, and the running of brothels are not. Sidestepping male or trans engagement in sex work, as well as debates about legalization or criminalization of sex work, the narratives that I analyze in this chapter reflect the increasing focus in U.S. policy on the eradication of "prostitution" as a necessary condition for the prevention of the spread of HIV and for the empowerment of women—and for receipt of U.S. grants. Rather than signaling women's subsumption into patriarchal structures, women's incorporation into the family symbolizes the culmination of their "empowerment."

As I discuss in the first part of this chapter, the 1993 film *Princess Street* portrays HIV prevention as most effectively carried out by sex workers who organize to educate themselves and insist on their clients' condom usage. The film affirms marriage, love, and art as alternatives to an economy driven by the "politics of the belly," as well as to what the film depicts as a debased

---

6. "*United States Leadership against HIV/AIDS*," 117 STAT 711.
7. Masenior and Beyrer, "The US Anti-Prostitution Pledge."
8. Chan, *Politics in the Corridor of Dying*, 30.

"tradition." However, *Princess Street* does not represent sex work as inherently degrading but depicts female sex workers' communal "empowerment" as leading to better HIV prevention. The later productions reflect U.S. funding mandates opposing sex work as form of "sexual victimization" and code the nongovernmental organization (NGO) as both support for and equivalent to the family as means of redemption. In "Amoin Séry," the naive female migrant who does not use condoms when she trades sex for money and gifts tests HIV-positive but, through the intervention of the NGO, is reincorporated into her polygamous household headed by a village chief who affirms a modern future entailing a reconfigured "traditional" male leadership. The 2001 *Amah Djah-Foulé* 1 concludes with the title character, Amah, still engaged in sex work. In the 2005 *Amah Djah-Foulé* 2, on the other hand, Amah's departure from sex work enables marriage and reproduction represented as rewards for her insistence on proper condom usage and for her embrace of individual entrepreneurialism carefully differentiated from sex work as improper, or not "real," labor.

PRINCESS STREET: CONDOM USAGE AS PREVENTION

Princess Street centers on a romance between Jean and Josie. Defying his father, a wealthy businessman and factory owner, Jean becomes a musician, a player of a stringed instrument, the kora. His lover Josie, a sex worker, joins his musical troupe and in the film's rousing conclusion marries him. Henri Duparc, the film's well-known Guinean director who trained in France but spent most of his professional life in Côte d'Ivoire, described *Princess Street* as actively embracing the pedagogical imperative underpinning Ivorian and much of African cinema. According to Duparc, *Princess Street* served as a counterpoint to what he considered generally inadequate governmental responses to AIDS, what he characterized as "a policy of burying one's head in the sand [la politique de l'autruche]."[9] Eschewing what he dismissed as the heavy-handed and ineffective techniques of existing HIV education campaigns, Duparc proposed an approach that addressed the public in familiar terms and educated through the seamless integration of HIV prevention into the film narrative: "People must be told [Il faut dire aux populations] that this illness exists and learn how to avoid it. This is why I render the subject banal [banaliser] and at the same time, pass along information about condoms to protect against the illness. Do

---

9. S. S. K. (S. Samba Koné) notes that "burying one's head in the sand [la politique de l'Autriche (*sic*)] is the worst of attitudes." S. S. K., "Sida: Le Hiv [*sic*] fait l'unité," *Fraternité Matin*, January 17, 1989, 21.

you think that the gigantic billboards that you see throughout our cities and our countrysides to warn people about the risks of AIDS have a real impact on our populations, the majority of which are not literate?"[10] Duparc implied that film or television more effectively conveyed educational messages to nonliterate populations than did written media. He associated "prostitution" with what he termed "other societal ills [maux], like corruption" and linked his film's challenge of stigmatization of AIDS with his efforts to challenge the stigmatization of sex workers: "I deliberately centered the film on that which society rejects: prostitution." Defending his use of humor in the film, he argued that it facilitated education and combated stigma: "By making people laugh, *Princess Street* contributes to raising awareness about the problem [of AIDS]. I work on the assumption [Je pars du principe] that a sense of humor always succeeds in combating intolerance."[11]

Although Duparc described his film as critical of official prevention campaigns, *Princess Street*'s approaches corresponded to modifications in approaches by the dominant global organizations responding to the epidemic. In 1986, the World Health Organization (WHO) formed the Control Programme on AIDS, renamed the Special Programme on AIDS and then the Global Programme on AIDS (GPA), and supported the creation of separate bureaucracies under the name National Programs for the Fight against AIDS [Programmes National de Lutte contre le Sida (PNLS)], which dealt with AIDS within the governments in each participating member country. Although intended to provide resources to underfunded health ministries and to raise government awareness about the epidemic,[12] WHO's GPA has been criticized for essentially reproducing colonial health models throughout sub-Saharan Africa; it imposed standardized, externally funded, autonomous, top-down structures and enforced the management of HIV/AIDS as primarily a medical issue, an approach that anthropologist Didier Fassin glosses as "hierarchy, medicalization, verticality, dependence."[13] Mandated decreases

---

10. Henri Duparc, "La Dérision contre l'intolérance," 15–16.

11. Elisabeth Lequeret, "Les Reines de la nuit," *Jeune Afrique* 1756, September 1–7, 1994, 46. Duparc, "La Dérision," 16.

12. Foreign governments and organizations, especially France and to an increasing extent the United States, provide the majority of funding for the national struggle against HIV/AIDS in the country. According to the Ivorian government, from 2006 to 2009, international funders provided 89% of funding to the struggle against HIV/AIDS; the Ivorian government, 8%. République de Côte d'Ivoire and Conseil National de Lutte contre le Sida, *Rapport National 2012*, 27.

13. Schoepf, "Culture, Sex Research and AIDS Prevention in Africa," 41; Kerouedan, "Lutter contre le sida," 204; Fassin, "Le Domaine privé," 755; Seidel and Vidal, "The Implications of 'Medical,'" 47; Viens, "Le GPA attendait." UNAIDS flatly contradicts this account of WHO's early approach to AIDS as primarily a medical issue. Knight, *UNAIDS: The First Ten Years*, 15.

in health-care spending following structural adjustment increased reliance on external funders in the fight against AIDS and reinforced the power of funders to demand "total submission" from targeted countries, including Côte d'Ivoire.[14]

According to the French Institute for Development Research, the hierarchical management of HIV prevention efforts proved ineffective in controlling the epidemic: "The progression of the pandemic that is clearly spreading in West Africa (with its epicenter in Côte d'Ivoire) highlights the limits of the first national PNLS education campaigns. The criticism regarding the excessive verticality [la trop grande verticalité] of National Programs thus has a rational basis."[15] By the early 1990s, in an attempt to address some of these critiques, WHO began to encourage broader-based support in the fight against HIV/AIDS, or what it termed *community mobilization*. In a periodization of approaches to HIV prevention, Vinh-Kim Nguyen identifies a first generation of programs centering on information, education, and communication, and then on social marketing campaigns designed to generate demand for condoms. A second generation shifted to what Nguyen describes as the "idiom of 'self help' and 'empowerment.'"[16] The 1992 slogan of WHO's World AIDS Day exemplifies the attempt to shift WHO's approach: "A Community Commitment." The French translation of the slogan, "Les Communautés s'engagent," or "Communities are committed," pronounces as ongoing the engagement that WHO hoped to instigate.

Princess Street critiques governmental distribution of free condoms to female sex workers and contrasts it with the community mobilization being fostered by global health policies. The film portrays the state's HIV prevention efforts as out of touch and absurdly unsuccessful. In one scene, a young girl uses condoms as sachets to fill with water and sell as drinks on the street (figure 5.1). As one of the sex workers, Double Coke (Delta Akissi, a star from *How's it going?* who also features in *AIDS in the City* and *Amah Djah-Foulé*), later scolds another young girl doing the same: "The condoms that the government gave us, that's what you're using to sell cold water! That is not good." In contrast, the film portrays sex workers' "community commitment" to encourage condom usage as effectively ensuring proper protection; the women both promote and enact the measures that the film insists are necessary to prevent the spread of HIV.

By 1991, the United States–based PSI began social marketing of Prudence-branded condoms, which feature prominently in the film. Eliding the extent to

---

14. Viens, "Le GPA attendait," 106.
15. Delaunay, Blibolo, and Cissé-Wone, "Des ONG et des associations," 72.
16. Nguyen, "Antiretroviral Globalism, Biopolitics, and Therapeutic Citizenship," 127.

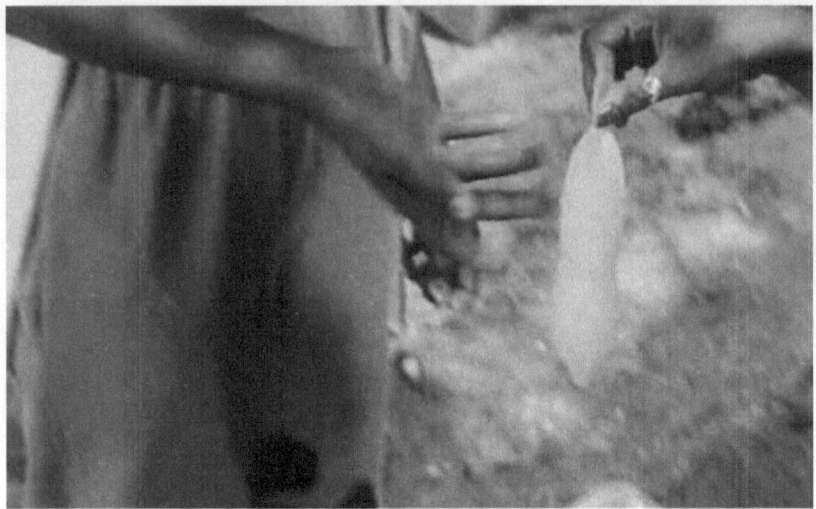

FIGURE 5.1. Condoms being used to sell drinks of water.

which the film epitomizes the kind of top-down social marketing campaigns that it critiques, *Princess Street* promotes condoms so conspicuously that critic André Videau characterized the film as "a sort of publicity spot in favor of condom usage."[17] In the film, sex workers promote condom usage with each other and their clients. As Josie hands Jean her basket filled with Prudence condoms, she reminds him that they are not for display but for "consummation and consumption [consommation]." When she encounters some other female sex workers on the street, Josie waves a Prudence condom packet and laughingly reminds them, "Have clients! Take them, but don't forget this!" In one of the last scenes of the film, Double Coke announces to the male clients lined up in front of the women's rooms that they must wear a condom. If they don't have one, she will sell them one for 50 francs.

The women provide each other essential information and, further, arrange for care of those who test HIV-positive. At the public hospital where the women test for HIV, the government's HIV prevention campaign poster hanging on the wall is almost illegible: "AIDS: Say no, protect yourself!" As useless in providing information as the poster is, the doctor simply dismisses those who have tested negative and sets apart those who have tested positive—though he does pull Josie aside to make an appointment to have sex with her later. Confronted with such inadequate state and biomedical responses,

---

17. Videau, *"Rue Princesse,"* 62.

the women offer each other the information and support that they need to survive.

Just before Josie and Jean's wedding, a group of women assemble for a meeting during which one of the women introduces a newcomer, Fatou, who will replace Josie. In 1991, the Ivorian Health Ministry launched the Prevention and Care Project for Sex Workers and Their Partners [Projet de Prévention et de Prise en charge des femmes libres et leurs Partenaires (PPP)] to provide health education, especially by peers, about HIV/AIDS in three districts in Abidjan.[18] The film does not link the sex workers to this project. It represents their meeting as organically centered on peer education, with the women gathered in a circle as the more experienced women advise Fatou about avoiding drugs and the police and about using condoms. As one of the women instructs Fatou, "You must always think of illness." Referring to Brigitte, who recently tested HIV-positive, the woman underscores the dangers of trying to earn extra money by agreeing to have sex without condoms: "She liked to work without condoms; now she has earned AIDS." DC-10—a role played by Maïmouna Koné who later starred as Jacky Sérapo (billed as Maï La Bombe) in the *AIDS in the City* series—underscores her friend's message: "My dear, you are right. That sex business, you can die for nothing, you can die for nothing [L'affaire de sexe là, tu peux mourir cadeau]." Despite the portrayal of AIDS as the result of individual choice and of the failure to choose to exercise proper precautions, during the meeting, the women agree that they will care for Brigitte.

In the film, formal economies and political processes are controlled by a hypocritical and corrupt governing elite, whether CEO, banker, doctor, politician, police, or white foreign men, all of whom enjoy and exploit, even as they stigmatize, the sex workers and their services. The coding of the female sex workers' "community commitment," then, is explicitly gendered and defined against these male elites whose overlapping networks of social, political, and economic influence are replicated in their similarly intersecting sexual networks. *Princess Street* depicts female sex workers forming their own associations and linkages to mitigate some of the inequities structuring their relationships with their clients. When Jean's father—a former client of Josie and a current client of Double Coke—physically attacks Josie, she blows a whistle, and all the women rush to her aid. After the police obey Jean's father's instructions and arrest Josie, the women all gather at the police station. Using their own stigmatization to challenge Jean's father's authority, as well as that of the commissioner and judge, the women threaten to go on television and

---

18. Vuylsteke and Jana, "Reducing HIV Risk," 204–5. Ghys et al., 252.

expose the men as clients. The police release Josie, and the women triumphantly leave the station.

Female sex workers band together to insist on condom usage, just as they join forces to protect each other from clients' physical violence and from threats by the police. The portrayal of sex workers organizing to protect and support each other celebrates their resourcefulness and generosity. Depictions of their mobilization figure the women not as passive recipients of prevention information and as sources of contamination but as ideal subjects and agents of HIV prevention. The film portrays the women's individual and communal initiatives, their grassroots efforts to demand condom usage and to care for each other, as pragmatic reactions given the inadequacy of governmental efforts—and as the most effective solution to the spread of the epidemic. The film suggests that although subjected to multiple forms of violence, the female sex workers can and do mobilize to educate each other and to redress failures around HIV prevention, as well as lack of care and support services for people who test HIV-positive.

Drawing from and reproducing global health agendas that affirm local communities and "women's empowerment," *Princess Street* displaces the burden of education for HIV and the costs of caring for the ill. The affirmation of female sex workers' ingenuity quickly blurs into affirmation of the individual and the assignment of responsibility for social welfare more broadly on individuals and "communities," and on unpaid female labor in particular. The film transforms economic and political marginalization into a romanticization of gendered agency and community and figures HIV prevention as a form of entrepreneurialism. "Times are hard," Double Coke reminds a client who complains that the condoms should be free. Passing the costs of prevention on to compliant male clients and adding a little to their profits, the women practice entrepreneurialism not only in their sex work but also in their prevention efforts.

"NOW I LOVE WITH MY HEART, NOT MY BELLY": ART, SEX, AND MARRIAGE

Duparc's previous 1992 short film, *Sweetheart*, urged HIV prevention and testing and sought to combat stigmatization of both HIV/AIDS and sex work. In *Sweetheart*, one of the female characters furiously reminds her judgmental household that she has "sold her belly [j'ai vendu mon ventre]" to put her brother through school and to feed the entire family. In an influential book on the African state, Jean-François Bayart refers to a phrase that he identifies as Cameroonian but that also circulates in Côte d'Ivoire: the "politics of the belly [politique du ventre]." For Bayart, the metaphor encapsulates the anxieties related to food shortages, as well as the corpulence and insatiability of the "big men [grands]" who ruthlessly amass prestige and riches. The politics of the belly are gendered, with the "big men" distributing patronage and benefits in highly stratified and hierarchal relations that Bayart argues operate as a form of African state politics (though his examples are generally taken from Francophone sub-Saharan contexts). In the few passages where he takes gendering into account, Bayart notes that mistresses and sexual liaisons function as "one of the cogs of the wheels of the postcolonial state," as symbols of the power of the big men. However, as he argues, far from accepting their position as dependents or "cogs," women, like young men, persistently challenge the senior "big men's" monopoly on the accumulation of wealth.[19]

Princess Street depicts sex work as instantiation of the gendered politics of the belly, with sex work by women driven by the belly—hunger and material needs—and the purchase of women's sexual services by male clients as an extension of the men's boundless appetites, a sign of their wealth and exercise of their authority and privilege. The film was released at the end of 1993, a year when the government of one of the seventeen most heavily indebted countries had acceded to additional structural adjustment programs. Poverty rates had more than tripled to 32.3% from 10% in 1985, and of 12 million unemployed, more than half were young people.[20] Against this backdrop, *Princess Street* rejects the view of sex work as fundamentally exploitative or victimizing to instead depict it as enabling young women to demand access to forms of accumulation not available to them. In other words, female sex work in *Princess Street* enables women to challenge their designated gendered roles as marginalized dependents.

Princess Street portrays Josie as a light-hearted free spirit who was compelled to engage in sex work but who resists categorization as victim. As Josie recounts to Jean, after she was orphaned, she was sent to live with an uncle who essentially acted as her pimp, sending her to have sex with his friends. As Josie laughingly explains, she decided to leave her uncle's household and "set up my own body [me mettre à mon corps]. So that's how I became the CEO of my body [C'est comme ça que je suis devenue PDG de mon corps]." Josie describes her decision to sell sex as an assertion of control over and a reclaiming of her body from patriarchal family authority and from economic

---

19. Bayart, *The State in Africa*, xviii, 241; Bayart, *L'État en Afrique*, 12, 150. Playing on the meaning of belly as womb, Lynn M. Thomas extends Bayart's insights to argue the centrality of the womb and reproductive politics in Kenyan political history. Thomas, *The Politics of the Womb*.

20. Akindès, "La Côte d'Ivoire depuis 1993," 16–17.

and sexual exploitation by her uncle and his friends. As CEO, she determines how her body circulates and sets the terms of exchange herself.

Vinh-Kim Nguyen describes how in Abidjan, after the economic crisis, "the self... became the subject of entrepreneurial remaking" through tactics that essentially "constituted the self as an object of transformation." Nguyen's discussion centers on young men in Abidjan who were economically marginalized after they graduated or could no longer afford to finish school. He describes male youths' self-refashioning as fare collectors on informal van transportation and as bodybuilders and security guards as "pragmatic, everyday economic tactics" enabling them to contribute to the maintenance of their households and, for a very few, to achieve some measure of financial stability.[21] In fashioning herself CEO of her body, Josie represents sex work as an alternative form of gendered and embodied urban self-making, a tactical transformation available to women to ensure survival and to access networks that would have otherwise been closed to them. By successfully claiming the title of CEO of her own body as corporation, Josie parodies the "big man," even as she contests her exclusion from the roles and privileges enjoyed by the male elite. Josie manages an array of clients, and to further capitalize on her earnings, she exchanges sex with a banker (the husband of Rokia, Jean's mother's best friend) at the African Bank Company [Société Africaine de Banque] for high interest rates on her deposits. Figured as a form of financial capital, sex enables Josie to profit from graft of the continent's bank, in other words, to gain entry into informal, if not illicit, systems of accumulation generally limited to the big men.[22]

While *Princess Street* portrays Josie's sex work as successfully challenging rather than reproducing her status as exploited dependent, the film's conclusion celebrates her union with Jean as an unambiguous rejection of the politics of the belly. The film carefully differentiates Josie's sex work with clients from the time she spends with Jean, who never pays her for her services. Whenever Josie is with a client, she affixes a sign on her door, "Taken [Occupé, or *engaged, busy*]," but when she goes out with Jean, she posts a sign that she has put the "factory [l'usine]" on "Work suspension." Josie goes with Jean to the purifying waters of the ocean where their sex—like their musical duet on the

---

21. Nguyen, *The Republic of Therapy*, 138, 152.
22. The African Bank Company is fictional, though the logo displayed on the building is that of the Togolese Interafrican Bank Company [Société Inter-Africaine de Banque]. Significantly, during demonstrations following the banning of a march authorized to begin in February 1992, forty-six vehicles identified as belonging to employees of the African Development Bank were destroyed. Francis Akindès describes the vehicles as "a heckled symbol of foreign presence on Ivorian soil [terre]." Akindès, "The Roots of the Political-Military Crisis," 15.

beach—is framed as an expression of pleasure and love not governed by the logic of work and economic transactions.

On the beach, Jean plays the kora as Josie sings and dances on the sand. They perform the film's theme song, which also opens the film and which they perform again together onstage after Josie becomes a part of Jean's musical troupe:

> Journeying is not easy, Mom.
> There is no honor in journeying.
>
> Son, if you go on a journey,
> do not forgot your people [relations],
> as their ties are above all others.
> There is no honor in journeying.[23]

The plaintive Malinké lyrics sung by Josie and the female dancers narrate the sorrow of departure on a journey. The song suggests palimpsests of long histories of gendered migration, including by traders and laborers in the precolonial period, to coffee and cocoa belt farms beginning in the 1920s, from the Upper Volta to the central and west Côte d'Ivoire during the period of French colonial forced labor, and continuing after its abolition in 1946.[24] The lyrics foreground the difficulties and the failed promises of these journeys, the call and response between mother and son reminders of those left behind. The song could also be read as a reference to Houphouët-Boigny's national development policies reliant on production of export crops and on labor from neighboring countries. During the first decades after independence, 80% of plantation laborers were immigrants, who during Houphouët-Boigny's presidency were promised health care, education, land, and the right to vote. By 1988, immigrants composed 28% of the population, 80% of whom were Malians and Burkinabé, and tensions between those figured as autochthonous and those figured as allogenes could no longer be contained after Houphouët-Boigny's death.[25]

Significantly, the song expresses sympathy for the suffering of the migrants and for the families they left behind. The refrain reflects the perspective of the adventurer, the traveler who laments the hardships of travel, but then it

---

23. Many thanks to Brahima Koné and to Mamadou Zongo for transcribing and translating the song.

24. Chauveau, "Question foncière," 102.

25. B. Campbell, "Defining New Development Options," 30; Akindès, "La Côte d'Ivoire depuis 1993," 4–5; Akindès, "The Roots of the Military-Political Crises," 10; Cutolo, "Modernity, Autochthony and the Ivorian Nation," 530.

shifts to the perspective of the mother addressed by the child, who addresses her in turn. When the troupe performs, the female dancers sing the entire song, concluding in the voice of the mother who gives her blessing to the son in the name of all the family. As the status of immigrants became an issue of increasingly violent contention, the song affirms a musical tradition emblematized by the kora and by the song itself, with the music and dance securing an artistic and romantic future for Jean and Josie, one that responds to the call of the song.

Despite Jean's father's attempts to intervene, both Josie and Jean abandon the role of CEO to marry. The film figures Josie's renouncement of sex work and of her role as CEO of her body as equivalent to Jean's refusal to take his place as CEO of his father's factory. In *Princess Street,* Jean and Josie's embrace of art and each other represents a turn to less corrupted forms of production that the film itself implicitly exemplifies. Significantly, when Josie first enters the theater, a demonstration of artists with signs reading "Artist equals unemployed [chômeur]" marches past. By conflating art and love, the film resolves the tension between its acknowledgment of the politics of the belly—the realities of material need and the power of the male elite—and the celebration of marriage and artistic performance as alternatives. Shortly before Josie and Jean's marriage, Double Coke reads Josie's future in tossed cowrie shells and poses the pragmatic question of how Josie and Jean will make a living after their marriage: "He takes women, and you take men, or you'll do it as a couple?" Josie responds, "We will do theater. Now I love with my heart and not my belly [ventre]."

"Doing theater" rather than "do[ing] it as a couple" substitutes art for sexual commerce, with Jean and Josie's sexual relations and artistic performances expressions of love removed from transactional economies driven by the belly. The belly as metonym for the material conditions compelling sex as work—and as a sign for the inequitable gendered networks of relations in which such work is embedded—is refigured as gift of reproductive future for Jean. As Josie declares during her wedding ceremony after Rokia accuses her of being a "prostitute" and therefore not fit for marriage, "My belly [ventre, which as in English also connotes *womb*] is not for sale—it is for Jean." The promise of the gift of reproductive future of Josie's womb contrasts starkly with the pregnancy of Rokia, Jean's mother's best friend, who in a convoluted plot strand concocts a "diabolical" plan with her husband for Jean to conceive a child with her. Jean refuses her proposition to have sex with her: "You're, as we say, a hot babe [super nana], but my mother's close friend [copine]. I think of you as an older person deserving respect [Je ne peux jamais vous regarder en face]." Rokia then consults a marabout, who, during a ritual supposed to help her get pregnant, drugs and rapes her as he flips his remote control to watch pornography on television. Unaware that she is already pregnant, Rokia drugs Jean and forces him to have sex with her. At the film's conclusion, pregnant by the marabout, Rokia is abandoned by her banker husband who leaves her for Kiki, whom Jean was supposed to marry as part of a "family arrangement" and whom Rokia had earlier instructed how to manipulate men for maximum financial and material benefits.

The film suggests that the upper-class older generation, men and women alike, seek to incorporate the younger in circuits of corrupted, quasi-incestuous heterosexual, reproductive, and economic exchanges, circuits that Jean and Josie's marriage repudiates. In the final scene, Josie counters Rokia's accusation that she is a prostitute and therefore should not be permitted to marry Jean: "Can you say who sells love and which man buys?" Insisting that her belly is not for sale, Josie distances herself and Jean from degraded forms of tradition and sexual and economic circulation impelled by the politics of the belly. Art, romantic love, marriage, and unpaid reproductive labor figured as the gift of the womb represent method of and reward for effective HIV prevention. Marriage with Jean symbolizes Josie's renouncement of sex work and the politics of the belly and a renewal of a tradition sharply distinguished from that represented by the fraudulent and corrupted marabout.

As an alternative to entrepreneurialism and proper condom usage, the film offers the generic conclusion of the romance—a wedding. The scene of Double Coke distributing condoms to waiting clients cuts to the film's conclusion, Josie and Jean's wedding, a celebration of love and art conflated with heterosexual romantic union. The editing of the sequences implies that the scenes offer analogous policy solutions and resolutions both for the female sex worker and for prevention of the spread of HIV. Significantly, the ceremony also reveals that the union is between Josie Kouamé and Jean Cissé—in other words, between a member of the Baoulé, a group with which Houphouët-Boigny identified and which he had self-interestedly cast as inherently fit to rule, and a Dioula, a category generally referring to Muslim Northerners increasingly defined as outsiders and foreigners from both within and outside Côte d'Ivoire.[26] Marriage therefore represents the promise of an artistic, an economic, and a political future facilitated by heteronormative, reproductively oriented romantic love.

Although marriage and rejection of sex work offer narrative closure, the film does not represent renunciation of sex work as a condition of HIV pre-

---

26. Akindès, "The Roots of the Political-Military Crisis," 12–13; Dembélé, "La Construction," 137.

vention and women's empowerment. In the scene where Josie affirms her love for Jean and her decision to depart from sex work, Double Coke counters, "I love money until my clients say, 'Grandmother, take a break [repose-toi]!' But I will not take a break, I will still be in the game [dedans]." A decade later, HIV prevention videos reject such humorous pragmatism. They portray the prevention of the spread of HIV and women's empowerment as necessitating the eradication of sex work depicted as sordid and demeaning.

"AMOIN SÉRY"

The main producer of "Amoin Séry," PSI, describes the video as educating viewers about the dangers of polygamy and multiple sexual partners. In 2000, PSI had produced a video with a similar message about multiple sexual partners, *The Seropositive People* [*Les Séropositifs*], in which a young female student represents the nexus of contamination—she has multiple sexual partners, including older wealthy men who help her pay for her studies. One of the men, a planter as well as a businessman, has an additional lover, his secretary, as well as a wife who has just become pregnant after having tried unsuccessfully for years. In addition, the female student has a lover, a fellow student, who has taken another lover. In the video, the female student tests HIV-positive, and the businessman's pregnant wife exhibits familiar signs—itchy sores—that suggest that she and potentially her baby will also test HIV-positive, along with the expanded network of the girl's sexual partners who comprise the seropositives in the plural of the video's title. In an interesting intertextual reference, the actor Bienvenu Neba, who plays the rich planter in *The Seropositives*, also plays the chief in the *AIDS in the City* series.

The 2003 *AIDS in the City* 3 series incorporates four independent segments, each four episodes long, including "Amoin Séry." This segment continues a storyline from the prior 1996 to 1997 versions of *AIDS in the City*, in which Amoin Séry, the fourth wife of a village chief, fled her village after accusations that she had deployed witchcraft to kill her cowife [rivale], the chief's third wife, who died after a prolonged illness. The 2003 segment begins with an intertitle "a few years later . . . ," referring to events depicted in the prior series. Opening with Amoin unable to pay rent to her landlord in Abidjan, the segment foregrounds Amoin's financial difficulties as a woman alone in the city.

"Amoin Séry" essentially renarrativizes the theme song from *Princess Street*, with Amoin's flight to Abidjan embedded within prior histories of gendered urban migration during and after French colonial rule. Amoin's flight to

Abidjan can be viewed as recapitulating the melodramatic figure that Onookome Okome terms the "good-time woman" of Nollywood videos derived from the literary figure of the "city woman" who has parallels in what Karen Jochelson identifies as a genre of Southern African literature centering on "the themes of the provocatively sexual 'loose town woman' who was promiscuous and enticed by money, and the evils of city life luring young men and women from the country to disease and personal destruction." The series also draws on and reproduces anxieties provoked by Abidjan as a self-styled cosmopolitan metropolis of "sexual liberation" and modernity."[27] These anxieties took on a different, intensified cast after the 2002 coup and subsequent division of the country—events that are only indirectly referred to in the 2003 series.

In Abidjan, Amoin struggles to earn enough money to survive through her work as a waitress in an outdoor bar [maquis]. The scenes of what are represented as her gradual corruption—she changes her dress and hair and learns that she must be "nice" to male clients—are intercut with scenes of the chief's second wife ill in the village and suffering from the same symptoms that killed the third wife. Eventually, the second wife's brother, a doctor, convinces the second wife to test for HIV. Scenes in which Amoin finishes a meal with a client, Mano Zell, and then drives with him to a hotel cut to the doctor informing the chief's second's wife that "in your blood . . . there is the AIDS virus" [figure 5.2]. The close-up of the second wife's shocked, tearful face cuts to the bar where Amoin speculates with another female waitress, Simone, about whether the client, Mano Zell, truly loves her, a conversation that suggests Amoin's innocence, naiveté, and redeemability, despite her requesting money in exchange for sex. From this scene, the camera cuts to Mano Zell who, in contrast to Amoin, lewdly describing his first sexual encounter with Amoin to a male friend:

> MANO ZELL: First, a little discreet meeting at a good restaurant. She ate well. She drank well. But watch out! It's not for free. [*Laughter*]. I said to her, "Listen, we're going to go take a rest somewhere." You know what she told me? "No, we don't know each other yet. Blah blah blah." My friend, is that my problem? I stopped a taxi—
> FRIEND: At maximum speed!
> MANO ZELL: At maximum speed—to the hotel! When we got there, I showed her what she's never seen before! [*Laughter*]

---

27. Okome, "Nollywood, Lagos, and the *Good-Time* Woman," 169; Jochelson, *The Colour of Disease*, 111; Nguyen, *The Republic of Therapy*, 159.

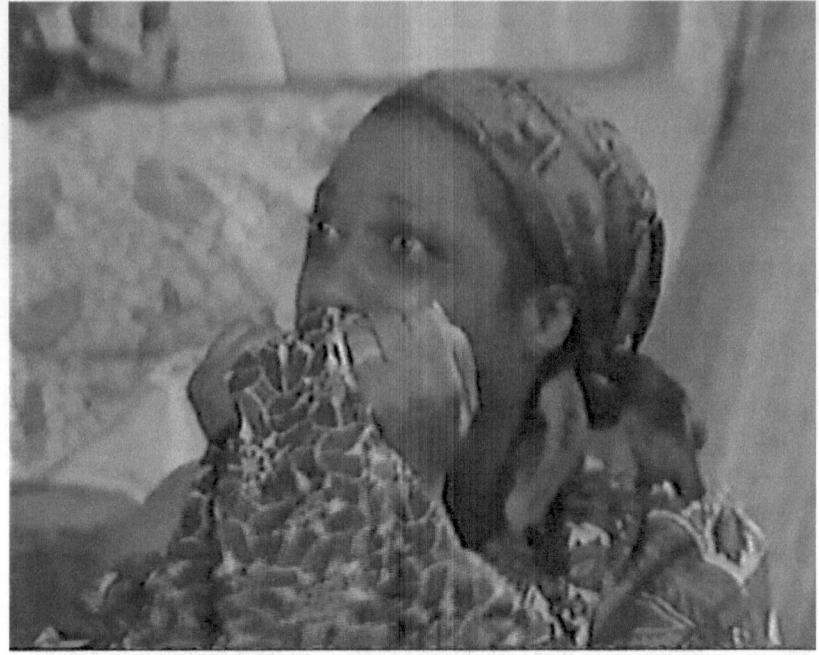

FIGURE 5.2. Second wife learns that "in your blood . . . there is the AIDS virus."

The episode depicts Amoin as a villager who repeatedly misunderstands the terms of the exchange governing her sexual relations with Mano Zell, including the need for condom usage. In the scene where the doctor informs the chief that his wife has tested HIV-positive, the doctor reminds the chief that the "the virus is transmitted primarily through unprotected sexual relations." The chief demands, "So, we can no longer make love in peace?" The doctor assures him that he can, "but you must use precautions." The scene cuts first to a quick pan of Mano Zell lying in bed, with Amoin calling off-screen, "Darling"; then it cuts to Amoin wrapped in a towel as she stands in the doorway:

> MANO ZELL: My darling, you were so good last night. You were awesome [formidable].
> AMOIN: For me, it's like that. When I'm with a man I like, I'm good. I have to make him happy. That's my secret.
> MANO ZELL: That's really good behavior [bon comportement]. Tell me, how many times did we do it [on a fait combien de coups]?
> AMOIN: I didn't count; we just did it.

MANO ZELL: I have a secret. When it's like that, the next morning, I count how many unused condoms are left. That way I know how many times [coups] we did it. [*He holds an unopened Prudence condom box*]. Amoin, no packet is open! That means—
AMOIN: We did it raw ["en live," without a condom], and it was really good. Mano Zell, you're a real man [un vrai gars].
MANO ZELL: Without condoms? Shit!
AMOIN: What's wrong? You seem mad.
MANO ZELL: No, but without condoms?

The segment codes Amoin as a naive villager for mistaking sex without condoms for proper behavior, for demonstration of masculinity, and for love. The series depicts Mano Zell as taking advantage of her naiveté; he lies to her about being the boss at his workplace, and when she asks for money to help pay for her bills after they have had sex, he angrily refuses. After Mano Zell abandons Amoin to have sex with her friend, Simone, Amoin begins to have sex with another client who pays her rent and gives her a cell phone.

The didactic, moralistic narrative apportions blame among women: The second wife represents the innocent victim. Continuing a narrative strand from the 1996–97 series, "Amoin Séry" identifies the deceased third wife and her extramarital affair with the husband of her friend (Jacky, the counselor) as having infected her cowives as well as her husband. When the HIV counselor asks Amoin if she has ever taken any risks, dramatic flashbacks underscore that her unprotected sex with the bar clients has either spread HIV to her male partners in Abidjan (who might then infect other partners, including Simone) if she has already been infected by the chief, or it will have caused her infection. As a solution to both the spread of HIV and the issue of care for people living with HIV, "Amoin Séry" advises the reconfiguration of the family and village.

WITCHCRAFT, MALE LEADERSHIP, AND THE VILLAGE: HIV/AIDS AND TRANSFORMATION OF "TRADITION"

The "Amoin Séry" segment parallels what it depicts as Amoin's naiveté with that of the chief, who has exiled Amoin from the village for witchcraft and who turns to traditional healers to cure his second wife. As anthropologists Jean and John L. Comaroff have argued, witchcraft represents not an expression of "traditional" practice in opposition to the "modern," but integral aspects of the contemporary world and attempts to grapple with and interpret the tensions and contradictions engendered by social and political upheavals.[28] Reiterating lessons from the 1996–1997 *AIDS in the City* episodes, "Amoin Séry" depicts the coding of HIV within the framework of "witchcraft [sorcellerie]" as an attempt to understand the inexplicable and intense suffering of the chief's wives. However, "Amoin Séry" represents such figuring of popular fears about HIV as dangerous and threatening manifestation of ignorance and of "traditional" practices to be addressed and corrected through education in modern science.

If the segment highlights the dangers of female financial and sexual independence and circulation in public spaces in the city, and if it associates the urban with moral and sexual corruption, it does not portray village life as an idyllic space of innocence reestablished or mourned. Rather, as in another *AIDS in the City* 3 segment, "The Story of the Fiancés," the rural emerges as a site of potential contamination and disease propagated by what the segments depicts as sexual promiscuity as well as polygamy. Moreover, the segment portrays rural locales as in the thrall of backward "fetishers," practitioners of indigenous medicine and "guardians of tradition" who, rather than recognize the symptoms of a new disease, unjustly accuse and banish women for witchcraft. What the segment represents as modern medicine prevails, as characters learn that the dangerous consequences of uncontained female sexuality do not manifest as witch's spell or curse [un sort] but rather as diseases and infections that must be treated by modern, not traditional, medicine.

Whereas the chief initially insists that as "father of the family and chief of the village," he cannot practice the so-called ABCs—abstinence, being faithful to one partner, and condom usage—the doctor eventually convinces him to go to the city with his first wife to test. Scenes of him undergoing counseling and receiving his positive HIV test results, and of his first wife receiving her negative results, are intercut with scenes of the second wife in the village refusing indigenous medicine and the fetishes of the traditional healers and insisting instead that the doctor's antibiotics have helped her while the healers have not. The video associates practices explicitly marked as "traditional" with the spread of HIV, but proper education leads to the supplanting of the traditional by the modern, with biomedicine triumphing over indigenous treatments, just as the chief realizes the dangers of practices such as polygamy: "We men think we are the happiest but we are running after useless risks. We expose our wives [nos femmes] to all sorts of dangers. We expose our lives and those of our wives [nos femmes] without even knowing."

---

28. Comaroff and Comaroff, "Introduction," xxviii–xxix.

In a series of coincidences characteristic of the melodramatic soap opera or telenovela, Jacky, who is from the same village as Amoin and the chief (and whose husband, Sérapo, who died of AIDS-related illnesses, had an affair with the chief's third wife), meets them separately and then arranges a reunion in which the chief asks for forgiveness and requests that Amoin return to the village. Amoin initially refuses but then tests HIV-positive herself. Like all the *AIDS in the City* segments, "Amoin Séry" elides the political and economic bases for the lack of treatment for HIV. In counseling Amoin, Jacky does not mention any treatment, except for opportunistic infections, and refers Amoin to NGOs for "psychosocial" issues. Jacky strongly encourages Amoin to return to the chief: "There are so many traps in the city." Jacky urges her to build a "support system [entourage]," especially as she gets sicker: "You must return to the village. It is your home." Amoin continues to resist, but after she falls ill and informs her lover that she has tested HIV-positive, he literally flees her house. Finally, she realizes she has no choice but to return to the village.

Amoin's return to the village offers the redemptive framework of the reconstituted patriarchal family into which Amoin is reintegrated, suitably chastened. As she tells Jacky on the way to the village, "In the end, I don't regret leaving the city at all." The chief, the benevolent patriarch, demonstrates his enlightenment by welcoming Amoin back and declaring that they will all take care of each other. Amoin then drops out of the narrative, which closes with the chief calling a meeting with the male village leaders and announcing that he himself is seropositive. After the chief's disclosure, the "guardian of tradition [le gardien de la tradition]" who had been berating the second wife for refusing his services finally acknowledges that AIDS has wrought irrevocable changes in the village: "Our ancestors are going to return to their tombs. What kind of sickness is this that does not respect tradition, that does not respect nobility! A village chief, sick with AIDS! Ay! Where is the world going?" The chief emphasizes the importance of adjusting to these changes: "AIDS didn't exist when our ancestors established our traditions. Today, we must live with new practices. We must protect ourselves. We must protect our families. We must protect our village. That is why, as chief, I will fight [me battrai], so no one in this village will be affected [touché] by AIDS through ignorance. We must speak of it. We must discuss it. We must fight [lutter]. We must evolve [évoluer]. This is how it will be henceforth [désormais]."

The narrative enlists "traditional" male leadership in an alliance against HIV as the chief proposes adapting tradition to the demands of the "modern" malady transmitted by ignorance. He serves as moral and political exemplar of what the segment celebrates as an enlightened modern patriarchy allied with biomedicine. The anaphora, the repeated imperative "We must . . ." compels viewers to share his vision of the future, one that requires "new practices" to preserve the future of the village and, by extension, the nation. In his appeal to fight and to evolve, the chief establishes contiguities between the struggle/fight against HIV/AIDS and the struggle against and adaptation to colonial rule when the French designated French-educated Africans as "the evolved [les évolués]." The chief's insistence on the need to adapt village "traditions" to a new form of disease codes HIV/AIDS as a depredation of the modern world. At the same time, the chief's declarations invoke the position of the évolués, those who in the past had attained certain privileged class status through guaranteed government administrative jobs following formal education in French. Such futures had been denied after the economic crisis and attending cutbacks in education and the state bureaucracy (see chapter 1), and had also been rendered even further out of reach after economic and political crises culminated in the country's first civil war beginning in 2002. The chief promises evolution as modern future for all who ally with him in the struggle against AIDS.

"Amoin Séry" depicts tradition as threatened by the modern, and it associates sex work with the corruption of the big city and with the spread of HIV as a "modern" malady. But it does not advocate a return to "tradition." On the contrary, the segment narrative implicates what it casts as "traditional" practices—polygamy, herbal medication, and reliance on fetishes—in the spread of HIV, the scapegoating of vulnerable women, and the inhibiting of proper treatment of opportunistic infections. In declaring his HIV-positive status and his willingness to join in the struggle against HIV/AIDS, the chief recognizes the need for traditional leadership to adapt to new challenges through "new practices." "Amoin Séry" endorses a colonial-era narrative of progress that recasts the village, not the city, as the preferred site of the redefinition of the modern but that requires the elimination of certain "traditions" to ensure continuity of patriarchal authority in the family and in the political and religious order. In particular, the segment reiterates familiar representations of polygamy after independence from the French, when, as Jeanne Toungara describes, President Houphouët-Boigny announced that "monogamy would be the only marital regime acceptable before the state," an announcement enforced by passage of a law formally privileging the nuclear family.[29] HIV prevention messages promoting monogamy reiterated these prior constructions, as well as those of the 1994 ministry devoted to women and the family, which viewed polygamy as hindering state-sanctioned monogamy and modern develop-

---

29. Loi 64–375 du 7 Octobre 1964; Toungara, "Changing the Meaning of Marriage," 57. In 2013, some provisions of this law were modified. See Afterword.

ment.³⁰ They further participated in ongoing debates about the role of the so-called traditional village in establishing Ivorian identity.

After the death of Houphouët-Boigny, in 1993, intellectuals supporting Henri Konan Bedié as Houphouët-Boigny's successor promoted conceptions of Ivoirité defining citizenship and national belonging by birth to "Ivorian parents belonging to one of the autochthonous ethnic groups of Côte d'Ivoire." Such a definition assumed affiliation with a home village under the authority of a chief who determined inclusion and political legitimacy.³¹ Both Houphouët-Boigny and Bedié identified as Baoulé, one of the supposedly autochthonous ethnic groups identified in colonial racial taxonomies. In producing the Baoulé as noble and destined to rule (in contrast to the Bété and Dioula), Houphouët-Boigny reproduced and revised colonial systems of classifications that linked definitions of ethnic difference to territory and that categorized groups in hierarchies—initially, according to their purported aptitude to being colonized. The production of discrete ethnic groups differentiated people who had for centuries been migrating, resettling, and intermixing, including through marriage. It also replaced the Muslim Mandé, who had been assigned the top position in colonial racial hierarchies, with the Baoulé to reinforce first Houphouët-Boigny's and then Bedié's political legitimacy.³²

In proposing a modified village leadership, the series carefully refrains from identifying a single ethnic group of the nation's future leaders. "Amoin Séry" confounds location of the title character's village. Amah is a Baoulé name given to girls born on Sunday, but the name Séry is Bété. During certain important scenes marked as "traditional"—for example, during the funeral procession for the second wife—villagers sing in Bété. Similarly, the griot announces in Bété that a village meeting has been canceled, and at the gathering where Amoin Séry is accused of practicing witchcraft against her cowife, the villagers mix French with Bété. But in a scene when the chief consults with his advisers, they insult and curse in Baoulé. The actors themselves are members of different groups—the chief is played by the well-known Bienvenu Neba, who is Alladian from Jacqueville.³³ In attempts to distance "Amoin Séry" from debates on the presidential elections—especially those on Ivoirité and the production of the Baoulé-Akan as naturally aristocratic rulers—the series blurs distinctions between Baoulé and Bété to suggest that the modern future that the series imagines does not hinge on a specific ethnic group for

---

30. MacLean, *Informal Institutions and Citizenship*, 134–35.

31. Babo, "Ivoirité and Citizenship in Ivory Coast," 204; Chauveau, "Question foncière," 102–3, 108; Dembélé, "Côte d'Ivoire," 43, 45–46.

32. Memel-Fotê, "Un Mythe politique," 23, 31; Chaveau and Dozon, "Au Coeur," 239, 241; Cutolo, "Modernity, Autochthony and the Ivorian Nation," 535.

33. Many thanks to Amani Konan for his helpful insights into these sections of the video.

leadership. However, significantly, the merging of the ethnic groups Baoulé and Bété does not encompass the Dioula, a category that incarnates the "allogene," collapsing all Northern Ivorian Muslims of different groups, as well as immigrants from Mali, Guinea, and Burkina Faso, as outsiders and foreigners.

Envisioning a revised traditional patriarchal leadership, the series reproduces and reinforces certain conceptions of ethnic difference and of gendered hierarchies as vital both to the struggle against HIV/AIDS and to the future of the nation. Jacky, the HIV counselor, plays a critical role in facilitating the reintegration of Amoin back into the village and family, both of which are figured as protecting women from sexual and financial exploitation, danger, and disease in the big city. There is no place for the female sex worker in the "evolved" nation any more than there is for the Dioula. Within the reconstituted family, the first wife will serve perhaps the most important role—one that is essential, assumed, and unstated. The family serves as both allegory and replacement for the state; in the absence of treatment or state services, the "support system" that Jacky urges Amoin and her husband to build will necessarily rely upon the first wife's assumption of much of the burden of maintenance of the household and of palliative care. In other words, the evolution of the village and of tradition that will enable restoration of the family and the reincorporation of the sex worker into the family as proper wife will depend on the NGO and on unpaid female labor for the care and support of people living with HIV/AIDS.

AMAH DJAH-FOULÉ: "PROTECT YOURSELF!"

The two versions of *Amah Djah-Foulé* perhaps most strikingly demonstrate the shift to depictions of abandonment of sex work as a necessary condition of empowerment and of HIV prevention. In 1992, the Côte d'Ivoire Retrovirus Project [Projet Rétrovirus Côte d'Ivoire (RETRO-CI)], in collaboration with the Ivorian Ministry of Health and the Belgian Institute of Tropical Medicine, created the Confidence Clinic [Clinique de Confiance] to provide sex workers and their "stable partners" education, care for sexually transmitted infections, and HIV counseling and testing. It also provided female sex workers free condoms.[34] The U.S. Centers for Disease Control (CDC) financed RETRO-CI, which commissioned *Amah Djah-Foulé*; and

---

34. From 2004 to 2010, the clinic was supported by Family Health International and the Belgian Institute of Tropical Medicine. It also received financial support from PEPFAR and the Belgian Directorate-General for Development Cooperation. Vuylsteke et al., "HIV and STI Prevalence," 1; Ghys et al., "Increase in Condom Use," 252.

PSI, a major recipient of financing from USAID, provided most of the funding for *Amah Djah-Foulé*, as it did for the "Amoin Séry" episode of *AIDS in the City* 3. Through *Amah Djah-Foulé*, producers intended to encourage condom and lubrication use, as well as HIV testing, among sex workers and to promote the Confidence Clinic. They also sought to challenge the stigmatization of female sex workers and of people living with HIV.[35] PSI distributed the first version of *Amah Djah-Foulé* to HIV organizations; to nongovernmental organizations (both within the country and throughout West Africa); to UNAIDS, UNICEF, CARE, among other multilateral organizations; and to its own regional offices. In addition, in 2001, *Amah Djah-Foulé* 1 was shown on Ivorian national television on World AIDS Day, December 1 at 11:00 p.m. and at 2:00 p.m. on December 2.[36] The second video, *Amah Djah-Foulé* 2, featuring the same cast and continuing the narrative from the previous video, was produced in 2005 and was broadcast and distributed in English and French throughout the region.

Amah Djah-Foulé 1 quickly establishes Amah as a good mother who has properly assimilated HIV prevention messages. The video intercuts scenes of Amah insisting on condom usage with her clients and with her "stable partner," Boni, as she simultaneously struggles to care for her young child. The video opens with Amah on the street. An SUV pulls up, and a man, Kokou, reaches out the window to grope her breasts. "How much?" he asks. "Whatever you want, as long as you use a condom," Amah responds. The series theme song offers commentary as the credits roll: "To do it right [bien], you have to protect yourself. / Or abstinence to protect yourself." The credits cut to Amah providing treats for her young son, who has just returned from school, as she worries about paying his school fees. In the next scene, she attempts to negotiate condom usage with Boni: "I love you, and you know it well. I already have a child and almost nothing from your job. You must understand me. . . . With condoms, we can also avoid STDs."

Like *Princess Street* and the *AIDS in the City* series, *Amah Djah-Foulé* 1 incorporates into its narrative the products and services that it promotes and that it depicts as preventing the spread of HIV. Amah prominently displays the Prudence brand on the condoms that she insists that her clients use. Another older sex worker, Fortuna (Delta Akissi), instructs Amah to use proper lubricants, not shea butter, and Fortuna brings her to the Confidence Clinic, where

---

35. With a 28-million-CFA budget, *Amah Djah-Foulé* 1 was produced by PSI through AIMAS [Ivorian Social Marketing Agency (Agence Ivoirienne de Marketing Social)], at the time ECODEV [Etude, Conseil, Formation et Développement], RETRO-CI, a project founded in 1987 by the CDC. Widmark, "The Success of Amah," 25, 30.

36. Widmark, "The Success," 22–23, 31.

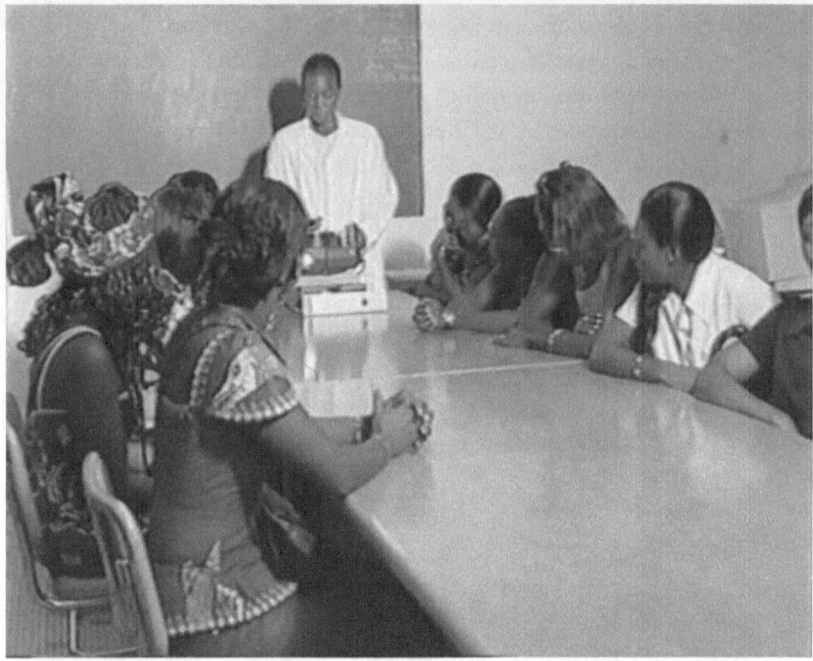

FIGURE 5.3. Doctor reminds women, "Trust is good, but Prudence is best."

she obtains additional free condoms and lubricants and gets tested for HIV. At the clinic, viewers of the video are educated alongside Amah, Fortuna, and other female sex workers, as they attend a slide presentation, also shown on-screen, which incorporates graphic close-up photographs of penises and vaginas oozing with sores from sexually transmitted diseases. As the doctor delivering the presentation reminds the women and viewers, "To avoid these, as well as AIDS, there is only one solution: condoms. You have to use condoms with everybody. I said: condoms with everyone, with boyfriends, and even with regular clients. Trust is good, but prudence [punning on the Prudence-brand condom] is the best" (figure 5.3).

Ultimately Amah is rewarded for heeding the Confidence Clinic's advice about condom usage and lubrication. Although Boni initially disapproves, Amah tests for HIV at the clinic, and at the close of the video, she learns that her results are negative. The couple celebrate together, and Boni promises to return to get tested himself. In contrast, Amah's client, Kokou, has sex with a young girl whom he pays twenty times more than Amah's usual rates not to use a condom—and contracts syphilis. Fortuna, whose partner and pimp, Prince, refuses to use condoms, tests HIV-positive. Initially, Fortuna considers her diagnosis a death sentence. She weeps: "I have a daughter. I will never see her get her diploma. I will never see her children. I won't see any of that. I killed myself working to help her." However, reflecting donor emphasis on "coming out" with HIV as "empowerment," the video represents the Confidence Clinic as enabling her to reunite with her daughter and to devote her life to saving others.[37]

The doctor at the Confidence Clinic promises Fortuna that the clinic will provide medication for AIDS-related infections and tries to persuade her to educate other women: "Some still ignore the danger of not protecting themselves and sleep with regular clients and boyfriends without condoms. So Fortuna, why not tell them about your experience? Why not help them?" Fortuna refuses, saying that she will be stigmatized if she acknowledges her HIV-positive status publicly, but without explanation the scene cuts to her addressing a crowd of women:

> I am Fortuna. There are some among you who know me. Others don't. It doesn't matter who you know. What is important is what I am going to tell you. Sometime in the past, I sometimes made love without condoms. Today, I am HIV positive. I don't know whether I got it from a client or my man. All I can tell you is always use condoms. Always, always. If you wish to have a safe life, always use condoms.

In *Amah Djah-Foulé*, the confession of the person living with HIV educates viewers who are positioned alongside the other sex workers listening and learning from Fortuna's testimony, which represents HIV as the result of individual failures to use condoms. Prevention then requires a simple step: condom usage. Serving as facilitator in the support group also offers an alternative to sex work, one that enables community education and reconciliation with the family. The first *Amah Djah-Foulé* closes with a woman on the street rejecting an offer to have unprotected sex for ten times the usual rates: "I may be a whore [pute], but I am not stupid. Me, I want to live." The later version shuttles between the futures that it suggests are available to the female sex worker: If she insists on condom usage and tests HIV-negative, she is rewarded with a proper heteronormative family defined as marriage with an employed man with whom she has a child. The video proposes an alternative if she does not consistently use condoms and therefore tests HIV-positive: peer counselor in the NGO.

---

37. Nguyen, "Counselling against HIV in Africa," S442.

SEX WORK AND "REAL" WORK AND "REAL" FAMILY

Produced in 2000, the first *Amah Djah-Foulé* concludes on an optimistically open-ended note, with Amah rewarded for her consistent condom usage and Boni promising both to be faithful to her and to test soon. The video does not even suggest departure from sex work as necessary for HIV prevention, much less as a manifestation of women's empowerment. Five years later, *Amah Djah-Foulé* 2 explicitly frames sex work as nonlabor and as an obstacle to marriage and to "real household" and "real family." PEPFAR began funding the Confidence Clinic in 2004, and the new version of the video conspicuously conforms to the U.S. government's funding mandates for eradicating prostitution. In the second *Amah Djah-Foulé*, after Amah's son Yao starts asking questions about "prostitution," Amah tries to apply for office jobs, but without certificates of formal education, she is told that she is not qualified, and her applications are rejected. When she goes to her former client Kokou for assistance, he crudely caricatures activists and scholars who maintain that sex work constitutes labor and a practical option, especially for women like Amah whose employment opportunities are limited. When Amah says that she has not come to sell sex but "to look for work," Kokou points out that she "already has work." His identification of "sex work" as work is represented as the self-interested and pernicious reasoning of the male elite, an unfaithful husband who has not learned his lesson from the previous video and who refuses to test for HIV. Amah responds by vehemently differentiating sex work from work: "That is not work. I am still young. I can find work. I can have a real household with my man [gars], have a real life, have children."

Kokou then urges Amah to accept an "arrangement" as his "second wife," in which case, as he claims, she will not have to work at all. He will find her a house and pay her bills in exchange for sex. This "arrangement" offers a stark contrast to the "real household," "real life," and reproductive future that the video promises can be attained through proper work. The video portrays Amah as rejecting sexual and economic exchanges that are figured as nonlabor and that entail financial dependence on men. Demonstrating exemplary individual initiative and gendered empowerment, Amah leaves the feckless Boni, who has been lazing about, playing video games, and who has also delayed testing for HIV. With the help of her friend Fortuna, Amah starts to sell food at an informal roadside stand (figure 5.4). The video depicts individual initiative and women's solidarity—local, community connections—as enabling entrepreneurialism unequivocally distinguished from sex work. This entrepreneurialism is marked as a sign of women's empowerment which facilitates establishment of the marriage and the real household that Amah desires.

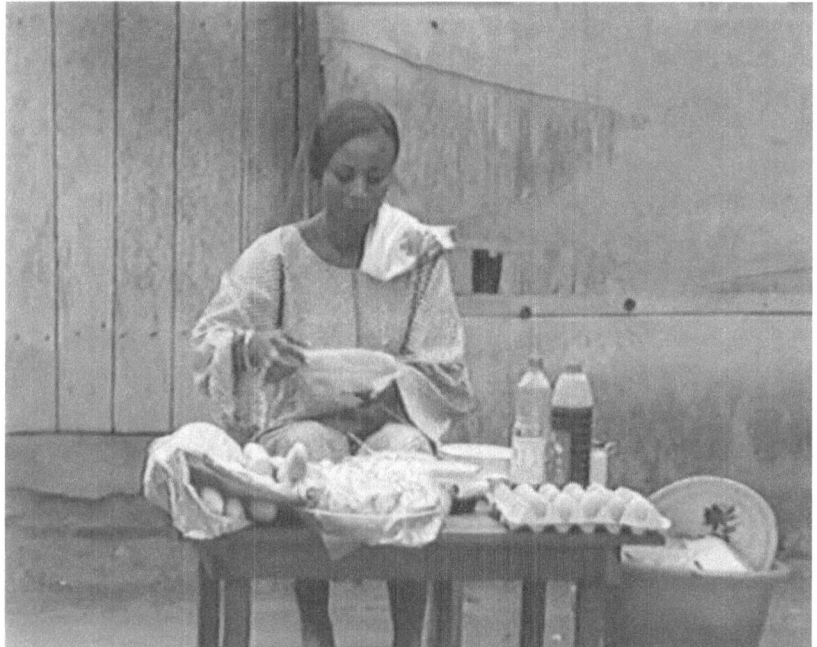

FIGURE 5.4. Amah as entrepreneur engaged in "real work."

Entrepreneurialism and departure from sex work make manifest the virtues of individual determination and initiative geared toward monogamous and reproductively oriented marriage.

In *Amah Djah-Foulé* 1, Amah's sex work financially supported Boni, who spent the money she gave him on other women. In *Amah Djah-Foulé* 2, Amah realizes that Boni "does nothing to help himself" and that he must learn to become a self-disciplined worker, as she has. After Amah leaves Boni, he cannot pay the rent that she has always covered. He tries to reconcile with Amah, who refuses, urging him, "You find work, no matter which. It's important. You cannot live on others. What example does that give for your son? Are you ready to change? Find work?" At the end of the video, Boni has finally taken action. He informs Amah that he has a job, and he and Amah return to the clinic where he tests and receives his HIV-negative results. The counselor reminds them, "To reduce risk, be faithful and use condoms," and in the next scene, the couple happily reunite in bed, joined by true love, not financial dependence.

While in the previous video, female sex work upended gender roles, in *Amah Djah-Foulé* 2's central tautology, women's empowerment enables and is enabled by renunciation of sex work and establishment of petty commerce that restores and stabilizes the gendered and familial order. *Amah Djah-Foulé* 2 characterizes the heteronormative reproductively oriented family—one that necessarily excludes HIV and sex work—as "real life" and "real household" framed as the reward for individual initiative, HIV testing, and real work. Finally, Boni is ready to assume the role of father, and Amah can act as proper mother. An intertitle just before the closing credits makes clear the connection between departure from sex work and establishment of the heteronormative family as desired resolution: "A year later, Amah definitively left prostitution and had a baby."

A parallel, contrasting narrative thread in *Amah Djah-Foulé* 2 focuses on Fortuna, who in the previous video had tested HIV-positive. Early in the second version, Fortuna's lover and pimp, Prince, also tests HIV-positive, and, after encouraging him to go to the Confidence Clinic for care, Fortuna promises to support him: "You accepted me with the virus. Today, I accept you." The video takes for granted that although the couple will remain together, they will not reproduce. The reconstitution of the family instead centers on resolving conflicts between Fortuna and her adolescent daughter, Sunshine, who was horrified to realize that her mother has been selling sex and later tested HIV-positive. The video attempts to counter stigmatization against both HIV and sex workers by depicting Fortuna's sale of sex, like Amah's, as a sign of her exemplary sacrificial maternity. Reiterating the familiar narrative of gendered rural-to-urban migration, Fortuna explains to Sunshine, "When I left the country to Abidjan, I couldn't find work. You are everything in my life. I sacrificed for you, for your studies, your future." Urging Sunshine to reconcile with Fortuna, Amah describes sex work as particularly difficult and debasing work: "You think that being a sex worker is easy? To sleep with anyone, no matter who [n'importe qui]? To accept being insulted by fools [imbeciles]? To give your body to dirty disgusting people?"

When Sunshine asks how Fortuna became HIV-positive, Amah responds, "I don't know. She made an error [erreur]." Analogous to Amah's entrepreneurialism, Fortuna's work in the Confidence Clinic offers a path of reconciliation and redemption from what the video represents as the degrading work of prostitution and subsequent lapse, or "error," leading to HIV infection. Amah encourages Sunshine to go see Fortuna at work, and in the video's last scene, Sunshine goes to the Confidence Clinic where she overhears a well-dressed and smiling Fortuna instructing a group of women that "HIV does not mean death" and that "it is best to avoid catching it. Always use condoms, always." The Confidence Clinic opened an NGO, "Place of Confidence [Espace Confiance]" to provide peer education to sex workers and their stable partners in November 2004 with the support of RETRO-CI, funded by the CDC and the Belgian Institute of Tropical Medicine.³⁸ In *Amah Djah-Foulé* 2, the NGO provides an alternative livelihood for Fortuna and serves as an indispensable pathway to receive medical care. Fortuna reminds the women that they should consult the Confidence Clinic: "No medicine can cure HIV, but with certain medicines, you can block it so that it cannot develop." She urges the women to go to the clinic to obtain more information from "specialists" about free treatment and care.

Eventually, Fortuna notices Sunshine listening in on the group and the two embrace as Sunshine declares, "I'm proud of you." The scene of Fortuna instructing the support group and her reconciliation with Sunshine immediately follows the scene where Amah and Boni embrace on a bed after having learned that Boni has tested HIV-negative (figures 5.5 and 5.6). The NGO provides the conditions of possibility for reconciliation of the family, as Fortuna and Prince support each other and Fortuna reunites with her daughter and becomes an agent of HIV prevention. Like the chief's public disclosure of his HIV status in the closing scene of "Amoin Séry," Fortuna's role as peer educator underscores the central role of what Vinh-Kim Nguyen, citing Nancy Rose Hunt, has described as "confessional technologies" that reflect the twin mandates of international agencies to "'break the silence'" and "'put a face on the epidemic.'"³⁹ Hunt traces the demand to "come out" in AIDS programming in Africa to gay activism and to feminist, Alcoholics Anonymous, and gay support groups in the United States and Western Europe. As Hunt argues, the consciousness-raising support group and the politicized act of challenging stigma and shame by "coming out" have, in the context of structural adjustment programs in Africa, translated into potent rhetoric that "slyly turns austerity into a virtue by suggesting empowerment," which facilitates accommodation and acquiescence to neoliberalism. Nguyen further details how in Côte d'Ivoire, international organizations' demand that people living with HIV "come out" produced new forms of subjectivity and undermined previously existing support networks, as people living with HIV came to recognize confession both in and out of support groups as an effective and necessary strategy to compete for scarce resources.⁴⁰

---

38. Bastien, "Espace Confiance," 6.
39. Nguyen, *The Republic of Therapy,* 32.
40. Hunt, "Among AIDS Derivatives in Africa." The support group for women living with HIV serves as a kind of counterpoint to the street forums like the well-known "Sorbonne" in Plateau, Abidjan. During Laurent Gbagbo's rule, the "Sorbonne" in Abidjan, as Aghi Bahi describes, constituted "spaces of street discussions essentially run [animés] by socially marginalized [des couches sociales defavorisés] young people (as speakers and listeners) who come to these places, the former to inform, enlighten, and teach, the latter to be informed, understand what is happening in the country, learn, and debate current events." The support group also

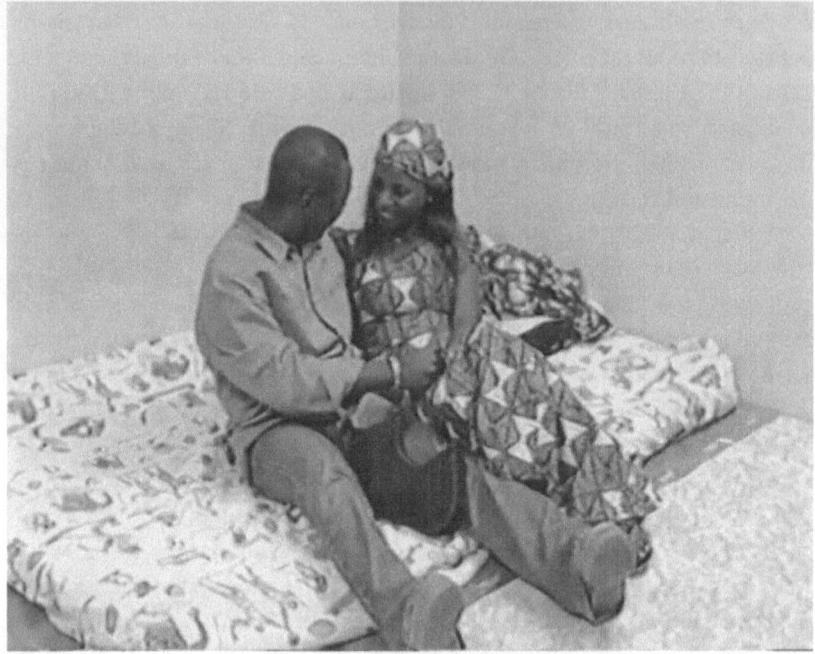

FIGURE 5.5. Amah and Boni celebrate.

Amah Djah-Foulé 1 and 2 position the viewer as transformed by the NGO support group, first as participant, educated alongside Amah and Fortuna, and then as onlooker, alongside Sunshine. The videos depict the NGO, like petty commerce, as enabling women's empowerment coded as renunciation of sex work. The support group not only provides life-saving information but also enables reconciliation and reunification of the family as the central strategy for the prevention of the spread of HIV. As the closing intertitle informs view-

---

serves as a contrast to the *grin*, a Malinké term derived from *galan* that refers to a kind of tea and, metonymically, to the talk, primarily by elites (royalty, counselors, and advisors), about the tea. Bahi, *L'Ivoirité mouvementée*, 212, 231. For historical context on the emergence of "voluntary associations," see Nguyen, *The Republic of Therapy*, 66–71. In the urban context in Côte d'Ivoire, *grins* now refers to informal meetings, mostly of Muslim men in Dioula neighborhoods who organized by age and social class in response to anti-Northerner hostility since the death of Houphouët-Boigny. The primarily male Muslim and Dioula political groups that continue to informally congregate in Abidjan, and the processes of politicization leading to informal networks of solidarity, in *AIDS in the City* translate into the gendered spaces of women's support groups. The groups are not divided along so-called ethnic lines; the shared identity is that of the woman living with HIV, an identity elaborated not to develop and assert political agendas but to affirm the importance of love as a source of individual empowerment. For more on how grins became incorporated into RDR organizing, see Banégas, "Briefing: Post-Election Crisis," 462.

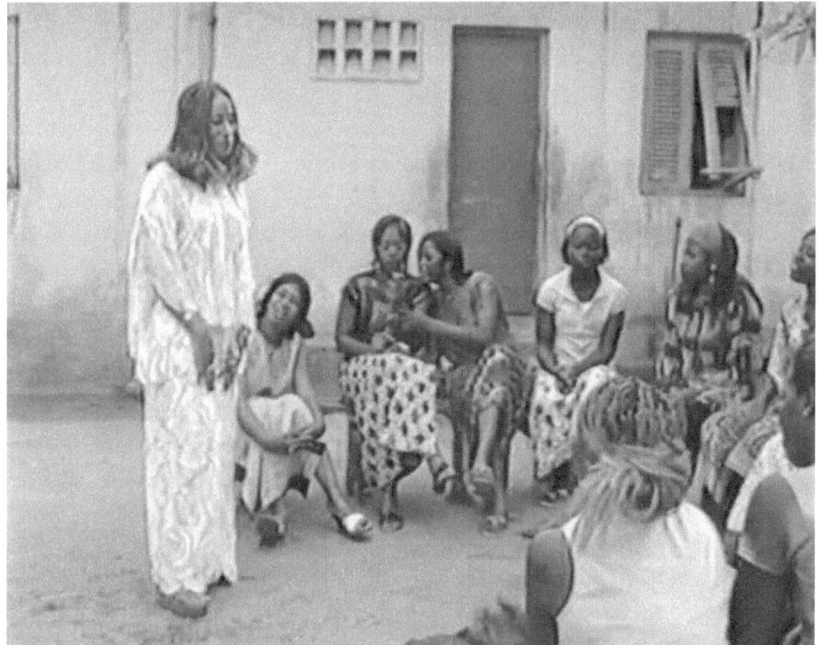

FIGURE 5.6. Fortuna instructs a support group about HIV/AIDS.

ers, "Fortuna lived from then on with her daughter Sunshine and still continues to fight against AIDS. Prince got himself medical care [se fait prendre en charge] and tries to live positively with the virus." Significantly, the NGO also participates in the production of the video as itself a form of HIV prevention.

CONCLUSION

The productions spanning over a decade offer contrasting representations of HIV prevention and sex work that negotiate both with the mandates of international financing and with the terms of ongoing political struggles. The 1993 *Princess Street* and the 2000 *Amah Djah-Foulé* 1 represent sex work as a viable option for women who provide each other with necessary information and support. But the later productions depict the NGO as empowering women to abandon sex work and establish monogamous families, the conditions of effective HIV prevention. The first Ivorian Civil War erupted in 2002, after an unsuccessful attempted coup against President Laurent Gbagbo. The 2003 "Amoin Séry" segment of *AIDS in the City* 3 links the reincorporation of the female sex worker into the patriarchal family with the promise of modern development overseen by a rehabilitated traditional political leadership that has overcome ethnic divisions. Produced after passage of PEPFAR, *Amah Djah-Foulé* 2 depicts the eradication of sex work and female entrepreneurialism as both enabled by and enabling women's empowerment defined as the establishment of "real" family and, in a familiar figuring, of a future embodied in the HIV-negative child.

Despite differences in treatment of sex work and the NGO, none of the films considers the state as a source of information, care, or support. Whatever the terms of "women's empowerment," whether through sex-worker mobilization and condom usage or departure from sex work, the film and videos depict that empowerment as achieved through individual, local, or NGO, not state initiatives. HIV prevention film and videos targeting sex workers and their clients work to shape definitions of proper sexualities, sexual behavior, and families. In their affirmation of individual empowerment, they depict the state as corrupt, ineffective, and ultimately unnecessary. They promote, instead, individual and what they depict as "community" enterprise and initiative, solutions that offer further rationales for cutbacks in state provision of services and care. All the productions after 1993 frame HIV prevention in exclusionary terms, with female sex work a source of danger and contamination for both women and their clients. Integration into the monogamous family and the NGO act as analogous forms of protection and reward for those who display proper individual initiative.

AFTERWORD

> Ecoutez les bons conseils de votre grande soeur[:]
> Les copines, n'écoutez pas les "on-dit"
> si vous ne faites rien y a rien [sic].
>
> Les amis, il faut des conditions pour faire du live.
> Si vous n'êtes pas sûrs de vous, utilisez le préservatif.
>
> Les amis, si vous ne pouvez pas vous abstenir, utilisez le préservatif
> pour éviter le SIDA, les IST et les grossesses non désirées.
>
> Les amis, prenez le temps de vous parler et
> de vous écouter. La vie se construit ensemble.
> —*SUPER GO*
>
> Listen to the good advice of your big sister[:]
> Girlfriends, don't listen to the talk [sic] if you
> don't do anything, you won't get anything.
>
> Friends, doing it raw [without a condom] requires conditions.
> If you are not sure of each other, use the condom.
>
> Friends, if you can't abstain, use the condom to
> avoid AIDS, STDs and unwanted pregnancies.
>
> Friends, take the time to speak to each other and
> to listen to each other. Life is built together.
> —*SUPER GIRL* POSTER[1]

THIS BOOK has situated prior media campaigns in the contexts of their dissemination in Côte d'Ivoire and has shown that many of the media reproduced pervasive tropes conflating political and reproductive legitimacy. The reconstitution of the family and the heterosexual romance worked as particularly powerful allegories for belonging to the modern nation and at the same time as substitutions for the state in retrenchment—with the family, the nongovernmental organization, and the corporation providing necessary services in place of the state. More-recent HIV prevention campaigns, such as *Super Girl* [*Super Go*], which urge the ABCs—abstinence, being faithful,

---

1. https://www.k4health.org/sites/default/files/Affiche%20Super%20Go.jpg.

and condom usage—continue to recapitulate the terms of both prior and contemporary political debates and reinforce their heternormative figurings of citizenship and national belonging. The campaign urges girls and their male sexual partners to instigate necessary changes in their sexual behavior and to forge companionate heterosexual relationships in the name of a future, a "Life" that is "built together." By way of conclusion—one that does not actually signal an end—I want to suggest how analyses of prior HIV prevention media might help to inform debates around more-recent campaigns, such as *Super Girl*, as well as to enable future prevention efforts.

The *Super Girl* campaign's major funders include the United States President's Emergency Plan for AIDS Relief (PEPFAR). In 2003, President George W. Bush announced that he planned to request $15 billion ($10 billion of it in "new money") over five years to combat HIV/AIDS. In his State of the Union Address, Bush characterized his proposal for PEPFAR in evangelical Christian terms: "a work of mercy beyond all current international efforts to help the people of Africa."[2] The legislation was signed into law, and beginning in 2004 PEPFAR set as a goal that 20% of total funding be allocated for prevention. In 2006, the legislation specified that one-third of all prevention funding be spent on abstinence-until-marriage programs. Between 2004 and 2013, PEPFAR directed $1.4 billion of funding in sub-Saharan Africa on programming that urged abstinence until marriage. Even after 2008, when stipulations requiring focus on the AB rather than the C of the ABCs were loosened, PEPFAR continued to channel millions to prevention campaigns promoting abstinence.

As critics have pointed out, PEPFAR's mandated emphasis on abstinence has not resulted in reductions in HIV transmission. Other scholars and activists have condemned PEPFAR's emphasis on abstinence and fidelity as a neoimperial foisting by the United States of evangelical Christian morality on targeted countries.[3] As a further case in point, on May 15, 2017, President Donald Trump reinstated the "Mexico City Policy," which had been suspended under former President Barack Obama. Renamed "Protecting Life in Global Health Assistance," the policy has been expanded to apply to all nongovernmental organizations (NGOs) receiving U.S. funding for global health. Simply

---

2. "2003 State of the Union Address," *Washington Post*, January 28, 2003. http://www.washingtonpost.com/wp-dyn/content/article/2005/10/19/AR2005101901529.html.

3. For an outline of such critiques, see Cynn, "The ABCs of HIV Prevention." A recent study measured changes in what it described as "five outcomes indicative of high-risk sexual behavior: number of sexual partners in the past twelve months for men and for women, age at first sexual intercourse for men and for women, and teenage pregnancies." It found "no evidence to suggest that PEPFAR funding was associated with population-level reductions in any of the five outcomes." Lo, Lowe, and Bendavid, "Abstinence Funding," 856.

put, for the first time, all recipients of U.S. government global health funding, including PEPFAR, are restricted from providing information about abortion, even if they use non–United States funding.

Another important strand of critique of prevention efforts centers on the focus on biomedical interventions, especially after passage of PEPFAR and its funding of antiretroviral treatment. Vinh-Kim Nguyen has persistently and convincingly explored how he came to realize that in Côte d'Ivoire, "calls for more biomedical interventions would neither fix the HIV problem nor remedy—and indeed might even exacerbate—the structural violence that underlay it."[4] Nguyen traces the hegemony of biomedicine in Côte d'Ivoire to postcolonial associations of biomedicine with technical progress and nation-building. In the 1980s, structural adjustment policies and lack of public health insurance rendered public hospitals increasingly inaccessible, and private infirmaries and injectionists and unregulated lay pharmacists emerged as important alternatives in Abidjan. As Nguyen describes, these informal care providers reused syringes to cut costs and dispensed antibiotics that relieved symptoms but did not eliminate infection of sexually transmitted infections (STIs), which thus became asymptomatic and more likely to spread. Nguyen proposes that if sex work and migration triggered the epidemic in Côte d'Ivoire, untreated STIs and reused syringes might account for Abidjan's high HIV prevalence.[5]

Alongside these critiques of dominant prevention approaches, I suggest the importance of attending to past and present HIV prevention media campaigns, especially as they continue to reflect political and economic conflicts about citizenship and the rights attributed to it. Initially launched in Côte d'Ivoire in 2009, the *Super Girl* campaign links its goals of "empower[ing] more girls" with its attempts to urge girls and young women to communicate with their male sexual partners and to practice the ABCs. Despite controversy, especially surrounding abstinence and fidelity-based approaches, the PEPFAR/USAID-financed campaign was renewed in 2015, along with affiliated multimedia campaigns targeting older heterosexual men.[6] In representing individual heterosexual behavior change bound to gendered "empowerment" as a solution to the spread of HIV, prevention media in its most recent incar-

---

4. Nguyen, "Therapeutic Modernism," 34–35.

5. Nguyen, "Therapeutic," 46. Using Mozambique as an example, James Pfeiffer critiques PEPFAR as deeply entangled in neoliberal policies, especially structural adjustment. Pfeiffer, "The Struggle for a Public Sector," 167.

6. *Super Girl* included Brother for Life, modeled after a South African campaign targeting men. It also included the mini-telenovela *Networks* [*Réseaux*], which was adopted from the South African program *Intersexions*. The six-episode show targeted younger women and older, married men, and began broadcasting in March 2014. https://healthcommcapacity.org/where-we-work/cote-divoire-project/.

nations evokes and builds on prior attempts to secure reproductive legitimacy as a pathway to political authority, land ownership, and voting rights.

The *Super Girl* campaigns were initiated just before the renewed civil war (2010–11) ended with the forced removal of President Laurent Gbagbo, who had refused to concede electoral victory to Alassane Ouattara. Reelected in 2015, Ouattara proposed a new Constitution, passed by voter referendum in 2016, that explicitly addresses the years of turmoil preceding its passage. The Constitution's preamble asserts that "we, people of Côte d'Ivoire . . . desirous of building a Nation that is fraternal, unified, united [solidaire], peaceful and prosperous and anxious to preserve political stability. . . . Approve and adopt freely and solemnly before the Nation and humanity the present Constitution as fundamental Law of the State." Among other measures, the Constitution establishes a vice presidency, as well as a National Chamber of Kings and Traditional Chiefs [La Chambre nationale des Rois et Chefs traditionnels]. It also addresses a central point of contention about Ouattara's own eligibility to be president. The Constitution declares that the president and the new vice president "must be exclusively of Ivorian nationality, born of a father or mother of Ivorian origin." The revision of the Constitution followed a 2013 revision of nationality laws granting citizenship through marriage to foreign men who married Ivorian women; existing law already granted Ivorian nationality to foreign women who married Ivorian men.[7]

Articles of the Constitution go on to enumerate rights that accrue to citizens and carefully distinguish universal from citizen rights: the Constitution accords the right to property to all and affirms the family as "the basic unit of society [La famille constitue la cellule de base de la société]." However, it limits the right to "free enterprise," "of decent work conditions and at equitable remuneration," and of free movement to citizens. Significantly, given prior conflicts, it also limits rural land ownership to "the State, public corporations, and Ivorian natural persons" [Seuls l'Etat [sic], les collectivités publiques et les personnes physiques ivoiriennes peuvent accéder à la propriété foncière rurale]."[8]

---

7. Le Projet de loi portant modification des articles 12, 13, 14 et 16 de la loi n 61–415 du 14 décembre 1961 portant Code de la Nationalité tel que modifié par les lois n 72–852 du 21 décembre 1972 et 2004–662 du 17 décembre 2004 et les décisions n 2005–03/PR du 15 juillet 2005 et n 2005–09/PR du 26 août 2005, Article 12 nouveau, http://www.assnat.ci/sites/default/files/PROJET%20DE%20LOI%20MODIFICATION%20ARTICLES%2012%2C%2013%2C%2014%20ET%2016.pdf.

8. République de Côte d'Ivoire, Projet de Loi Portant Constitution de la République de Côte d'Ivoire, October 12, 2016, Preamble, Arts. 11, 12, 13, 15, 21, 31, 34, 52, 78, 175. http://www.gouv.ci/doc/accords/1476446768projet_de_loi_portant_constitution_rci.pdf.

Ivorian law delineates the circumstances of birth, reproduction, and marriage that determine citizenship and eligibility to political power as well as entitlement to enumerated rights. In advising the adoption of certain sexual behavior and family formations as critical to the building of a communal life, HIV prevention media dovetails with neoliberal economic agendas and the biopolitical project of determining the conditions of national belonging. Tracking convergences and divergences between HIV prevention campaigns, foreign-funder mandates, and nation-building clearly remains an ongoing project. So too does the project of contending with how heteronormative reproduction and family continue to figure as central to the foundation of a "unified, united, peaceful and prosperous" nation, and to the Constitution of "the people of Côte d'Ivoire."

HIV prevention media is inscribed in, and at the same time continually re-inscribes, histories that precede the epidemic. It retains the trace of these histories even as it insistently retains its focus on constructing a future presumed both desirable and shared. The bodies, families, and behaviors that the media delineates as a condition for—and an enactment of—the future that it imagines, therefore, has larger implications than how effectively the media works to instigate behavior change. HIV prevention media calls for inquiries that extend beyond these frameworks and for the imagining of more open-ended futures that extend beyond those offered, that are yet to come.

BIBLIOGRAPHY

Abbott, Frederick M. and Jerome H. Reichman. "The Doha Round's Public Health Legacy: Strategies for the Production and Diffusion of Patented Medicines under the Amended TRIPS Provisions." *Journal of International Economic Law* 10, no. 4 (2007): 921–87.

Abitbol, Eliette. "La Famille conjugale et le droit nouveau du mariage en Côte d'Ivoire." *Journal of African Law* 10, no. 3 (1966): 141–63.

Abolou, Camille Roger. *Les Français populaires africains.* Paris: L'Harmattan, 2012.

Abu-Lughod, Lila. "Egyptian Melodrama: Technology of the Modern Subject?" In *Media Worlds: Anthropology on New Terrain,* edited by Faye D. Ginsburg, Lila Abu-Lughod, and Brian Larkin, 115–33. Berkeley: University of California Press, 2002.

Afshar, Haleh and Carolyne Dennis. *Women and Adjustment Policies in the Third World.* London: Macmillan, 1991.

Agamben, Giorgio. *Homo Sacer: Sovereign Power and Bare Life.* Translated by Daniel Heller-Roazen. Stanford: Stanford University Press, 1998.

Akindès, Francis. "La Côte d'Ivoire depuis 1993: La réinvention risquée d'une nation." In *Côte d'Ivoire: La réinvention de soi dans la violence,* edited by Francis Akindès, 3–38. Dakar: CODESRIA, 2011.

———. *The Roots of the Military-Political Crises in Côte d'Ivoire.* Uppsala, Sweden: Nordiska Afrikainstitutet, 2004.

Akindes, Simon. "The Hip Hop Generation: Ghana's Hip Life and Ivory Coast's Coupé-Decalé." By Siddhartha Mitter. *Afropop Worldwide,* May 3, 2012. http://afropop.org/articles/the-hip-hop-generation-ghanas-hip-life-and-ivory-coasts-coupe-decale.

———. "Playing It 'Loud and Straight': Reggae, Zouglou, Mapouka, and Youth Insubordination in Côte d'Ivoire." In *Playing with Identities in Contemporary Music in Africa,* edited by Mai Palmberg and Annemette Kirkegaard, 86–103. Uppsala, Sweden: Nordiska Afrikainstitutet, 2002.

Allen, Rika. "Art Activism in South Africa and the Ethics of Representation in a Time of AIDS." *Critical Arts* 23, no. 3 (2009): 396–415.

Allen, Robert C. *Speaking of Soap Operas.* Chapel Hill: University of North Carolina Press, 1985.

Amad, Paula. "Visual Riposte: Looking Back at the Return of the Gaze as Postcolonial Theory's Gift to Film Studies." *Cinema Journal* 52, no. 3 (2013): 49–74. doi: 10.1353/cj.2013.0015.

Amondji, Marcel. *Côte d'Ivoire: La dépendance et l'épreuve des faits.* Paris: L'Harmattan, 1988.

———. *Félix Houphouët et la Côte-d'Ivoire: L'envers d'une légende.* Paris: Karthala, 1984.

Andrade-Watkins, Claire. "France's Bureau of Cinema—Financial and Technical Assistance 1961–1977: Operations and Implications for African Cinema." In *African Experiences of Cinema,* edited by Imruh Bakari and Mbye B. Cham, 112–27. London: British Film Institute, 1996.

Andreasen, Alan. *Marketing Social Change: Changing Behavior to Promote Health, Social Development, and the Environment.* San Francisco: Jossey Bass, 1995.

———. *Social Marketing in the 21st Century.* Thousand Oaks, CA: Sage, 2006.

Anoh, Amoakon, Raïmi Fassassi, and Patrice Vimard. *Politique de population et planification famille en Côte d'Ivoire.* Paris: Centre français sur la population et le développement, 2002.

Arnold, David. *Imperial Medicine and Indigenous Societies.* Manchester and New York: Manchester University Press, 1988.

Babo, Alfred, "*Ivoirité* and Citizenship in Ivory Coast: The Controversial Policy of Ethnicity." In *Citizenship in Question: Evidentiary Birthright and Statelessness,* edited by Benjamin N. Lawrance and Jacqueline Stevens, 200–216. Durham: Duke University Press, 2017.

Babo, Alfred and Yvan Droz. "Conflits fonciers: De l'ethnie à la nation: Rapports interethniques et 'ivoirité' dans le sud-ouest de la Côte-d'Ivoire." *Cahiers d'Études africaines* 48, no. 192 (2008): 741–63.

Bahi, Aghi. "Jeunes et imaginaire de la modernité à Abidjan." *Caderno de Estudos Africanos* 18/19 (2010): 56–67.

———. *L'Ivoirité mouvementée: Jeunes, médias et politique en Côte d'Ivoire.* Cameroon: Langaa RPCIG, 2013.

———. "Narration, tradition et modernité dans le discours filmique de *Comment ça va?*: Une émission de la télévision ivoirienne." PhD diss., Université Lumière Lyon II, 1994.

Bakari, Imruh. "Algiers Charter on African Cinema (1975)." Reprinted in *African Experiences of Cinema,* edited by Imruh Bakari and Mbye B. Cham, 25–26. London: British Film Institute, 1996.

Banégas, Richard. "Briefing: Post-Election Crisis in Côte d'Ivoire: The *Gbonhi* War." *African Affairs* 110, no. 440 (2011): 457–68.

Barbé, Thierry and Dominique Kerouedan. "Santé publique et privée: L'état et le citoyen en Côte d'Ivoire." *Sociologie Santé* 13 (1995): 18–30.

Barlet, Olivier. *African Cinemas: Decolonizing the Gaze.* London: Zed Books, 2000.

Barnard, Rita. "On Laughter, the Grotesque, and the South African Transition: Zakes Mda's *Ways of Dying.*" *NOVEL: A Forum on Fiction* 37, no. 3 (2004): 277–302.

Barrera, Vivian and Denise D. Bielby. "Places, Faces, and Other Familiar Things: The Cultural Experience of Telenovela Viewing among Latinos in the United States." *The Journal of American Popular Culture* 34, no. 4 (2001): 1–18.

Barry, Kathleen L. *Female Sexual Slavery.* New York: New York University Press, 1984.

Barz, Gregory and Judah M. Cohen, eds. *The Culture of AIDS in Africa: Hope and Healing Through Music and the Arts*. Oxford: Oxford University Press, 2011.

Bastien, Vincent. *Espace Confiance: Des services orientés vers la santé sexuelle*. Paris: Sidaction, 2013.

Bayart, Jean-François. *L'État en Afrique: La politique du ventre*. Paris: Librairie Arthème Fayard, 1989.

———. *The State in Africa: The Politics of the Belly*. Translated by Mary Harper, Christopher Harrison, and Elizabeth Harrison. London: Longman, 1993.

Bayer, Ronald. "Perinatal Transmission of HIV Infection: The Ethics of Prevention." *Clinical Obstetrics and Gynecology* 32, no. 3 (1989): 497–505.

Beall, Reed and Randall Kuhn. "Trends in Compulsory Licensing of Pharmaceuticals Since the Doha Declaration: A Database Analysis." *PLoS Medicine* 9, no. 1 (2012): 1–9.

Beinart, William and Marcelle C. Dawson, eds. *Popular Politics and Resistance Movements in South Africa*. Johannesburg: Wits University Press, 2010.

Bekelynck, Anne. "Le Rôle des entreprises privées dans la lutte contre le VIH/sida en Côte d'Ivoire: Des vecteurs d'une utopie sociale aux partenaires d'une action publique." *Lien social et politiques* 72 (2014): 129–49.

Benveniste, Annie. "Côte-d'Ivoire: Télévision extra-scolaire pour l'éducation des adultes ruraux: Bilan critique." *Revue Tiers-Monde* 20, no. 79 (1979): 465–78.

Bertrand, Jane T., Kevin O'Reilly, Julie Denison, Rebecca Anhang, and Michael Sweat. "Systematic Review of the Effectiveness of Mass Communication Programs to Change HIV/AIDS-Related Behaviors in Developing Countries." *Health Education Research* 21, no. 4 (2006): 567–97.

BFM TV. "Le Discours de Simone Veil en 1974 à l'Assemblée Nationale." http://www.bfmtv.com/politique/texte-le-discours-de-simone-veil-en-1974-a-l-assemblee-nationale-1198272.html.

Bibollet-Ruche, Frédéric, Anh Galat-Luoung, Gérard Cuny, Pascale Sarni-Manchado, Gérard Galat, Jean-Paul Durand, Xavier Pourrut, and Francisco Veas. "Simian Immunodeficiency Virus Infection in a Patas Monkey (*Erythrocebus patas*): Evidence for Cross-Species Transmission from African Green Monkeys (*Cercopithecus aethiops sabaeus*) in the Wild." *Journal of General Virology* 77 (1996): 773–81.

Blondy, Alpha. "SIDA dans la cité," recorded 1991, track 5 on *SOS Guerre Tribale*. EMI France, compact disc.

Bloom, Peter J. *French Colonial Documentary: Mythologies of Humanitarianism*. Minneapolis: University of Minnesota Press, 2008.

Boddy, Janice. *Civilizing Women: British Crusades in Colonial Sudan*. Princeton: Princeton University Press, 2007.

Boone, Catherine. "Africa's New Territorial Politics: Regionalism and the Open Economy in Côte d'Ivoire." *African Studies Review* 50, no. 1 (2007): 59–81.

Boone, Catherine and Norma Kriger. "Multiparty Elections and Land Patronage: Zimbabwe and Côte d'Ivoire." *Commonwealth and Comparative Politics* 48, no. 2 (2010): 173–202.

Booth, Karen M. "A Magic Bullet for the 'African' Mother?: Neo-Imperial Reproductive Futurism and the Pharmaceutical 'Solution' to the HIV/AIDS Crisis." *Social Politics: International Studies in Gender, State and Society* 17, no. 3 (2010): 349–78.

Bourgault, Louise M. *Playing for Life: Performance in Africa in the Age of AIDS*. Durham: Carolina Academic Press, 2003.

Boutin, Béatrice Akissi and Jérémie Kouadio N'Guessan. "Citoyenneté et politique linguistique en Côte d'Ivoire." *Revue française de linguistique appliquée* 18, no. 2 (2013): 121–33.

Brooks, Peter. *The Melodramatic Imagination: Balzac, Henry James, Melodrama, and the Mode of Excess*. New Haven: Yale University Press, 1976.

Brown, Wendy. "Neoliberalized Knowledge." *History of the Present* 1, no. 1 (Summer 2011): 113–29.

Bujra, Janet. "Sex Talk: Mutuality and Power in the Shadow of HIV/AIDS in Africa." In *Gender and AIDS: Critical Perspectives from the Developing World*, edited by Jelke Boesten and Nana K. Poku, 159–76. Burlington, VT: Ashgate, 2009.

Butler, Judith. "Mbembe's Extravagant Power." *Public Culture* 5, no. 1 (1992): 67–74.

Campbell, Bonnie. "Defining New Development Options and New Social Compromises in the Context of Reduced Political Space: Reflections on the Crisis in Côte d'Ivoire." *African Sociological Review* 7, no. 2 (2003): 29–44.

———. "Political Dimensions of the Adjustment Experience in Côte d'Ivoire." In *Critical Political Studies: Debates and Dialogues from the Left*, edited by Abigail B. Bakan and Eleanor MacDonald, 156–78. Montreal: McGill-Queen's University Press, 2002.

Campbell, Joseph W. *The Emergent Independent Press in Benin and Côte d'Ivoire: From Voice of the State to Advocate of Democracy*. Westport, CT: Praeger, 1998.

Center for Reproductive Rights. "The World's Abortion Laws Map 2013 Update." http://reproductiverights.org/sites/crr.civicactions.net/files/documents/AbortionMap_Factsheet_2013.pdf.

Centers for Disease Control and Prevention. "Current Trends Recommendations for Assisting in the Prevention of Perinatal Transmission of Human T-Lymphotropic Virus Type III/Lymphadenopathy-Associated Virus and Acquired Immunodeficiency Syndrome." *Morbidity and Mortality Weekly Report* 34 (December 6, 1985): 721–26. https://www.cdc.gov/mmwr/preview/mmwrhtml/00033122.htm.

Centre Africain de Recherche et d'Intervention en Développement and Johns Hopkins Bloomberg School of Public Health/Center for Communication Programs. *Communication pour le changement de comportement dans le domaine du VIH/SIDA en Côte d'Ivoire: Analyse des stratégies et de la réponse de 1985 à 2004, rapport final*, March 2005.

Chan, Jennifer. *Politics in the Corridor of Dying: AIDS Activism and Global Health Governance*. Baltimore: Johns Hopkins University Press, 2015.

Charbonneau, Bruno. *France and the New Imperialism: Security Policy in Sub-Saharan Africa*. Abingdon: Taylor & Francis Group, 2008.

"La Charte d'Alger du cinéma africain: Pour un cinéma responsable, libre et engagé." *Afrique littéraire et artistique* 35 (1978): 165.

Chauveau, Jean-Pierre. "La Part baule [sic]: Effectif de population et domination ethnique: Une perspective historique." *Cahiers d'Études africaines* 27, no. 105/106 (1987): 123–65.

———. "Question foncière et construction nationale en Côte d'Ivoire: Les enjeux silencieux d'un coup d'État." *Politique africaine* 78 (2000): 94–125.

Chauveau, Jean-Pierre and Jean-Pierre Dozon. "Au Coeur des éthnies ivoiriennes... l'état." In *L'État contemporain en Afrique*. Paris: L'Harmattan, 1987.

Clift, Elaine and World Health Organization. *Information, Education and Communication: Lessons from the Past, Perspectives for the Future*. Geneva: World Health Organization, 2001. http://apps.who.int/iris/handle/10665/67127.

Le Code Civil. "Mariage." Loi 64-375 du 7 octobre 1964.

———. "Mariage." Loi 64-375 du 7 octobre 1964 modifiée par la loi no. 83-800 du 2 août 1983.

Le Code Pénal. Loi 81-640 du 31 juillet 1981.

Cogneau, Denis and Rémi Jedwab. "Commodity Price Shocks and Child Outcomes: The 1990 Cocoa Crisis in Côte d'Ivoire." *Economic Development and Cultural Change* 60, no. 3 (2012): 507–34.

Cohen, David William. "The Banalities of Interpretation." *Public Culture* 5, no. 1 (1992): 57–59.

Comaroff, Jean. "Beyond Bare Life: AIDS, (Bio)Politics, and the Neoliberal Order." *Public Culture* 19, no. 1 (2007): 197–219.

———. "The Diseased Heart of Africa: Medicine, Colonialism and the Black Body." In *Knowledge, Power and Practice: The Anthropology of Medicine and Everyday Life*, edited by Shirley Lindenbaum and Margaret Lock, 305–29. Berkeley: University of California Press, 1993.

Comaroff, Jean and John Comaroff. "Introduction." In *Modernity and Its Malcontents*, edited by Jean Comaroff and John Comaroff, xi–xxxvii. Chicago: University of Chicago Press, 1993.

Connell, Raewyn and Nour Dados. "Where in the World Does Neoliberalism Come From? The Market Agenda in Southern Perspective." *Theory and Society* 43, no. 2 (March 2014): 117–38.

Connor, Edward M., Rhoda S. Sperling, Richard Gelber, Pavel Kiselev, Gwendolyn Scott, Mary Jo O'Sullivan, Russell VanDyke, Mohammed Bey, William Shearer, Robert L. Jacobson, Eleanor Jimenez, Edward O'Neill, Brigitte Bazin, Jean-Francois Delfraissy, Mary Culnane, Robert Coombs, Mary Elkins, Jack Moye, Pamela Stratton, and James Balsley, for the Pediatric AIDS Clinical Trials Group Protocol 076 Study Group. "Reduction of Maternal-Infant Transmission of Human Immunodeficiency Virus Type 1 with Zidovudine Treatment." *New England Journal of Medicine* 331 (1994): 1173–80.

Contamin, Bernard and Yves-A. Fauré. *La Bataille des entreprises publiques en Côte d'Ivoire: L'histoire d'un ajustement interne*. Paris: Karthala and ORSTOM, 1990.

Cooper, Frederick. "Possibility and Constraint: African Independence in Historical Perspective." *The Journal of African History* 49, no. 2 (2008): 167–96.

Coronil, Fernando. "Can Postcoloniality Be Decolonized? Imperial Banality and Postcolonial Power." *Public Culture* 5, no. 1 (1992): 89–108.

Coulibaly, Luzéni. "Les Traits principaux de nouveau droit ivoirien de la famille." *Revue juridique et politique, indépendance et coopération* 21 (1967): 76–95.

Crook, Richard C. "Côte d'Ivoire: Multi-Party Democracy and Political Change: Surviving the Crisis." In *Democracy and Political Change in Sub-Saharan Africa*, edited by John A. Wiseman, 11–44. New York: Routledge, 1995.

Currier, Ashley and Thérèse Migraine-George. "Queer Studies/African Studies: An (Im)possible Transaction?" *GLQ: A Journal of Lesbian and Gay Studies* 22, no. 2 (2016): 281–305.

Cutolo, Armando. "Modernity, Autochthony and the Ivorian Nation: The End of a Century in Côte d'Ivoire." *Africa* 80, no. 4 (2010): 527–52.

Cynn, Christine. "The ABCs of HIV Prevention in Uganda and Côte d'Ivoire." *Transformations* 21, no. 2 (Fall 2009/Winter 2010): 102–22.

———. "*AIDS in the City*: Melodrama and the Social Marketing of HIV Prevention in Francophone West Africa." *Camera Obscura* 32, no. 1 (2017): 33–61.

"Débats sur les communications de Mm. Coulibaly et Vangah." *Revue juridique et politique, indépendance et coopération* 21 (1967): 101–4.

Decoteau, Claire Laurier. *Ancestors and Antiretrovirals: The Biopolitics of HIV/AIDS in Post-Apartheid South Africa*. Chicago: University of Chicago Press, 2013.

Delaunay, Karine. "Réflexions sur les dynamiques socio-politiques de la lutte contre le sida en Côte d'Ivoire." In *Organiser la lutte contre le sida: Une étude comparative sur les rapports État/société civile en Afrique,* edited by Marc-Éric Gruénais, 113–18. Paris: L'Agence nationale de recherche sur le sida, 1999.

Delaunay, Karine A., Didier Blibolo, and Katy Cissé-Wone. "Des ONG et des associations: Concurrences et dépendances sur un 'marché du sida' émergent (cas ivoirien et sénégalais)." In *Organiser la lutte contre le SIDA,* edited by Marc-Éric Gruénais, 69–89. Paris: l'Agence nationale de recherche sur le sida, 1999.

Delaunay, Karine, Jean-Pierre Dozon, Gabin Kponhassia, and Philippe Msellati. "Prémices et déroulement de l'Initiative (1996–2000): Une première analyse." In *L'Accès aux traitements du VIH/sida en Côte d'Ivoire: Évaluation de l'initiative Onusida/ministère ivoirien de la Santé publique,* edited by Philippe Msellati, Laurent Vidal, and Jean-Paul Moatti, 13–61. Paris: l'Agence nationale de recherche sur le sida, 2001.

De Lauretis, Theresa. *Technologies of Gender: Essays on Theory, Film, and Fiction.* Bloomington: Indiana University Press, 1987.

Dembélé, Ousmane. "La Construction économique et politique de la catégorie 'étranger' en Côte d'Ivoire." In *Côte d'Ivoire: L'année terrible: 1999–2000,* edited by Marc Le Pape and Claudine Vidal, 123–72. Paris: Karthala, 2002.

———. "Côte d'Ivoire: La fracture communautaire." *Politique africaine* 89 (2003): 34–48.

Deniaud, François. "'Chaussette de vie,' ou une biographie africaine de la protection." In *La Paradoxe de la marchandise authentique: Imagination et consommation de masse,* edited by Jean-Pierre Warnier, 119–43. Paris: l'Harmattan, 1994.

———. "Jeunes et préservatifs à Abidjan: Une recherche d'ethno-prévention du sida et des MST." In *Les Sciences sociales face au SIDA: Cas africains autour de l'exemple ivoirien,* edited by Jean-Pierre Dozon and Laurent Vidal, 89–108. Paris: OSTROM, 1995.

Deniaud, François and Kitia Touré. "Présentation de documents audiovisuels sur la prévention du SIDA." In *Les Sciences sociales face au SIDA: Cas africains autour de l'exemple ivoirien,* edited by Jean Pièrre Dozon and Laurent Vidal, 123–26. Paris: ORSTROM, 1995.

Désalmand, P. "Une Aventure ambiguë, le programme d'éducation télévisuelle (1971–1982)." *Politiques Africaines* 24 (1986): 91–103.

Desgrées-Du-Loû, Annabel, Philippe Msellati, Ida Viho, Angèle Yao, Delphine Yapi, Pierrette Kassi, Christiane Welffens-Ekra, Laurent Mandelbrot, and François Dabis. "Contraceptive Use, Protected Sexual Intercourse and Incidence of Pregnancies among African HIV-Infected Women: DITRAME ANRS 049 Project, Abidjan 1995–2000." *International Journal of STDs and AIDS* 13, no. 7 (2002): 462–68.

De Turégano, Teresa Hoefert. "The New Politics of African Cinema at the French Ministry of Foreign Affairs." *French Politics, Culture and Society* 20, no. 3 (2002): 22–32.

Deutsche Gesellschaft für Internationale Zusammenarbeit and Kreditanstalt für Wiederaufbau. *Les Séries télévisées dans l'éducation sur le VIH: Atteindre les populations grâce au divertissement populaire.* Eschborn, Germany, 2009.

———. *TV Soap Operas in HIV Education: Reaching Out with Popular Entertainment.* Eschborn, Germany: German HIV Practice Collective, 2011.

Deutscher, Penelope. "The Inversion of Exceptionality: Foucault, Agamben, and 'Reproductive Rights.'" *South Atlantic Quarterly* 107, no. 1 (2008): 55–70.

Diawara, Manthia. *African Cinema: Politics and Culture.* Bloomington: Indiana University Press, 1992.

Dilger, Hansjörg. "Targeting the Empowered Individual: Transnational Policy Making, the Global Economy of Aid and the Limitations of Biopower in Tanzania." In *Medicine, Mobility, and Power in Global Africa: Transnational Health and Healing*, edited by Hansjörg Dilger, Abdoulaye Kane, and Stacey Langwick, 60–91. Bloomington: Indiana University Press, 2012.

Doane, Mary Ann. *The Desire to Desire: The Woman's Film of the 1940s*. Bloomington: Indiana University Press, 1987.

Dodd, Rebecca. "AIDS Soap Opera Generates Massive Interest." *AIDS Analysis Africa* 5, no. 6 (1995): 16.

Doezema, Jo. "Ouch! Western Feminists' 'Wounded Attachment' to the 'Third World Prostitute.'" *Feminist Review* 67 (2001): 16–38.

———. *Sex Slaves and Discourse Masters: The Construction of Trafficking*. New York: Zed Books, 2010.

Doolittle, Russell F. "The Simian-Human Connection." *Nature* 339, no. 6223 (1989): 338–39.

Dozon, Jean-Pierre. *Les Clefs de la crise ivoirienne*. Paris: Karthala, 2011.

———. "La Côte d'Ivoire entre démocratie, nationalisme et ethnonationalisme." *Politique africaine* 78, no. 2 (2000): 45–62.

Dozon, Jean-Pierre and Didier Fassin. "Raison épidémiologique et raisons d'État. Les Enjeux socio-politiques du SIDA en Afrique." *Sciences sociales et santé* 7, no. 1 (1989): 21–36.

Duggan, Lisa. *The Twilight of Equality? Neoliberalism, Cultural Politics, and the Attack on Democracy*. Boston: Beacon Press, 2003.

Duparc, Henri. "La Dérision contre l'intolérance." By Clément Tapsoba. *Écrans d'Afrique* 8 (1994): 14–17.

Easterly, William. "What Did Structural Adjustment Adjust? The Association of Policies and Growth with Repeated IMF and World Bank Adjustment Loans." *Journal of Developmental Economics* 76, no. 1 (2005): 1–22.

Égly, Max. *Télévision didactique: Entre le kitsch et les systèmes du troisième type?* Paris: Edilig, 1984.

———. "L'utilisation de la télévision scolaire au Niger en Côte d'Ivoire et au Sénégal." *International Review of Education* 32, no. 3 (1986): 338–46.

Elmendorf, A. Edward, Cecilia Cabañero-Verzosa, Michele Lioy, and Kathryn LaRusso. "Behavior Change Communication for Better Health Outcomes in Africa: Experience and Lessons Learned from World Bank–Financed Health, Nutrition and Population Projects." World Bank, Africa Region, Human Development Working Paper Series, no. 92 (2005).

Elsaesser, Thomas. "Tales of Sound and Fury: Observations on the Family Melodrama." In *Imitations of Life: A Reader on Film and Television Melodrama*, edited by Marcia Landy, 68–91. Detroit, MI: Wayne State University Press, 1991.

"Epidemiological Notes and Reports: Pneumocystis Pneumonia—Los Angeles." *Morbidity and Mortality Weekly Report* 30, no. 21 (June 5, 1981): 250–52.

Epprecht, Marc. *Heterosexual Africa? The History of an Idea from the Age of Exploration to the Age of AIDS*. Athens: Ohio University Press, 2008.

Epstein, Helen. *The Invisible Cure: Why We Are Losing the Fight against AIDS in Africa*. New York: Picador, 2007.

Esacove, Anne. *Modernizing Sexuality: U.S. HIV Prevention in Sub-Saharan Africa*. New York: Oxford University Press, 2016.

Evans, Stella and Stephen Klees. *ETV Program Production in the Ivory Coast.* Washington, DC: Academy for Educational Development and the Stanford University Institute for Communication Research for the Agency for International Development, Bureau for Africa, 1976.

Everett, Anna. *Returning the Gaze: A Genealogy of Black Film Criticism, 1909–1949.* Durham: Duke University Press, 2001.

Family Health International. *Behavior Change Communication (BCC) for HIV/AIDS: A Strategic Framework.* USAID, 2002. http://www.hivpolicy.org/Library/HPP000533.pdf.

Farmer, Paul. *AIDS and Accusation: Haiti and the Geography of Blame.* Berkeley: University of California Press, 1992.

———. "An Anthropology of Structural Violence." *Current Anthropology* 45, no. 3 (June 2004): 305–25.

———. "On Suffering and Structural Violence: A View from Below." *Race/Ethnicity: Multidisciplinary Global Contexts* 3, no. 1 (Autumn 2009): 11–28.

Fassin, Didier. "Le Domaine privé de la santé publique: Pouvoir, politique et sida au Congo." *Annales: Histoire, Sciences Sociales* 4 (July–August 1994): 745–75.

———. *When Bodies Remember: Experiences and Politics of AIDS in South Africa.* Berkeley: University of California Press, 2007.

Fauré, Yves A. "Côte d'Ivoire: Analysing the Crisis." In *Contemporary West Africa States*, edited by Donal B. Cruise O'Brien, John Dunn, and Richard Rathbone, 59–73. Cambridge: Cambridge University Press, 1989.

———. "Democracy and Realism: Reflections on the Case of Côte d'Ivoire." *Africa: Journal of the International African Institute* 63, no. 3 (1993): 313–29.

Foucault, Michel. *The History of Sexuality, Volume 1: An Introduction.* Translated by Robert Hurley. New York: Vintage, 1990.

———. *"Society Must Be Defended": Lectures at the Collège de France, 1975–1976.* Edited by Mauro Bertani and Alessandro Fontana. Translated by David Macey. New York: Picador, 2003.

Fowler, Mary Glenn, Lynne Mofenson, and Michelle McConnell. "Editorial: The Interface of Perinatal HIV Prevention, Antiretroviral Drug Resistance, and Antiretroviral Treatment: What Do We Really Know?" *JAIDS: Journal of Acquired Immune Deficiency Syndromes* 34, no. 3 (2003): 308–11.

Freud, Sigmund. *Jokes and Their Relation to the Unconscious.* Translated and edited by James Strachey. New York: Norton, 1963.

Gaber, Sabrina and Preeti Patel. "Tracing Health System Challenges in Post-Conflict Côte d'Ivoire from 1893 to 2013." *Global Public Health: An International Journal for Research, Policy and Practice* 8, no. 6 (2013): 698–712.

Gbanou, Sélom Komlan. "De la Planche à la bande: Les voies modernes de l'oralité africaine: De la scène à la cassette." In *Interfaces between the Oral and the Written/ Interfaces entre l'écrit et l'oral: Versions and Subversions in African Literature 2*, edited by Ricard Alain and Flora Veit-Wild, 43–60. New York: Rodopi, 2005.

Genova, James E. *Cinema and Development in West Africa: Film as a Vehicle for Liberation.* Bloomington: Indiana University Press, 2013.

Ghys, Peter D., Mamadou O. Diallo, Virginie Ettiègne-Traoré, Kouamé Kalé, Oussama Tawil, Michel Caraël, Moussa Traoré, Guessan Mah-bi, Kevin M. De Cock, Stefan Z. Wiktor, Marie Laga, and Alan E. Greenberg. "Increase in Condom Use and Decline in HIV and Sexually Transmitted Diseases among Female Sex Workers in Abidjan, Cote d'Ivoire, 1991–1998." *AIDS* 16, no. 2 (2002): 251–58.

GIZ, KfW. *Les Séries télévisées dans l'education sur le VIH: Atteindre les populations grâce au divertissement populaire*. Eschborn: Germany, 2009.

Gledhill, Christine. "Speculations on the Relationship between Soap Opera and Melodrama." *Quarterly Review of Film and Video* 14, no. 1/2 (1992): 103–24.

Goldfarb, Brian. *Visual Pedagogies: Media Cultures in and beyond the Classroom*. Durham: Duke University Press, 2002.

Green-Simms, Lindsey. "Occult Melodramas: Spectral Affect and West African Video-Film." *Camera Obscura* 27, no. 2 (2012): 25–59.

Grünkemeier, Ellen. *Breaking the Silence: South African Representations of HIV/AIDS*. Rochester, New York: James Curry, 2013.

Guenou, Ghislaine. *Impact d'une campagne de sensibilisation télévisée: "SIDA dans la cité 2."* Abidjan: ICAO/ISCOM, 1997.

Guillaume, Agnès and Annabel Desgrées Du Loû. "Fertility Regulation among Women in Abidjan, Côte d'Ivoire: Contraception, Abortion or Both?" *International Family Planning Perspectives* 28, no. 3 (2002): 159–66.

Haffner, Pierre. *Essai sur les fondements du cinéma africain*. Abidjan-Dakar: Nouvelles éditions africaines, 1978.

Hahn, Beatrice H., George M. Shaw, Kevin M. De Cock, Paul M. Sharp. "AIDS as a Zoonosis: Scientific and Public Health Implications." *Science* 287, no. 5453 (2000): 607–14.

Hanefeld, Johanna. "Patent Rights vs. Patient Rights: Intellectual Property, Pharmaceutical Companies and Access to Treatment for People Living with HIV/AIDS in Sub-Saharan Africa." *Feminist Review* 72, no. 1 (2002): 84–92.

Harrison, Graham. *Neoliberal Africa: The Impact of Global Social Engineering*. London: Zed Books, 2010.

Harrow, Kenneth W. *Postcolonial African Cinema: From Political Engagement to Postmodernism*. Bloomington: Indiana University Press, 2007.

Harvey, David. *A Brief History of Neoliberalism*. Oxford: Oxford University Press, 2005.

Hattiger, Jean-Louis. "Humour et pidgin: L'exemple du français populaire d'Abidjan." In *Humoresques: L'humour d'expression française*, volume 2. 175–80. Nice: Z'éditions, 1990.

Hawkridge, David. *General Operational Review of Distance Education*. International Bank for Reconstruction and Development/World Bank, 1987.

Hirsch, Jennifer S. and Holly Wardlow. "Introduction." In *Modern Loves: The Anthropology of Romantic Courtship and Companionate Marriage*, edited by Jennifer S. Hirsch and Holly Wardlow, 1–31. Ann Arbor: University of Michigan Press, 2006.

Hoad, Neville. *African Intimacies: Race, Homosexuality, and Globalization*. Minneapolis: University of Minnesota Press, 2007.

———. "Arrested Development or the Queerness of Savages: Resisting Evolutionary Narratives of Difference." *Postcolonial Studies* 3, no. 2 (2000): 133–58.

———. "Miss HIV and Us: Beauty Queens against the HIV/AIDS Pandemic." *CR: The New Centennial Review* 10, no. 1 (Spring 2010): 9–28.

Houphouët-Boigny, Félix. *Anthologie des discours 1946–1978*. Abidjan: CEDA, 1978.

Hunt, Nancy Rose. *A Colonial Lexicon: Of Birth Ritual, Medicalization, and Mobility in the Congo*. Durham: Duke University Press, 1999.

———. "Among AIDS Derivatives in Africa." *Journal of the International Institute* 4, no. 3 (1997). http://hdl.handle.net/2027/spo.4750978.0004.301.

Hunter, Mark. *Love in the Time of AIDS: Inequality, Gender, and Rights in South Africa*. Bloomington: Indiana University Press, 2010.

Iliffe, John. *The African AIDS Epidemic: A History*. Athens: Ohio University Press, 2006.

International Monetary Fund. *External Evaluation of the ESAF: Report by a Group of Independent Experts*. Washington, DC, 1998.

———. *Republique de Côte d'Ivoire: Stratégie de relance du développement et de réduction de la pauvreté*, 2009. https://www.imf.org/~/media/Websites/IMF/imported-publications.../cr09156f.ashx.

Jochelson, Karen. *The Colour of Disease: Syphilis and Racism in South Africa, 1880–1950*. New York: Palgrave, 2001.

Kaleeba, Noerine, Joyce Namulando Kadowe, Daniel Kalinaki, and Glen Williams. *Open Secret: People Facing Up to HIV and AIDS in Uganda*. London: ActionAid, 2000.

Kalipeni, Ezekiel, Susan Craddock, and Jayati Ghosh. "Mapping the AIDS Pandemic in Eastern and Southern Africa: A Critical Overview." In *HIV and AIDS in Africa: Beyond Epidemiology*, edited by Ezekiel Kalipeni, Susan Craddock, Joseph R. Oppong, and Jayati Ghosh, 58–69. Malden, MA: Blackwell Publishing, 2004.

Kalipeni, Ezekiel, Susan Craddock, Joseph R. Oppong, and Jayati Ghosh, eds. *HIV and AIDS in Africa: Beyond Epidemiology*. Malden, MA: Blackwell Publishing, 2004.

Kane, Thomas T., Mohamadou Gueye, Ilene Speizer, Sara Pacque-Margolis, and Danielle Baron. "The Impact of a Family Planning Multimedia Campaign in Bamako, Mali." *Studies in Family Planning* 29, no. 3 (September 1998): 309–23.

Kaplan, E. Ann. *Looking for the Other: Feminism, Film, and the Imperial Gaze*. New York: Routledge, 1997.

———. "Theories of Melodrama: A Feminist Perspective." *Women and Performance* 1, no. 1 (1983): 40–48.

Karim, Quarraisha Abdool. "Heterosexual Transmission of HIV—The Importance of a Gendered Perspective in HIV Prevention." In *HIV/AIDS in South Africa*, edited by S. S. Abdool Karim and Q. Abdool Karim, 243–61. Cambridge: Cambridge University Press, 2005.

Kaye, Anthony. "The Ivory Coast Educational Television Project." In *Educational Television: A Policy Critique and Guide for Developing Countries*, edited by Robert F. Arnove, 140–79. New York: Praeger, 1976.

Kerouedan, Dominique Marie. "Lutter contre le sida en Afrique de l'Ouest: Quelles perspectives en cette fin de siècle?" *Santé Publique* 10, no. 2 (1998): 203–18.

Klaas, Brian. "From Miracle to Nightmare: An Institutional Analysis of Development Failures in Côte d'Ivoire." *Africa Today* 55, no. 1 (2008): 109–26.

Klees, Steven J. "Cost Analysis of Non-Formal ETV Systems: A Case Study of the 'Extra-Scolaire' System in the Ivory Coast." Washington, DC: USAID, 1977.

Knight, Lindsay. *UNAIDS: The First Ten Years: 1996-2007*. Geneva: UNAIDS, 2008. http://data.unaids.org/pub/report/2008/jc1579_first_10_years_en.pdf.

Knoppers, Bartha Maria and Isabel Brault. *La Loi et l'avortement dans les pays francophones*. Montréal: Les Éditions Thémis, 1989.

Knoppers, Bartha Maria, Isabel Brault, and Elizabeth Sloss. "Abortion Law in Francophone Countries." *The American Journal of Comparative Law* 38, no. 4 (1990): 889–922.

Koffi, Michel. "La Tradition ivoirienne de la comédie." *CinémAction* 106 (2003): 146–47.

Koly, Souleymane. "'Le Kotèba parle de l'Afrique d'aujourd'hui.'" Interview by Julien Le Gros, *Africultures: Les mondes en relation*, August 3, 2014. http://africultures.com/souleymane-koly-le-koteba-parle-de-lafrique-daujourdhui-12347/.

Konaté, Yacouba. "Abidjan: Malentendu, poésies et lieux propres." *Outre-Terre* 2, no. 11 (2005): 319–28.

———. "Génération zouglou." *Cahiers d'Études africaines* 42, no. 168 (2002): 777–96.

Koné, Hugues and Janet Jenkins. "The Programme for Educational Television in the Ivory Coast." *Educational Media International* 27, no. 2 (1990): 86–93.

Koné, Hugues and Justine Agness. "La Communication dans la lutte contre le SIDA en Côte d'Ivoire: Éléments de stratégies." In *La Communication pour le développement durable en Afrique*, edited by Hugues Koné and Jacques Habila Sy. Abidjan: Presses Universitaires de Côte d'Ivoire, 1995.

Kwahulé, Koffi. *Pour une critique du théâtre ivoirien contemporain*. Paris: L'Harmattan, 1997.

Lafage, Suzanne. "'Français façon la [sic], y a pas son deux!' Ou Les chroniques de Moussa dans l'hebdomadaire *Ivoire-Dimanche*." In *Humoresques: L'humour d'expression française*, volume 2, 175–80. Nice: Z'éditions, 1990.

Land, Mitchell. "Ivoirien [sic] Television, Willing Vector of Cultural Imperialism." *The Howard Journal of Communications* 4, nos. 1 & 2 (1992): 10–27.

Larkin, Brian. *Signal and Noise: Media, Infrastructure, and Urban Culture in Nigeria*. Durham: Duke University Press, 2008.

Lasker, Judith N. "The Role of Health Services in Colonial Rule: The Case of the Ivory Coast." *Culture, Medicine, and Psychiatry* 1, no. 3 (September 1977): 277–97.

Laurent, Suzanne. "Formation, information et développement en Côte d'Ivoire." *Cahiers d'Études africaines* 10, no. 39 (1970): 422–68.

Lenglet, Frans B. "Educational Television in Ivory Coast." In *Mass Communication, Culture and Society in West Africa*, edited by Frank Okwu Ugboajah, 153–64. Munich: Hans Zell Publishers, 1985.

Le Pape, Marc and Claudine Vidal. "Libéralisme et vécus sexuels à Abidjan." *Cahiers internationaux de sociologie* 76 (Jan.–June 1984): 111–18.

Lo, Nathan C., Anita Lowe, and Eran Bendavid. "Abstinence Funding Was Not Associated with Reductions in HIV Risk Behavior in Sub-Saharan Africa." *Health Affairs* 35, no. 5 (2016): 856–63.

Lutz, Tom. "Men's Tears and the Roles of Melodrama." In *Boys Don't Cry?: Rethinking Narratives of Masculinity and Emotion in the U.S.*, edited by Milette Shamir and Jennifer Travis, 185–204. New York: Columbia University Press, 2002.

MacKinnon, Catharine. "Trafficking, Prostitution and Inequality." *Harvard Civil Rights Civil Liberties Law Review* 46, no. 2 (2011): 271–309.

MacLean, Lauren M. *Informal Institutions and Citizenship in Rural Africa: Risk and Reciprocity in Ghana and Côte d'Ivoire*. Cambridge: Cambridge University Press, 2010.

Mahieu, François Régis. "Variable Dimension Adjustment in the Côte d'Ivoire: Reasons for Failure." *Review of African Political Economy* 22, no. 63 (March 1995): 9–26.

Marshall-Fratani, Ruth. "The War of 'Who Is Who': Autochthony, Nationalism, and Citizenship in the Ivoirian Crisis." *African Studies Review* 49, no. 2 (2006): 9–43.

Masenior, Nicole Franck and Chris Beyrer. "The US Anti-Prostitution Pledge: First Amendment Challenges and Public Health Priorities." *PLoS Med* 4, no. 7 (2007): e207. https://doi.org/10.1371/journal.pmed.0040207.

Mayne, Judith. *The Woman at the Keyhole: Feminism and Women's Cinema*. Bloomington: Indiana University Press, 1990.

Mbembe, Achille. "The Banality of Power and the Aesthetics of Vulgarity in the Postcolony." Translated by Janet Roitman. *Public Culture* 4, no. 2 (1992): 1–30.

———. "Notes provisoires sur la postcolonie." *Politique Africaine* 60 (1995): 76–109.

———. *De la postcolonie. Essai sur l'imagination politique dans l'Afrique contemporaine*. Paris: Karthala, 2000.

———. *On the Postcolony*. Translated by A. M. Berrett, Janet Roitman, Murray Last, and Steven Rendall. Berkeley: University of California Press, 2001.

———. "*On the Postcolony*: A Brief Response to Critics." Translated by Nima Bassiri and Peter Skafish. *African Identities* 4, no. 2 (2006): 143–78.

———. "Le Potentat sexuel: À propos de la sodomie, de la fellation et autres privautés postcoloniales. En partenariat avec le quotidien *Le Messager* paraissant à Douala au Cameroun." *Africultures: Les mondes en relation* (2006). http://africultures.com/le-potentat-sexuel-a-propos-de-la-sodomie-de-la-fellation-et-autres-privautes-postcoloniales-4296/.

———. "Prosaics of Servitude and Authoritarian Civilities." Translated by Janet Roitman. *Public Culture* 5, no. 1 (1992): 123–45.

McClintock, Anne. *Imperial Leather: Race, Gender and Sexuality in the Colonial Contest*. New York: Routledge, 1995.

McGovern, Mike. *Making War in Côte d'Ivoire*. Chicago: University of Chicago Press, 2011.

McNeill, Fraser G. "'Condoms Cause Aids': Poison, Prevention and Denial in Venda, South Africa." *African Affairs* 108, no. 432 (2009): 353–70.

Memel-Fotê, Harris. "Un Mythe politique des Akan en Côte d'Ivoire: Le sens de l'État." In *Mondes akan: Identité et pouvoir en Afrique occidentale*, edited by Pierluigi Valsecchi and Fabio Viti, 21–42. Paris: L'Harmattan, 2000.

Meyer, Birgit. "'Praise the Lord': Popular Cinema and Pentecostalite Style in Ghana's New Public Sphere." *American Ethnologist* 31, no. 1 (2004): 92–110.

Mikell, Gwendolyn. *African Feminism: The Politics of Survival in Sub-Saharan Africa*. Philadelphia: University of Pennsylvania Press, 1997.

Ministère de la Santé et de l'Hygiène Publique, PEPFAR, and Johns Hopkins University. *Stratégie Nationale de Communication pour le Changement de Comportement en matière de prise en charge des personnes vivant avec le VIH/SIDA en Côte d'Ivoire*, 2006.

Modleski, Tania. *Loving with a Vengeance: Mass-Produced Fantasies for Women*. 2nd ed. New York: Routledge, 2008.

Moghadam, Valentine M. "The 'Feminization of Poverty' and Women's Human Rights." SHS Papers in Women's Studies/Gender Research, no. 2 (July 2005). http://www.unesco.org/new/fileadmin/MULTIMEDIA/HQ/SHS/pdf/Feminization_of_Poverty.pdf.

Morand, Catherine. "*SIDA dans la cité*: Une série TV passionne les Ivoiriens." *Jeune Afrique* 1791 (May 4–10, 1995): 44.

Morley, David and Kevin Robins. *Spaces of Identity: Global Media, Electronic Landscapes and Cultural Boundaries*. New York: Routledge, 1995.

Moussa, Zio. *Les Médias et la crise politique en Côte d'Ivoire*. Accra, Ghana: Fondation pour les Médias en Afrique de l'Ouest, 2012.

Msellati, Philippe, Anne Juillet-Amari, Joanne Prudhomme, Hortense Aka-Dago Akribi, Djénéba Coulibaly-Traore, Marc Souville, Jean-Paul Moatti, and Côte d'Ivoire HIV Drug Access Initiative Socio-Behavioural Evaluation Group. "Socio-economic and Health Characteristics of HIV-infected Patients Seeking Care in Relation to Access to the Drug Access Initiative and to Antiretroviral Treatment in Côte d'Ivoire." *AIDS* 17, supplement 3 (2003): S63–68.

Mulvey, Laura. "Visual Pleasure and Narrative Cinema." *Screen* 16, no. 3 (1975): 6–18.

Nattrass, Nicoli. *Mortal Combat: AIDS Denialism and the Struggle for Antiretrovirals in South Africa*. Pietermaritzburg, South Africa: University of KwaZulu-Natal Press, 2007.

Ndjio, Basile. "Evolués and Feymen: Old and New Figures of Modernity in Cameroon." In *Readings in Modernity in Africa*, edited by Peter Geschiere, Birgit Meyer, and Peter Pels, 205–14. Bloomington: International African Institute and Indiana University Press, 2008.

Newell, Sasha. *The Modernity Bluff: Crime, Consumption, and Citizenship in Côte d'Ivoire*. Chicago: University of Chicago Press, 2012.

Nguyen, Vinh-Kim. "Antiretroviral Globalism, Biopolitics, and Therapeutic Citizenship." In *Global Assemblages: Technology, Politics, and Ethics as Anthropological Problems*, edited by Aihwa Ong and Stephen J. Collier, 124–44. Malden, MA: Blackwell Publishing, 2005.

———. "Counselling against HIV in Africa: A Genealogy of Confessional Technologies." *Culture, Health and Sexuality* 15, supplement 4 (2013): S440–52.

———. "Therapeutic Modernism: Medical Pluralism, Local Biologies, and HIV in Côte d'Ivoire." In *Troubling Natural Categories: Engaging the Medical Anthropology of Margaret Lock*, edited by Naomi Adelson, Leslie Butt, and Karina Kielmann, 34–57. Montreal: McGill-Queen's University Press, 2013.

———. *The Republic of Therapy: Triage and Sovereignty in West Africa's Time of AIDS*. Durham: Duke University Press, 2010.

———. "Uses and Pleasures: Sexual Modernity, HIV/AIDS, and Confessional Technologies in a West African Metropolis." In *Sex in Development: Science, Sexuality, and Morality in Global Perspective*, edited by Vincanne Adams and Stacy Leigh Pigg, 245–68. Durham: Duke University Press, 2005.

Ngwena, Charles G. "Reforming African Abortion Laws and Practice: The Place of Transparency." In *Abortion Law in Transnational Perspective: Cases and Controversies*, edited by Rebecca J. Cook, Joanna N. Erdman, and Bernard M. Dickens, 166–86. Philadelphia: University of Pennsylvania Press, 2014.

Noar, Seth M. "A 10-Year Retrospective of Research in Health Mass Media Campaigns: Where Do We Go from Here?" *Journal of Health Communication* 11, no. 1 (2006): 21–42.

Noar, Seth, Philip Palmgreen, Melissa Chabot, Nicole Dobransky, and Rick S. Zimmerman. "A 10-Year Systematic Review of HIV/AIDS Mass Communication Campaigns: Have We Made Progress?" *Journal of Health Communication* 14, no. 1 (2009): 15–42.

Nutall, Sarah. *Entanglement: Literary and Cultural Reflections on Post-Apartheid*. Johannesburg: Wits University Press, 2009.

Office of the United Nations High Commissioner for Human Rights and the Joint United Nations Programme on HIV/AIDS. *International Guidelines on HIV/AIDS and Human Rights*. Second International Consultation on HIV/AIDS and Human Rights, Geneva, 23–25 September 1996. New York: United Nations, 1998, HR/PUB/98/1.

Okagbue, Osita. *African Theatres and Performances.* London: Routledge, 2007.

Okome, Onookome. "Nollywood, Lagos, and the *Good-Time* Woman." *Research in African Literatures* 43, no. 4 (2012): 166–86.

O'Manique, Colleen. "Global Neoliberalism and AIDS Policy: International Responses to Sub-Saharan Africa's Pandemic." *Studies in Political Economy* 73 (2004): 47–68.

———. *Neoliberalism and AIDS Crisis in Sub-Saharan Africa: Globalization's Pandemic.* New York: Palgrave Macmillan, 2004.

Ong, Aihwa. *Neoliberalism as Exception: Mutations in Citizenship and Sovereignty.* Durham: Duke University Press, 2006.

Oppong, Christine, M. Yaa, P. A. Oppong, and Irene K. Odotei. *Sex and Gender in an Era of AIDS: Ghana at the Turn of the Millennium.* Accra, Ghana: Sub-Saharan Publishers, 2006.

Pagézy, Hélène. "Le Théâtre *koteba* comme support de messages pour la prévention du sida au Mali." In *Anthropologie et sida: Bilan et perspectives,* edited by Jean Benoist and Alice Desclaux, 323–29. Paris: Karthala, 1996.

Parker, Richard G., Delia Easton, and Charles H. Klein. "Structural Barriers and Facilitators in HIV Prevention: A Review of International Research." *AIDS* 14, supplement 1, no. 1 (2000): S22–32.

Patton, Cindy. *Inventing AIDS.* New York: Routledge, 1990.

Paulme, Denise. "Typologie des contes africains du Décepteur (A Typology of African Trickster Tales)." *Cahiers d'Études africaines* 15, no. 60 (1975): 569–600.

Pauvert, Jean-Claude and Max Egly. *Le "Complexe" de Bouaké, 1967–1981.* Paris: Association des anciens fonctionnaires de l'Unesco, 2001.

Pégatiénan, Jacques H. and Didier A. Blibolo. *Impact socio-économique à long terme du VIH/SIDA sur les enfants et les politiques de réponse: Le cas de la Côte d'Ivoire.* Fonds des Nations-unies pour l'enfance, Bureau Côte d'Ivoire, 2002. https://www.unicef.org/evaldatabase/files/2002_Senegal_AIDS_rec_347660.pdf.

PEPFAR. "Côte d'Ivoire Country Operational Plan (COP) 2017: Strategic Direction Summary." March 2017. https://www.pepfar.gov/documents/organization/272009.pdf.

Perez, Hiram. "*Alma Latina*: The American Hemisphere's Racial Melodramas." *S&F Online* 7, no. 2 (Spring 2009): 1–4. http://sfonline.barnard.edu/africana/perez_01.htm.

Pfeiffer, James. "Condom Social Marketing, Pentecostalism, and Structural Adjustment in Mozambique: A Clash of AIDS Prevention Messages." *Medical Anthropology Quarterly* 18, no. 1 (2004): 77–103.

———. "The Struggle for a Public Sector: PEPFAR in Mozambique." In *When People Come First: Critical Studies in Global Health,* edited by João Biehl and Adriana Petryna, 166–81. Princeton: Princeton University Press, 2013.

Poku, Nana K. "Poverty, Debt and Africa's HIV/AIDS Crisis." *International Affairs* 78, no. 3 (2002): 531–46.

Population Services International. "PSI: Approaches." http://www.psi.org/work-impact/approaches/.

———. "PSI at a Glance." http://www.psi.org/about/at-a-glance/.

———. "Social Marketing: Evidence Base." http://www.psi.org/research/evidence/psi-social-marketing-evidence-base/.

Pourrut, X., A. Galat-Luong, and G. Galat. "Associations du Singe vert avec d'autres espèces de Primates au Sénégal." *Revue de médecine vétérinaire* 147 (1996): 47–58.

Povinelli, Elizabeth A. *Economies of Abandonment: Social Belonging and Endurance in Late Liberalism*. Durham: Duke University Press, 2011.

Price, Neil. "The Performance of Social Marketing in Reaching the Poor and Vulnerable in AIDS Control Programmes." *Health Policy and Planning* 16, no. 3 (2001): 231–39.

Proteau, Laurence. *Passions scolaires en Côte d'Ivoire: École, État et société*. Paris: Karthala, 2002.

Pype, Katrien. *The Making of the Pentecostal Melodrama: Religion, Media and Gender in Kinshasa*. New York: Berghahn Books, 2012.

Quayson, Ato. "Obverse Denominations: Africa?" *Public Culture* 14, no. 3 (2002): 585–88.

Raulin, H. "Le Droit des personnes et de la famille en Côte d'Ivoire." In *Le Droit de la famille en Afrique noire et à Madagascar*, edited by Kéba M'Baye, 221–41. Paris: G.-P. Maisonneuve et Larose, 1968.

Reed, Daniel B. "'C'est le wake up! Africa': Two Case Studies of HIV/AIDS Edutainment Campaigns in Francophone Africa." In *The Culture of AIDS in Africa: Hope and Healing through Music and the Arts*, edited by Gregory Barz and Judah M. Cohen, 180–92. New York: Oxford University Press, 2011.

République de Côte d'Ivoire, Ministère de l'éducation nationale, Secrétariat d'état chargé de l'enseignement primaire et de la télévision éducative. *Actualisation du programme d'éducation télévisuelle, 1973–1976*. Abidjan, May 1973.

République de Côte d'Ivoire and Conseil National de Lutte contre le SIDA. *Rapport National 2012*, 2012.

Rhine, Kathryn A. *The Unseen Things: Women, Secrecy, and HIV in Northern Nigeria*. Bloomington: Indiana University Press, 2016.

Robinson, Rachel Sullivan. *Intimate Interventions in Global Health: Family Planning and HIV Prevention in Sub-Saharan Africa*. Cambridge: Cambridge University Press, 2017.

Rony, Fatimah Tobing. *The Third Eye: Race, Cinema, and Ethnographic Spectacle*. Durham: Duke University Press, 1996.

Santelli, John S., Ilene S. Speizer, and Zoe R. Edelstein. "Abstinence Promotion under PEPFAR: The Shifting Focus of HIV Prevention for Youth." *Global Public Health: An International Journal for Research, Policy and Practice* 8, no. 1 (2013): 1–12.

Schiller, Nina Glick, Stephen Crystal, and Denver Lewellen, "Risky Business: The Cultural Construction of AIDS Risk Groups." *Social Science and Medicine* 38, no. 10 (1994): 1337–46.

Schoepf, Brooke Grundfest. "AIDS." In *A Companion to the Anthropology of Politics*, edited by David Nugent and Joan Vincent, 37–54. Malden, MA: Blackwell, 2004.

———. "Assessing AIDS Research in Africa: Twenty-Five Years Later." *African Studies Review* 53, no. 1 (2010): 105–42.

———. "Culture, Sex Research and AIDS Prevention in Africa." In *Culture and Sexual Risk: Anthropological Perspectives on AIDS*, edited by Hans Ten Brummelhuis and Gilbert Herdt, 29–52. Amsterdam: Gordon and Breach Publishers, 1995.

Schoepf, Brooke G., Claude Schoepf, and Joyce Millen. "Theoretical Therapies, Remote Remedies: SAPs and the Political Ecology of Poverty and Health in Africa." In *Dying for Growth: Global Inequality and the Health of the Poor*, edited by Jim Y. Kim, Joyce V. Millen, Alec Irwin, and John Gershman, 91–126. Monroe, ME: Common Courage Press, 2000.

Schumann, Anne. "A Generation of Orphans: The Socio-Economic Crisis in Côte d'Ivoire as Seen through Popular Music." *Africa: The Journal of the International African Institute* 82, no. 4 (2012): 535–55.

Seidel, Gill and Laurent Vidal. "The Implications of 'Medical,' 'Gender in Development' and 'Culturalist' Discourses for HIVAIDS Policy in Africa." In *Anthropology of Policy: Critical Perspectives on Governance and Power*, edited by Cris Shore and Susan Wright, 59–87. New York: Routledge, 1997.

Séry, Dédy and Tapé Gozé. "Jeunesse, sexualité et sida à Abidjan." In *Les Sciences sociales face au SIDA: Cas africains autour de l'exemple Ivoirien*, edited by Jean Pierre Dozon and Laurent Vidal, 83–86. Paris: ORSTOM, 1995.

Shapiro, David and Dominique Meekers. "Target Audience Reach of the *SIDA Dans La Cité* AIDS Prevention Series in Côte d'Ivoire." *Social Marketing Quarterly* 6, no. 4 (2000): 21–30.

Shapiro, D., D. Meekers, and B. Tambashe. "Exposure to the 'SIDA dans la Cité' AIDS Prevention Television Series in Côte d'Ivoire, Sexual Risk Behaviour and Condom Use." *AIDS Care* 15, no. 3 (2003): 303–14.

Sharp, Paul M. and Beatrice H. Hahn. "Origins of HIV and the AIDS Pandemic." *Cold Spring Harbor Perspecti.ves in Medicine* 1, no. 1 (2011): 1–22.

Singer, Linda. *Erotic Welfare: Sexual Theory and Politics in the Age of Epidemic*, edited by Judith Butler and Maureen MacGrogan. New York: Routledge, 1993.

Singhal, Arvind and Everett M. Rogers. *Entertainment-Education: A Communication Strategy for Social Change*. Mahwah, NJ: Lawrence Erlbaum Associates, 1999.

Siomopoulos, Anna. "Political Theory and Melodrama Studies." *Camera Obscura* 21, no. 2 (2006): 178–83.

Sow, Alioune. "Alternating Views: Malian Cinema, Television Serials, and Democratic Experience." *Africa Today* 55, no. 4 (2009): 51–70.

Spivak, Gayatri Chakravorty. "Can the Subaltern Speak?" In *Can the Subaltern Speak?: Reflections on the History of an Idea*, edited by Rosalind C. Morris. New York: Columbia University Press, 2010.

Stepan, Jan. "Preface." In *La Loi et l'avortement dans les pays francophones*, by Bartha Maria Knoppers and Isabel Brault. Montréal: Éditions Thémis, 1989.

Stillwaggon, Eileen. *AIDS and the Ecology of Poverty*. New York: Oxford University Press, 2005.

Suret-Canale, Jean. *French Colonialism in Tropical Africa 1900–1945*. New York: Pica Press, 1971.

Susser, Ida. *AIDS, Sex, and Culture: Global Politics and Survival in Southern Africa*. Malden, MA: Wiley Blackwell, 2009.

Tallon, Brigitte. "Le Français de Moussa." *Capitales de la Couleur* 9 (1984): 148–55.

Tamale, Sylvia. *African Sexualities: A Reader*. Cape Town: Pambazuka Press, 2011.

Tambashe, B. Oleko, Ilene S. Speizer, Agbessi Amouzou, and A. M. Rachelle Djangone. "Evaluation of the PSAMAO 'Roulez Protégé' Mass Media Campaign in Burkina Faso." *AIDS Education and Prevention* 15, no. 1 (2003): 33–48.

Tapsoba, Clément. "La Dérision contre l'intolérance." *Ecrans d'Afrique* 8 (1994): 14–17.

———. "*Sida dans la cité II/AIDS in the City*." *Ecrans d'Afrique* 17–18 (1996): 88–90.

Tcheuyap, Alexie. "Comedy of Power, Power of Comedy: Strategic Transformations in African Cinemas." *Journal of African Cultural Studies* 22 (2010): 25–40.

———. *Postnationalist African Cinema*. Manchester: Manchester University Press, 2011.

Thackway, Melissa. *Africa Shoots Back: Alternative Perspectives in Sub-Saharan Francophone African Film.* Bloomington: Indiana University Press, 2003.

Thomann, Matthew. "HIV Vulnerability and the Erasure of Sexual and Gender Diversity in Abidjan, Côte d'Ivoire." *Global Public Health* 11, nos. 7–8 (2016): 994–1009.

———. "Zones of Difference, Boundaries of Access: Moral Geography and Community Mapping in Abidjan, Côte d'Ivoire." *Journal of Homosexuality* 63, no. 3 (2016): 426–36.

Thomas, Lynn M. "Gendered Reproduction: Placing Schoolgirl Pregnancies in African History." In *Africa after Gender?* edited by Catherine M. Cole, Takyiwaa Manuh, and Stephan F. Miescher, 48–62. Bloomington: Indiana University Press, 2007.

———. "Modernity's Failings, Political Claims, and Intermediate Concepts." *The American Historical Review* 116, no. 3 (2011): 727–40.

———. *The Politics of the Womb: Women, Reproduction, and the State in Kenya.* Berkeley: University of California Press, 2003.

Thonneau Patrick, Yao Djanhan, Murielle Tran, Christianne Welfens-Ekra, Marcelin Bohoussou, and Emile Papiernik. "The Persistence of a High Maternal Mortality Rate in the Ivory Coast." *American Journal of Public Health* 86 (1996): 1478–79.

Thornton, Robert J. *Unimagined Community: Sex, Networks, and AIDS in Uganda and South Africa.* Berkeley: University of California Press, 2008.

Toungara, Jeanne M. "The Apotheosis of Côte d'Ivoire's Nana Houphouët-Boigny." *The Journal of Modern African Studies* 28, no. 1 (1990): 23–54.

———. "Changing the Meaning of Marriage: Women and Family Law in Côte d'Ivoire." In *African Feminism: The Politics of Survival in Sub-Saharan Africa,* edited by Gwendolyn Mikell, 53–76. Philadelphia: University of Pennsylvania Press, 1997.

———. "Inventing the African Family: Gender and Family Law Reform in Cote d'Ivoire." *Journal of Social History* 28, no. 1 (1994): 37–61.

Touré, Khadidia. "Telenovelas Reception by Women in Bouaké (Côte d'Ivoire) and Bamako (Mali)." *Visual Anthropology* 20, no. 1 (2007): 41–56.

Touré, Kitia. "Sida et liberté." *Présence Africaine Volume Spéciale: Cinémas et libertés: Contribution au thème de FEPASCO* 93 (1993): 81–87.

———. *Destins parallèles.* Abidjan: Nouvelles Éditions Ivoiriennes, 1995.

Touré, Kolo and Henri Munier. "Primary Education by Television in the Ivory Coast." *UNESCO Chronicle* 21, no. 11 (1975): 308–14.

Touré, Saliou. *L'Ivoirité, ou, l'esprit du nouveau contrat social du Président Henri Konan Bédié, Actes du forum Curdiphe du 20 au 23 mars 1996. Abidjan. Ethics.* Curdiphe: Presses Universitaires d'Abidjan, 1996.

Tozzo, Émile A. "La Réforme des médias publics en Afrique de l'Ouest: Servir le gouvernement ou le citoyen?" *Politique africaine* 1, no. 97 (2005): 99–115.

Treichler, Paula A. *How to Have Theory in an Epidemic: Cultural Chronicles of AIDS.* Durham: Duke University Press, 1999.

Trouillot, Michel-Rolph. "The Vulgarity of Power." *Public Culture* 5, no. 1 (1992): 75–81.

Tudesq, André-Jean. *Les Médias en Afrique.* Paris: Ellipses, 1999.

———. "Problems of Press Freedom in Côte d'Ivoire." In *Press Freedom and Communication in Africa,* edited by Festus Eribo and William Jong-Ebot. Trenton, NJ: Africa World Press, 1998.

———. "La Télévision en Côte d'Ivoire." *African Media Cultures: Transdisciplinary Perspectives/ Cultures de médias en Afrique: Perspectives transdisciplinaires*, edited by Rose Marie Beck and Frank Wittmann, 241–62. Köln: Rüdiger Köppe Verlag, 2004.

Ukadike, Nwachukwu Frank. *Black African Cinema*. Berkeley: University of California Press, 1994.

UNAIDS. *25th Meeting of the UNAIDS Programme Coordinating Board, Geneva Switzerland. Conference Room Paper. Second Independent Evaluation 2002–2008 Country Visit to Côte d'Ivoire*. Geneva, 2009.

———. *90-90-90: An Ambitious Treatment Target to End the AIDS Epidemic*. Geneva: Joint United Nations Programme on AIDS, 2014. http://www.unaids.org/sites/default/files/media_asset/90-90-90_en.pdf.

———. *2011–2015 Strategy: Getting to Zero*. Geneva: Joint United Nations Programme on AIDS, 2010. http://www.unaids.org/sites/default/files/sub_landing/files/JC2034_UNAIDS_Strategy_en.pdf.

———. *Condom Social Marketing: Selected Case Studies*. Geneva: UNAIDS, 2000. http://www.unaids.org/sites/default/files/media_asset/jc1195-condsocmark_en_0.pdf.

———. *Data: 2017*. Geneva, 2017. http://www.unaids.org/sites/default/files/media_asset/20170720_Data_book_2017_en.pdf.

UNAIDS and WHO. *Côte d'Ivoire: Epidemiological Fact Sheet on HIV/AIDS and Sexually Transmitted Infections, 2000 Update*. http://pdf.usaid.gov/pdf_docs/Pnacl531.pdf.

UNAIDS, WHO, and UNDP. *Policy Brief: Using TRIPS Flexibilities to Improve Access to HIV Treatment*. Geneva, 2011. http://www.unaids.org/sites/default/files/media_asset/JC2049_PolicyBrief_TRIPS_en_1.pdf.

UNDP, UN-HABITAT, and Urban Management Program, Regional Office for Africa. *HIV/AIDS and Local Governance in Sub-Saharan Africa*. Occasional Paper 1, June 2002.

UNESCO. *Globalization and Women's Vulnerabilities to HIV and AIDS*. Paris: Division for Gender Equality, 2010. http://unesdoc.unesco.org/images/0019/001915/191501e.pdf.

UN Inter-agency Group for Child Mortality Estimation. *Levels and Trends in Child Mortality*. New York: UN Children's Fund, 2017. https://www.unicef.org/publications/files/Child_Mortality_Report_2017.pdf.

United States Leadership against HIV/AIDS, Tuberculosis, and Malaria Act of 2003. Public Law 108-25, 117 STAT 711, May 27, 2003. https://www.congress.gov/108/plaws/publ25/PLAW-108publ25.pdf.

Useche, Bernardo and Amalia L. Cabezas, "The Vicious Cycle of AIDS, Poverty, and Neoliberalism." In *The Wages of Empire: Neoliberal Policies, Repression, and Women's Poverty*, edited by Amalia L. Cabezas, Ellen Reese, and Marguerite Waller, 16–27. Boulder: Paradigm, 2007.

Vangah, Désiré. "Le Statut de la femme mariée dans le nouveau droit de la famille en Côte d'Ivoire." *Revue juridique et politique, indépendance et coopération* 21 (1967): 96–101.

Vaughan, Megan. *Curing Their Ills: Colonial Power and African Illness*. Stanford: Stanford University Press, 1991.

Vidal, Laurent. "Images du sida dans le regard d'un quotidien ivoirien (1988–1994)." *Politique Africaine* 56 (1994): 158–63.

Videau, André. "*Rue Princesse*: Film ivoirien de Henri Duparc." *Hommes et Migrations* 1180 (1994): 62.

Viens, Pierre. "'Le GPA attendait des PNLS une soumission totale. . . .'" *Le Journal du sida* 86–87 (1996): 106–8.

Vléï-Yoroba, Chantal. "Droit de la famille et réalités familiales: Le cas de la Côte d'Ivoire depuis l'indépendance." *Clio: Femmes, Genre, Histoire* (1997): 1–6. http://journals.openedition.org/clio/383.

Vogel, Ronald J. *Cost Recovery in the Health Care Sector: Selected Country Studies in West Africa.* World Bank Technical Paper Number 82. Washington, DC, May 1988. http://documents.worldbank.org/curated/en/431061468774699528/pdf/multi-page.pdf.

Vuylsteke, Bea, Gisèle Semdé, Lazare Sika, Tania Crucitti, Virginie Ettiègne Traoré, Anne Buvé, and Marie Laga. "HIV and STI Prevalence among Female Sex Workers in Côte d'Ivoire: Why Targeted Prevention Programs Should Be Continued and Strengthened." *Plos One* 7, no. 3 (2012): 1–6.

Vuylsteke, Bea and Smrajit Jana. "Reducing HIV Risk in Sex Workers, Their Clients and Partners." In *HIV/AIDS Prevention and Care in Resource-Constrained Settings: A Handbook for the Design and Management of Programs*, edited by Peter R. Lamptey and Helene D. Gayle, 187–210. Arlington, VA: Family Health International, 2001. https://pdf.usaid.gov/pdf_docs/pnacy892.pdf.

Warner, Michael. *Publics and Counterpublics*. New York: Zone Books, 2002.

Watney, Simon. "The Spectacle of AIDS." In *Lesbian and Gay Studies Reader*, edited by Henry Abelove, Michèle Aina Barale, and David M. Halperin, 202–11. New York: Routledge, 1993.

Wendland, Claire L. "Animating Biomedicine's Moral Order: The Crisis of Practice in Malawian Medical Training." *Current Anthropology* 53, no. 6 (2012): 755–88.

———. "Research, Therapy, and Bioethical Hegemony: The Controversy over Perinatal AZT Trials in Africa." *African Studies Review* 51, no. 3 (2008): 1–23.

WHO. *Côte d'Ivoire: Estimated Number of People Needing Antiretroviral Therapy (0–49 years), 2005*. http://www.who.int/hiv/HIVCP_CIV.pdf.

———. *HIV/AIDS: Mother-to-Child Transmission of HIV*, November 29, 2016. http://www.who.int/hiv/topics/mtct/about/en/.

WHO and UNAIDS. *HIV in Pregnancy: A Review*, 1998. http://www.unaids.org/sites/default/files/media_asset/jc151-hiv-in-pregnancy_en_1.pdf.

WHO, UNICEF, UNFPA, World Bank Group, and United Nations Population Division Maternal Mortality Estimation Inter-Agency Group. *Maternal Mortality in 1990–2015: Côte d'Ivoire*. http://www.who.int/gho/maternal_health/countries/civ.pdf.

Widmark, Annica. "The Success of Amah." M.A. thesis, Malmö University, 2002.

Williams, Linda. "Melodrama Revised." In *Refiguring American Film Genres: Theory and History*, edited by Nick Browne, 42–88. Berkeley: University of California Press, 1998.

———. *Playing the Race Card: Melodramas of Black and White from Uncle Tom to O. J. Simpson*. Princeton: Princeton University Press, 2002.

Wondji, Christophe. "La Fièvre jaune à Grand-Bassam (1899–1903)." *Revue française d'histoire d'Outre-Mer* 59, no. 215, 2e trimestr (1972): 205–39.

Woods, Dwayne. "The Politicization of Teachers' Associations in the Côte d'Ivoire." *African Studies Review* 39, no. 3 (1996): 113–29.

World Bank. *Data, Côte d'Ivoire*, World Bank, 2018. http://data.worldbank.org/country/cote-divoire.

———. *Republic of Ivory Coast: Staff Appraisal Report, Third Education Project*. Projects Department, Education Division: Western Africa Regional Office, 1979. http://documents.banquemondiale.org/curated/fr/612641468262484464/text/multi-page.txt.

———. *World Bank, Project Performance Audit Report: Ivory Coast First Education Project (Loan 667-IVC)*, May 8, 1980. http://documents.banquemondiale.org/curated/fr/682961468025499798/pdf/multi-page.pdf.

WTO, General Council. *Implementation of Paragraph 6 of the Doha Declaration on the TRIPS Agreement and Public Health, Decision of the General Council of 30 August 2003*, September 1, 2003. WT/L/540 and Corr. 1. https://www.wto.org/english/tratop_e/trips_e/implem_para6_e.htm.

Wynchank, Anny. "Persistance du théâtre populaire traditionnel en Afrique." In *New Theatre in Francophone and Anglophone Africa*, edited by Anne Fuchs, 49–59. Amsterdam: Editions Rodopi, 1999.

Yang, Suzanne. "Speaking of the Surface: The Texts of Kaposi's Sarcoma." In *Homosexuality and Psychoanalysis*, edited by Tim Dean and Christopher Lane, 322–48. Chicago: University of Chicago Press, 2001.

Yao, Koudajo Faustin. "Communication Technology Transfer for Development: Issues from the Ivory Coast Educational Television Program." PhD diss., Stanford University, 1983. ProQuest Dissertations and Theses.

Zoungrana, Cécile Marie, Benjamin Zanou, Amani Koffi, Lanssina Touré, B. Oleko Tambashe, and Rob Eiger. *La Prévention du Sida en Côte d'Ivoire: Rôle des médias de masse et de la série Sida dans la Cité 2 dans les attitudes générales vis-à-vis du Sida et les comportements à risque.* SFPS, PSI/ECODEV. Abidjan, 1999.

INDEX

Abidjan, 12, 28, 30, 33, 36, 85, 102, 124, 185; Awareness Center, 148; SOTRA (Société des Transports Abidjanais), 133–35, 135n69; University Hospital Center, 32

Abitbol, Elliette, 98n7

abortion, 109–10, 128, 132

abstinence, 3, 12, 47, 188, 193, 203–4; funders' mandates, 12, 204; and PEPFAR, 12, 204

Abu-Lughod, Lila, 12–13

"Adams the Driver": 13, 152, 154–55; heterosexual reproductivity, 156; marriage rewards self-management, 140, 156; melodrama, 16, 141; social marketing pedagogy, 153

Africa: Algeria, 106; Burkina Faso, 7, 23, 101n6, 121n54, 124–26, 181, 192; elite planters, 98; Francophone "educated natives [*évolués*]," 62; Ghana, 36; Guinea, 16, 192; Kenya, 143, 179n19; Mali, 28, 52, 181, 192; Mozambique, 205n5; Niger, 55, 126n59 (*see also* Nollywood); poverty and lack of services, 111, 151; Rwanda, 18n2; South Africa, 1n3, 10n30, 21, 166n59, 185, 205; stereotyped as primitive and depraved, 28–30, 32; stereotyped as primitive, innocent, but corrupted, 29; stereotypes of sexuality, 30, 132; Tanzania, 143, 152n49; Uganda, 45n91; Upper Volta (*see* Burkina Faso); western "heart of darkness" discourse, 21; Zaire, 32. *See also* Cameroon

"African AIDS": construction of, 30, 32; and heterosexuality, 132; racialized and sexualized definition, 14, 21, 30, 49

African banks: African Bank Company, 180; African Development Bank, 180n22; Inter-African Bank Company, 280

African cinema, 9, 65, 85n113; and decolonization, 9; film and video scholarship, 11; foreign producers of, 11; Francophone, 9, 9n256, 146; Nollywood videos, 80, 141n11, 144, 185; Pan African Federation of Filmmakers (FEPACI), 9; pedagogy and, 156n51, 173

Agamben, Giorgio: biopolitics and the modern state, 5; and *homo sacer,* 56, 108; state of exception, 5, 15; suspension of law in states of emergency, 105–8, 137

AIDS in the City, 121, 127–28, 157–59; dangers of, 128–29, 136, 158–59; *Gestures or Life* and, 96, 101–5, 111; and HIV-positive women, 96, 101, 109–13; as HIV prevention, 5, 122, 127, 158; HIV transmission not reduced by, 204–5; illegality of, 96, 106–12, 129; as infanticide, 108–9, 130, 136; pressure to abort and human rights,

229

128; religious prohibitions, 96, 112; and state of emergency, 105–6, 109–13, 137; U.S. policy, 10, 105–6, 128, 205. *See also* PEPFAR; perinatal transmission; PMI; USAID

AIDS in the City 1, 121, 136; and abortion, 121, 124; CNLS prevention clip, 157–58; and condom usage, 121; culpable promiscuity, 132, 137; fidelity, 121; foreign funders' mandates, 121–22; heterosexual family as prophylaxis, 121; pregnant HIV-infected woman destroys families, 120–23; reproductive and political legitimacy, 137

AIDS in the City 2, 121, 123, 136; and abortion, 121, 124; culpable promiscuity, 123, 132, 137; enlightened male authorities, 124–25; foreign funders' mandates, 121–22; gender struggle, 124; pregnant HIV-infected women destroy families, 120–23, 132; reproductive and political legitimacy, 137

AIDS in the City 3, 96, 121, 136; marriage rewards self-management, 140; melodrama, 141; narratives of redemption, 137, 140. *See also* "Adams the Driver"; "Amoin Séry"; "Fatoumata: HIV-Positive Mother"; "The Story of the Fiancés"

AIMAS (Agence Ivoirienne de Marketing Social) 147, 193n35

Allen, Robert C., 142n14, 168

Alpha Blondy, 67n81, 147–48; *AIDS in the City* theme song, 147

Amad, Paula, 25

Amah Djah-Foulé 1 and *2*, 16, 169, 170, 173, 175, 192–93, 200

Amah Djah-Foulé 1, 16; condoms, lubrication, and testing, 193–95; and the Confidence Clinic, 193–96, 198; entrepreneurialism and empowerment, 196–98, 202; eradication of sex-work, 202; marriage rewards HIV-negative test, 195; sex-work demeaning, 16, 196; social marketing of products and services, 193–94

Amah Djah-Foulé 2: confessional technologies, 199–200; entrepreneurialism and empowerment, 196–99, 202; funders' mandates, 196; and NGOs, 199, 200–201; restoring gendered order, 196, 198; sex-work as obstacle to "real family," 196, 198; sex-work viable option for women, 201; stigmatization of HIV-positive people and sex workers, 198

"Amoin Séry," 169, 173, 183–84, 186–87: Baoulé and Bété combined in name, 191; corruption of the big city, 185, 188–90, 192; foreign funders' mandates, 170; the "good-time woman" of melodrama, 185; multiple partners, 139, 184; polygamy, 184, 186–88; reintegration into patriarchal family, 189, 192, 201–2; rural village 188–92; sexual naiveté, 187; traditional healers, 187–88; unprotected sex, 187; witchcraft, 188, 191

Andreasen, Alan, 146

Assamoi, Léon N'Cho, 15, 53; also known as Old Headscarf, 50–51, 84–85, 90–92

Association of Ivorian Women (Association des Femmes Ivoiriennes), 99

Atchié, Paul, 84–85

austerity: and development, 14, 21–22; empowerment, 199; funder-mandated, 3; Houphouët-Boigny and 35; *Moussa* on, 34, 38, 49; rejection of sexual austerity, 34, 50, 78–79, 85; self-discipline and, 92; sexual and economic, 14, 22, 28, 50, 73; submission to, 50; and structural adjustment, 4, 27, 73, 94

Awareness Center, 148, 156

Ayé, Jean-Pierre, 27n35, 108

Bailly, Diégou, 24, 67n81, 93n120

Bakary, Bamba, 93

Bakhtin, Mikhail, 25

Barrera, Vitoria, 143

Bayart, Jean-François, 178–79. *See also* "politics of the belly"

Bayer, Ronald, 103

Béchio, Jean-Jacques, 73–74

Bedié, Henri Konan, 128, 129n64, 167: as Houphouët-Boigny's successor, 122–23, 191; identified as Baoulé, 191; and *Ivoirité*, 123, 191

behavior change communication (BCC). *See under* HIV/AIDS prevention media

Belgium, aid to Côte d'Ivoire, 57n29, 143, 192, 199

Bielby, Denise D., 143

Big Questions, The: and the "AIDS episode" of *How's it going*, 67, 79; close-ups of sores and growths, 69; condom use, 67, 69; Minister of Health appears on, 72

biomedical authority, 16; hegemonic, 205; and social marketing, 157; submission to,

97, 136; and technical progress, 205; and traditional medicine, 188
biopolitics, 5; and HIV prevention media, 6; politicization, 105; postcolonial, 108–9; and reproduction, 107; zero-sum calculus, 110
Brooks, Peter, 139, 165
Brown, Wendy, 3

CAFP (Centres d'Animation et de Formation Pédagogique), 58
Cameroon: influence of Cameroonian comedy, 25, 93; "politics of the belly," 178–79; public ceremonies in, 26. *See also* Guignol; Kankan, Jean-Michel; Nbo, Daniel
Campbell, Joseph W., 22, 61n53
capitalism: and economic development, 27n35, 98; global markets, 8; reliance on foreign capital, 19; sex work as capital, 180. *See also* structural adjustment
CARE, 193
CARID (Centre Africain de Recherche et d'Intervention en Développement), 47
CATEL (Compagnie Africaine de Télévision; African Television Company), 57
CETV (Complexe d'Éducation Télévisuelle), 55
Chauveau, Jean-Pierre, 19, 166n60
CHI (Centre hospitalier universitaire), 109
Christianity: disease prevention and morality, 97, 204; white religious, technological, medical authority, 102–3
CIDA (Canadian International Development Agency), 57n29
CNLS (Comité national de lutte contre le Sida): and condoms, 69; education campaign, 45, 67, 77, 157; and *Gestures or Life*, 101; and *How's it going?*, 77; WHO funding for, 45. *See also* PNLS; WHO
Coca-Cola Africa Foundation, 147
Comaroff, Jean, 6, 148, 164n57, 187
Comaroff, John K., 187
condoms, 11, 39, 42–43, 45, 115, 153, 188; believed to cause AIDS, 83n106; and "healthy carriers," 114; and *How's it going?*, 8; *Moussa* on, 39, 41; initially only available at pharmacies, 68n83, 76; NGOs and, 69, 86n114, 177; and *Princess Street*, 175, 177; RAP-MC's "Young People, Put on a Condom," 86n114; use conforms to "proper" gender roles, 76;

Wintin Wintin's comic misunderstanding of, 86–87; women demand partners use, 75–77, 86–87, 124. *See also* Prudence condoms
Confidence Clinic, 192–95; *Amah Djah-Foulé 1* promotes, 192–95, 198; foreign funders, 192–93, 196; and "Place of Confidence" NGO, 198–99; and sex-workers, 192–94, 198–99
Contamin, Bernard, 20
Coulibaly, Luzéni, 98, 99n12
Craddock, Susan, 145

Dadié, Bernard Binlin, 52, 93n119
Decoteau, Claire, 11
Delaunay, Karine, 123, 151n48
Désalmand, Paul, 61
Deutscher, Penelope, 105–8
Dioula, 153, 192; *Gestures or Life* theme song, 102; *grins*, 199n40; Moussa as Dioula immigrant, 23n21; Muslim Northerners, 167, 183, 192; status of, 167, 191. *See also* Dioula *under* languages of Côte d'Ivoire; *Moussa*, Tiébé, Alain Djédjé
diseases: cancer, 31; diarrhea, 18n20, 111, 152; gonorrhea (clap), 31, 43, 155; malaria, 18, 18n2, 67n81, 111; "numerous epidemics," 42; pneumonia, 29, 111; and poverty, 111; STDs, 41, 155, 193, 203; syphilis, 32, 194; yaws, 32n54. *See also* HIV/AIDS epidemic
Dosso, Mireille, 46
Dosso, Mousso. *See* Tiébé, Alain Djédjé
Drive Protected, 152, 154
drug use: and AIDS, 32–33, 42; campaign against addiction, 66; and homosexuality, 33, 42; prevention and repression of, 66–67; users socially excluded, 6, 16, 32, 132, 137, 140, 168; and sex-workers, 35, 41
Duggan, Lisa, 3
Duparc, Henri, 169, 170n4; and health education, 173–74; *Sweetheart*, 178. See also *Princess Street* (*Rue Princesse*)

ECODEV (Étude, Conseil, Formation et Développement), 193n35
economic issues and crises, 19–20, 55, 61, 78, 170, 180–81; devalued currency, 122; export crops, 4, 19, 61, 78, 122, 181; failure to enter "free market," 151; gendered effects of crises, 170, 180; internal

migration, 78, 19, 41, 66, 107n27, 151, 169, 181, 184, 198, 205; "Ivorian miracle," 19; Keynesian economics and the welfare state, 149; oil crisis, 4, 19; periods of instability, 4, 50, 94, 150; World Bank and IMF assistance, 19–20. *See also* capitalism; poverty; structural adjustment

education, 62–63, 78: educated natives [évolués], 62, 190; educational capital, 62; educational television and national identity, 64; entrance exams, 61, 63; foreign funderd, 55; and French models, 56n25, 63n63; literacy, 55; Ministry of Education, 53, 55, 56; Ministry of Youth and Popular Education, 55; Radio-Télé-Bac, 55; and visual arts, 9, 11. *See also* PETV; SYNESCI; SYNARES

elections, 61, 123; contested presidential elections 60, 129n64, 191; first multi-party, 15, 50, 78; single party, 35, 60

Elsaesser, Thomas, 160

empowerment: and austerity, 199; coming out with HIV as, 195; entrepreneurialism and, 197, 200, 202; gendered, 4, 16, 170–71, 196, 205; love as source of, 199n40; and self-help, 175, 196; and sex-workers, 173, 192, 196, 200; unassisted, 202; women's, 12, 170, 172, 178, 184, 196, 200, 202

epidemiology: categories and risk groups, 13, 140; HIV surveillance system, 45n90

Epprecht, Marc, 30, 132–33

Esacove, Anna, 5n13, 11n33

ethnic groups: Akan, 10n3, 60; Akan-Baoulé, 167; Alladian, 191; Baoulé, 157, 166–67, 183, 191; Baoulé-Bété, 192; Bété, 7, 85n110, 157, 166–67, 191–92; Dioula, 7, 23n21, 85n110, 157, 166, 167n63, 183, 191–92, 199n40; Ebrié, 165; intermarriage between, 166–67, 183, 191; Malinké, 157; Mandé, 191, 199; and opposing political parties, 167. *See also* languages in Côte d'Ivoire

ethnonationalism, 4, 6, 123. *See also* Ivoirité

European Union, 101

excluded groups, 6, 100, 140n5, 167; bisexuals, 140; drug users, 6, 16, 96, 132, 137, 140, 168; foreigners, 6, 128; "homosexuals" gays, 6, 16, 96, 132–33, 137, 140, 168; Muslims, 6, 167; Northerners, 6; "prostitutes" ("whores"), 16, 96, 132–33, 137, 168

FAC (Fonds d'aide et de coopération), 57n29

family: central Ivorian organizing unit, 97; conjugal, 96, 98–99, 105, 136; heteronormative family as prophylaxis, 13, 87, 97, 115–16, 119, 121, 170, 202; HIV-positive persons incorporated into, 114–15, 189; monogamous nuclear, 98, 153; "properly" gendered, 34. *See also* heteronormativity; monogamy; polygamy

Family Health International, 170n4, 192n34

Fassin, Didier, 174. *See also* AIDS denialism

"Fatoumata: HIV-Positive Mother," 96–97, 129–36; against abortion, 96, 129–30, 134; at-risk people excluded, 97, 132–34; and biomedical and patriarchal authority, 96, 133, 135; harmful traditional remedies, 131, 135; HIV-positive women and the reward of family, 96, 129; monogamous reproductive heteronormativity, 132–33; perinatal transmission, 132–35; and private sector, 134–35; responsible living with HIV, 130; testing and treatment for pregnant women and partner, 96, 129, 133–34; treatment access, 134; virtuous motherhood, 132; women's support group, 131, 195

feminist theory, 11–12; against neoliberalism, 141; and behavioral approaches to prevention, 141

fidelity and family as prophylaxis, 12, 40, 47, 77, 87, 99, 121, 131–32, 156, 188; PEPFAR and, 12, 204–5. *See also* infidelity; marriage

foreign donors and prevention media, 5, 21, 77, 88, 92, 100–101, 113, 147, 166n59; against abortion, 121–22; dictate policies, 4, 6, 9–11, 22, 207; foreign/state collaboration, 54, 57n29, 174n12; *Moussa* on, 22, 27, 34, 38, 41; nuclear families and self-discipline, 45, 39, 49; resistance to, 15, 38, 49, 51

Foucault, Michel: biopolitics, 5, 20; homosexuality, 30; "node," 150; state discipline, 5

FPA (français populaire d'Abidjan), *See under* languages of Côte d'Ivoire

FPI (français populaire ivoirien). *See under* languages of Côte d'Ivoire

FPI (Front Populaire Ivoirien; Ivorian Popular Front): supported by the Bété, 167. *See also* Gbagbo, Laurent

France and colonial Côte d'Ivoire: "educated natives [évolués]," 62, 190; forced labor, 7, 98, 181; hierarchies of ethnic groups, 7, 166–67, 91; independence and post-inde-

INDEX • 233

pendence relations, 8, 19, 35, 57, 60, 62, 64, 83, 98, 108, 181; internal migration, 181; market for French goods, 7; North-South divisions in, 7, 64; penal laws and reproductivity, 105–6; and the monogamous nuclear family, 97
France: Institute for Development Research, 175; ORSTOM (*Office de la Recherche Scientifique et Technique d'Outre-Mer*), 5, 7n29, 86n114
Fraternité Hebdo, 22, 26–27
Fraternité Matin, 22, 27n35: on abortion, 108; on AIDS transmission, 44, 74–75, 81, 169; on forbidding women with HIV to reproduce, 159n52; on infidelity and promiscuity, 81; on living in fear, 68n82; and PETV, 60, 63 reportage of early AIDS cases, 35, 169; on R. F. K., 67, 67n81; on teachers' salaries, 62; on "second offices," 75n96; on transvestites, 38n67. *See also* Lebry, Léon Francis; Moussa, Alfred Dan
Freud, Sigmund, 83

Gadeau, Germain Coffi, 52
GATT (General Agreement on Tariffs and Trade), 151
Gbagbo, Laurent, 60, 129n64, 199n40, 201; forced removal of, 206; and the FPI, 167
Gbanou, Sélom Komlan, 24–25
gendered issues and sexualities, 2–4, 6–7, 367, 130; challenging binaries, 6; comic staging of gender conflict, 15, 51, 92; drag queens, 37–8; and koteba satire, 51–52; modernity and, 36–37; precarity, 17, 170, 184–85; recalcitrant male heterosexuality. 51; rural-urban migration, 41; transvestites, 21, 37–38
Germany: Gesellschaft für Technische Zusammenarbeit (GTZ), 147; Kreditanstalt für Wiederaufbau (KfW), 121n54, 147
Gestures or Life, 96, 101, 119, 132, 156; abortion for pregnant HIV-positive women, 103–5, 111, 113, 158; avoids political topics, 136; corporate benevolence, 118; foreign funders, 101; "healthy carriers," 114, 116–18; HIV-positive women in families, 114, 117–18; "In the Name of Love," 114–17; "My Name Is 'Life,'" 119; perinatal transmission, 15, 101–05, 108–11, 113; "Reasons for Fear," 101–2, 110–14; "That Happens Only to Others," 114, 117–18; women living with HIV, 96, 114
Ghosh, Jayati, 145
Gledhill, Christine, 142
government: civil-service cutbacks, 73–74; l'Office national de la promotion rurale, 58; Medium-Term Plan for AIDS prevention, 77; Ministry for AIDS Control, 147; Ministry of the Civil Service, 73–74; Ministry of Culture, 101; Ministry of Education, 53, 55, 56; Ministry of Health, 39, 67, 70, 72n84, 147, 177, 192; Ministry of Health and Public Hygiene, 134; Ministry of Information, 54; Ministry of Primary and Televisual Education, 56; Ministry of Youth and Popular Education, 55
GPA (Global Program on AIDS), 174
Gramsci, Antonio, 26, 26n31
Groguhet, Léonard, 52, 65; compared to Hugo, Voltaire, and Molière, 93; criticizes civil service absenteeism, 74; honored by government, 923; in *How is it going?*, 67–68, 75, 84; inspiration for *Moussa*, 65n75; promotes state policies with humor, 42, 65, 92–93; targets women as vectors, 75; and *Wintin Wintin and Old Headscarf*, 84
Guéï, Robert, 129n64
Guignol, 14, 24–25, 27; gendered male, 25; *The Guignols of Abidjan*, 25; *See also* Gbanou, Sélom Komlan; Kankan, Jean-Michel; *Moussa*: as Guignol; Ndo, Daniel

Haiti, 29
health care, 7–8: child and maternal mortality, 111–12; community or individual management of, 148, 178; and enlightened corporate benevolence, 117–19, 134–35; funder-mandated cutbacks, 4, 10, 175; INLS (Institut national de santé publique), 77; marketization of, 148; and state of emergency, 105–8, 110–12; state sheds responsibility for, 14, 34, 110, 178; traditional medicine, 44, 129, 136, 188. *See also* Houphouët-Boigny; PMI
heteronormativity: enforcing (hetero)sexual morality, 36; and families, 17, 97, 100, 140, 170; and female reproductivity, 137; heterosexual monogamy, 11, 17, 140; in prevention efforts, 3, 11, 13, 17, 137; reproductive heterosexual normativity,

153, 157–58, 167; romantic family, 116, 166; and self-management, 95; and state 98–100

Hirsch, Jennifer H., 159

HIV/AIDS epidemic, 18, 21, 30, 37, 41, 78, 80n103, 100, 135n70, 139, 158, 205; adult HIV/AIDS prevalence, 1, 15–16; AIDS denialism, 21n13, 49, 83, 83n106, 84; AIDS as imaginary or invented, 33–34, 45, 48, 83, 152; and blood transfusion, 32, 40–41, 44, 119; "coming out" about HIV, 195, 199; contesting the origins of, 28–34, 41; as curse, 124–26, 128, 132, 137, 138, 188; as disease of homosexuals, 21, 27, 29, 31–33, 36–37, 118; as disease of whites, 14, 21–22, 28–37; early cases of, 29, 35, 95, 159; fear of contamination, 95, 111, 117, 150; "healthy carriers," 114, 115, 116–17; Kaposi's sarcoma, 69, 80n101; marriage as protection, 40, 47, 68, 77, 87, 121, 133; medical authority, 16, 26, 33, 82, 133, 136–37, 140, 156; partner notification, 103, 105, 114–15, 123–24, 131, 156; perinatal transmission, 15, 100–101, 110–11, 124, 132, 134–35, 139, 164, 166; prevalence among pregnant women, 15, 100–101; as punishment, 15, 50, 69, 72, 83, 84, 92, 125, 132, 138; spread exacerbated by IMF policies, 150; and state of emergency, 105–8, 110–14, 137; stigmatization of HIV-positive people, 115–16, 117n48, 124, 133; symptoms legible on body, 69–78, 80, 124, 157, 184, 194

HIV/AIDS epidemic, problems addressing: delayed or inadequate government response, 2, 47, 173; focus on managing women's reproduction, 95–96, 137; health-care cuts, 3; high cost of patented drugs, 112n45, 160, 166; neoliberal emphasis on self-management, 22, 95

HIV/AIDS prevention media, 49, 78, 95, 117, 129, 144, 152, 159, 170, 175; abstinence, fidelity, and monogamy, 12, 47, 121, 204–5; *AIDS, The Big Meeting*, 67; "AIDS is there . . . It Kills" campaign, 82–84, 103, 123, 128, 132, 134, 160, 161, 167, 195; *The Big Questions*, 67, 69, 72n84; behavior change communication (BCC), 3, 5, 13, 16–17, 40, 44, 47–48, 68, 70, 72, 75, 82, 84, 100, 127–29, 132, 138, 141, 144–51, 152n50, 153, 156, 158, 165, 168, 204, 207; and corporate benevolence, 116–18, 134–35; *Drive Protected*, 152, 154–55; enlightened benevolence and the family, 116–17;

fear arousal, 129, 157; foreign funders, 10, 46, 100, 113, 121, 207; graphic images, 48, 194; individual responsibilization, 3, 105, 138; NGOs, 138, 202; paternalistic authority over women, 16, 84, 96, 105, 136; peer counseling and education 130–31, 133, 177, 195, 198–201; *Right to Health*, 40–41, 72n84; romantic heterosexual love, 138, 160, 170; satirical programs, 15, 25; state campaigns, 4, 6, 8–9; and success and failure to effect change, 6–7, 11, 138, 156; *Super Girl*, 3, 203, 205; women as mouthpieces for, 92, 95

HIV/AIDS, testing and treatment of, 100, 112n44, 121, 124, 134, 159, 163n56; access to, 16, 63, 112–13, 122, 134–36, 159–60, 164–66, 168; antiretrovirals, 112, 134–35, 151; AZT (azidothymidine), 100, 112–13, 112n44; high cost of patented drugs, 112, 151, 159, 163–64; Confidence Clinic, 192–98; NGOs and, 100, 124; testing, 105, 114, 136, 139–40, 151–52, 156–7, 159, 161, 166, 196, 198; testing without treatment, 123, 177

homo sacer, 56

homosexuality, 13, 28, 30, 119, 132–33; associated with anal sex, 32–35, 37, 38, 45n88, 119–20; associated with HIV, 31–32, 133, 169n1; associated with development, 21, 28–29, 33, 34, 36–38; foreign and white, 29–30, 34, 36–38, 87, 133; Ivorian *milieu*, 30; social exclusion, 6, 97, 132, 134, 137; supposedly nonexistent in Africa, 30, 87, 132

Houphouët-Boigny, Félix, 8, 14, 20, 34–35, 50, 60, 78; austerity measures, 20, 34–35, 94; the Baoulé, 60n48, 167, 183, 191; and colonial mode of governance, 8, 34; co-opts dissent via media, 94; "Days of Dialogue," 53, 61, 78; death of, 94, 101, 122, 137, 150, 181, 191; development and progress, 49, 98, 181; father of the nation, 76, 122; and *How's it going?*, 65–6, 76, 94; and Ivorian ethnic groups, 166; and monogamy, 98–100, 190; *Moussa* and, 21–22, 34–35, 49; and paternalistic state, 4, 8, 14, 19–21, 27, 35, 49, 60, 64, 76, 94, 98, 122; strategies to retain power, 19, 21–22, 61n53, 62, 94; tolerance of satire, 53, 65, 93n120, 94; weakening power, 10, 20, 50, 94

How's it going?, 51, 53, 63, 65–66, 68–71, 73–74, 78–79, 81–83, 94; AIDS as invented, 83; "AIDS: The Illness of the

Century" episode, 15, 50, 67–69, 74–78; comic males defy HIV warnings, 51, 68, 70; and condoms, 68–69, 71, 81–82; female satiric targets, 51, 75, 82; "Joke to Kill" episode, 15, 77–83; male control of female sexuality, 79, 81–82; punitive moralism in, 69–70, 72, 75; sexual and economic austerity, 50, 73–74, 78

Hunt, Nancy Rose, 199

hygiene, 8, 135n69; discourse of, 40; hygienic interventions, 150; unhygienic conditions, 65

IMF (International Monetary Fund), 19–20, 35, 122, 151

India, 97, 143

infidelity, 51, 68, 75n96, 81, 84, 96, 128, 131–32, 96; "second office," 68, 74. *See also* fidelity

Ivoire Dimanche, 18n2, 42, 67, 73–75, 93n120; on abortion, 108–9, 129n62; on AIDS, 32, 40, 43–46, 169n174; effects of structural adjustment on the poor, 27; on *How's it going?*, 65–66, 74–75; interviews Léonard Groguhet, 52, 65–66; and *Right to Health* HIV/AIDS message, 40; on *Wintin Wintin and Old Headscarf*, 53, 85

Ivoirité: Bedié and, 107n27, 122–23, 191; disqualifies Ouattara, 123, 129n64; ethnonationalist claims, 6, 123; Muslim Northerners as foreign, 123n56, 167; stigmatization of foreigners and immigrants, 123, 128; vs. Houphouët-Boigny's rhetoric of unity and inclusion, 123

Ivoir'Soir, 22n15

Jenkins, Janet, 63

Jeune Afrique, 42, 121n52, 174n10

Johns Hopkins University, 48n95, 135n69, 143

jokes: about AIDS, 47, 49–50, 79; "AIDS: Imaginary Syndrome to Discourage Lovers," 32–33, 45, 46, 48, 83–85; AIDS not a joke, 33, 46–47, 49, 67, 83; and fear of AIDS, 80–84; Freud and jokes as male sexual aggression, 83–84; puns, 32, 33, 36, 48n94, 81n105, 83, 85, 87, 121, 194; and serious message, 24n23

Kakou, Odehouri, 69
Kalipeni, Ezekiel, 145
Kankan, Jean-Michel, 25, 93

Kassy, Roger Fulence (R. F. K.), 66n77, 67; Alpha Blondy on, 67n81

Koly, Souleymane, 52

Koné, Hugues, 63

Koné, Maïmouna, 177

Koné, S. Samba, 42, 173n9

koteba performance, 15; gendered targets of, 51–52; in health education, 52; *How's it going*, 51; in Mali, 51–52; *Wintin Wintin and Old Headscarf*, 51

Koteba Theater, 52

languages of Côte d'Ivoire: Attié, 85; Baoulé, 65, 85, 191; Dioula, 41n76, 102, 152; French speakers vs. non-speakers, 64; French the official language, 8, 24, 64; indigenous languages, 8, 22, 64; Malinké, 152–53, 181, 199n40, 200; Popular Ivorian French, (FPI), 14, 23, 52; "Moussa's French," 14, 23, 23n21, 24, 36, 52; *nouchi*, 14, 23, 33, 44n86, 52, 52n8, 85; Popular French of Abidjan (FPA), 14, 23, 23n21; pidgins, 23; untranslatable puns and idiomatic FPI, 31, 36, 41n76, 43n84, 44n86, 81n105, 88, 92. *See also* PETV

laws of Côte d'Ivoire: on abortion, 104–8; citizenship, 206–7; Civil Code, 98–99; the new Constitution, 206–7; conjugal family, 98; customary law (statut coutumier), 98, 126; French law (statut civil français), 98; and Napoleonic Penal Code, 106

Larkin, Brian, 80; aesthetics of outrage, 144; on melodrama, 141n11, 155

Lebry, Léon Francis, 27nn35–36, 44n87, 45, 74–75, 159n53, 169n1

Le Pape, Marc, 30

MacLean, Lauren M., 97

Mady, Alphonse Djédjé, 39–43, 45

Maï La Bombe. *See* Koné, Maïmouna

marriage, 12, 87, 74, 98–99, 140, 166, 183, 196, 204; citizenship through, 206–7; class and generational conflict over, 159–61, 183; companionate, 5, 140, 157, 159, 204; divorce, 98n7; ethnic intermixing, 166, 191; and HIV-infected partners, 115, 161, 163; monogamous reproductivity, 5, 16, 138, 140, 159–60, 166–67, 173, 183, 197, 207; and national reunification, 140, 207; as redemption for sex-workers, 170–73,

183–84, 195; telenovela marriage plot, 167; testing before, 157–59, 161; vs. "politics of the belly," 172–73, 178, 182–83; *See also* family; monogamy; patriarchy; polygamy

M'Bala, Roger Gnoan, 77

Mbembe, Achille, 1, 22, 37; on Gramsci and Bakhtin, 24–6; on postcolonial entanglements, 1–2

melodrama, 153–55, 157: and aesthetics of outrage, 144; and *AIDS in the City*, 143–63; feminist scholarship on, 141–42; Hollywood cinematic vocabulary, 140–41, 160, 164–65; the melodramatic mode, 139–41, 143, 163–64, 168, 185; and moral legibility, 139, 165; and representations of suffering, 80, 144; social marketing of prevention, 138–68; in the telenovela, 16, 121, 140–41, 165, 189; visual conventions of, 159–61, 164

men, 38, 43, 75: comedic triumph over female sexual partner, 51, 94; defying HIV prevention messages, 15, 50–51, 92; heterosexual masculinity, 38, 44, 76–77, 92; infidelity of, 68, 75n96, 80–81, 99; jokes and misogynistic aggression, 84; lacking sexual self-control, 72, 74, 77, 179; male prostitution, 36, 37, 38n67, 172

Mianhoro, Joseph, 23

migration and immigration, 8, 19, 41, 78, 107n27, 151, 181, 205: immigration, prostitution, and disease, 41, 169; rural-to-urban, 41, 66, 184, 198; trigger for epidemic, 205

military coups, 129n64, 150, 201

Miremont, Auguste, 22–23, 53

Modeleski, Tanya, 140

modernity: 2, 64, 97, 159, 185; in Abidjan, 21, 28, 36, 49, 55n22, 185; and biopolitics, 5, 109; and development, 21, 49; HIV and 14, 19, 169; *Moussa* on, 21–22, 23n21, 28, 36–37; as narrative of development and progress, 36–38, 108–9, 190; and national identity, 49, 64; and prostitution, 169; television and, 55, 64; and tradition, 153; white, 14, 19, 21–22, 36–37

Molière, 32, 93

monogamy, 97–99, 137, 190: and capitalist modernity, 97–99, 157, 190–91; gender subordination, 99, 133; and heterosexual reproductivity, 100, 153, 157, 168, 197; nation-building, 100, 140, 153; prevention media and, 5, 11–12, 72, 133, 140, 170, 190–91, 201–2

Monsieur Zézé, 44n86

Moussa, 14, 23–27, 32–33, 36, 38, 41, 43–44; on AIDS as foreign or imaginary, 28–29, 33–34, 83; anxiety about, 28; and condom usage, 39–41, 43; contained dissent, 19, 34; disputes AIDS origin accounts, 39; and elites' view of the poor, 23, 27; and foreign funders' policies, 27, 35, 38; as Guignol, 24–25; on HIV/AIDS crisis, 19, 32–33, 39, 43; on Houphouët-Boigny, 19, 21, 22, 25, 35; laughter ratifying state domination, 25–26, 35; moralistic approach to HIV/AIDS prevention, 49, 72; *Moussa the Taxi Driver* (films), 23n21; "Moussa's French," 23–24, 36; as naïve, childlike villager in big city, 21, 26, 28; on prostitution, 36–39, 41; on racialized and sexual definitions of Africa and AIDS, 14, 19, 32–33; satirizes AIDS education, 31, 33; on self-discipline, 14, 21, 49; on sexual and economic austerity, 14, 22, 28, 33–36, 38, 49; vulgar humor in, 14, 25–27, 33, 41; white modernity and corruption, 21–22, 35–36

Moussa, Alfred Dan, 26–27

music in prevention media: *AIDS in the City*, 127, 147–48, 166; *Gestures or Life*, 102; *Princess Street*, 181–82; RAP-MC's condom-promotion song, 86n114; Waby Spider's "AIDS," 67

Muslims: Dioula, 167, 192; excluded from Ivorian society, 6, 27, 123, 123n56, 167n63, 183, 191–92; the good Muslim wife, 118; Moussa as Muslim Northerner, 23n21, 27; Muslim/Christian contrasts, 102; representing "tradition," 156

My Family, 143

Ndijio, Basile, 62

Ndo, Daniel, 25, 25n26

Neba, Bienvenu, 184, 191

neocolonialism and neoimperialism, 20, 60n48, 204

neoliberalism, 2–3, 16, 20, 111n41, 149, 150n44, 179, 199; approaches to HIV/AIDS, 8, 11, 16, 95; globalization, 111n41, 149n40; individual responsibility, 22, 95, 149; privatization, 20, 149; technologies of domination, 141. *See also* privatization; structural adjustment

Newell, Sasha, 24, 86
NGOs, 17; depicted in prevention media, 130, 135–36, 157, 160, 168; limitations imposed on, 121–22; reliance on, 95, 161–75; and social marketing of behavior change, 149, 168; source of HIV/AIDs testing, treatment, and care, 100, 138, 168; source of information, 12, 45, 95; submission to, 96, 137
Nguyen, Vinh-Kim, 11, 20n6, 30, 180, 199; on biomedical interventions, 112n45, 205; confessional technologies, 199; on controlling HIV/AIDS epidemic, 175, 205
Niang, Abdoulaye, 23
Nollywood videos, 80, 141n11, 144, 185
nouchi, 14, 33, 44n86, 53, 85. See also *Moussa*
Nuttall, Sarah, 6

Okagbue, Osita, 52
Okome, Onookome, 185
"Old Headscarf." *See* Assamoi, Léon N'Cho
O'Manique, Colleen, 5n13, 11, 111n41, 145n26
Oscar (Malian performer), 38
Our Health, 42, 68
Ouattara, Alassane, 122–23, 206; possibly Burkinabé, 123, 129n64, 206; struggles for presidency, 122, 129n64, 206. *See also* Ivoirité

Patton, Cindy, 21, 132n66, 146n31
patriarchal authority, 76, 84, 119, 171, 179; enlightened and benevolent, 189, 192; in the family, 16, 96, 100, 136–37, 140, 149, 157, 172, 189–90, 202; and heteronormativity, 133, 140; Houphouët-Boigny and, 4, 8, 14, 19–21, 27, 35, 49, 60, 64, 76, 94, 98, 122; and "traditional" leadership, 37, 190, 192
PDCI (Parti democratique de la Côte d'Ivoire), 19, 23, 167; single-party rule, 4, 7, 8, 10, 19, 21, 22, 25, 35, 53, 61–62. *See also* Houphouët-Boigny
PEPFAR (U.S. President's Emergency Plan for AIDS Relief), 4, 12, 20, 171–72, 192n34, 196, 203–5; and neoliberal policies, 204, 205n5; on prostitution, 16, 171–72, 202
Pérez, Hiram, 141
perinatal transmission, 15, 95–96, 100–105, 122; and abortion, 15, 100, 100n15, 110, 122, 134, 158; *See also* "Fatoumata: HIV-Positive Mother"
personal responsibility and self-control, 4, 16, 22, 40, 95, 101, 139, 168, 170; and neoliberalism, 3, 14, 149
PETV (Le Programme d'éducation télévisuelle), 8, 53, 58–63, 79; demise of, 59–60, 64; and foreign funders, 53, 55, 57, 61; mission, 54, 59n40; as nation-building instrument, 57, 59
Pfeiffer, James, 146, 205n5
PMI (Centres de protection maternelle et infantile), 109, 135
PNLS (Programme National de Lutte contre le Sida), 45, 45n90, 78, 174, 175; foreign funders, 77; Medium-Term Plan, 46; Short-Term Plan, 46n90, 175
"politics of the belly" ("la politique du ventre"): alternatives to, 182–3; Bayart on, 178–79; and "big men," 179–80; gendered, 179, 179n19, 182–83; independence from, 178, 180; poverty and sex work, 172, 179, 182–83
polygamy, 98, 100, 118, 170; coded as "traditional," 139, 156, 170, 190; and French colonial government, 98, 190, 170; Houphouët-Boigny and, 98–99, 139; Muslims and, 117–18, 156, 170, 173, 190; prevention media and, 117–18, 156, 170, 173, 184, 188, 190; as risk factor, 139, 184, 188; and state-sanctioned monogamy, 190
population, 15, 107n27, 109
postcolonial dynamics, 4, 11, 106–8, 113: "entanglement," 2, 4, 6, 25; educational programming, 4, 6; female reproductivity and national identity, 107–9
poverty, 111, 122, 151; feminization of, 150n44; increases in, 151, 179; and structural adjustment, 136, 179
PPP (Projet de Prévention et de Prise en charge des femmes libres et leurs Partenaires), 177
Price, Neil, 148
Princess Street, 173, 175, 179, 183, 201; condoms and HIV prevention, 173, 175, 177–79; foreign funders, 16, 170, 170n4; marriage, love, and art alternatives to sex work, 172–73, 182, 184; prevention carried out by sex workers, 172, 178
privatization: 3, 20, 61, 149

prostitution, 36–38, 43, 169, 171, 179; foreign funders and, 171–72; high-risk sexual partners, 40–1, 169n1; HIV associated with, 133, 169; male, 36–37, 172; social exclusion of sex-workers, 16, 97, 132–33, 137, 182–83; trans, 37–38, 172; as white innovation, 36–38; and white modernity, 21, 36; "whores" (les putes), 37, 123, 133, 195. *See also* sex workers

Proteau, Laurence, 62–63

Prudence condoms, 148–49, 151, 153–54: and *AIDS in the City,* 121n52, 148–49, 153, 184–92; Alpha Blondy sings about, 148; and *Amah Djah-Foulé,* 193–4; and *Gestures or Life,* 114, 115; and *Princess Street,* 175–76

PSI (Population Services International), 128, 148; and *AIDS in the City,* 10–11, 16, 120, 137, 147; and AIMAS (Ivorian Agency of Social Marketing), 147, 149, 193n35; and *Amah Djah-Foulé,* 192–93; foreign funders, 16, 120–22, 137, 150, 170; and social marketing of family planning, 146, 152, 175; and Prudence condoms, 121n52, 148–49, 153–55, 175–76; videos and telenovelas, 96, 128, 169–70, 184, 193

public health, 118, 112n45, 122; and behavior change, 5, 10, 30, 42, 48, 48n95, 77n8, 144–45, 205; individual responsibility for, 42, 138, 168; social marketing of, 165, 168

queer theory, 11, 12n3

Radio-Télé-Bac, 55

RDR (Rassemblement des Républicains), 123, 199n40

Red Ribbon, 88

reproduction, 98, 109n34, 136, 153, 156; female reproductivity and family, 100; HIV-positive women and reproduction, 132, 156; normative gender roles and, 130, 136; omen reduced to reproductive life, 108, 130

RETRO-CI (Projet Rétrovirus de Côte d'Ivoire), 147, 192–93

Right to Health (*Droit à la santé*), 40

RTI (Radiodiffusion Télévision Ivoirienne), 52–54, 64n72, 147

Sabido, Miguel, 142–43

satire, 50, 53, 93; entangled with state, 53, 92–93

Seropositive People, The (*Les Séropositifs*), 184

sexual activities: anal sex, 32–35, 37, 38, 45n88, 119–20; commodification of, 86; cross-dressing, 37; female same-sex relations, 31; inadequate self-discipline, 41; limiting, 40; male same-sex relations, 31, 119; pornography, 183; and reproduction, 96, 98n7; "second offices," 74–75, 119; sexual networks (multiple partners), 80n103

sexualities: colonial stereotype of African sexuality, 132; containing female sexuality and reproduction, 100, 188; degradation of elite male status, 74; gendered normativities, 2, 11; identitarian, 29–31; racialized normativity, 11, 29, 33; restraint as sanitation, 40

sex workers, 42, 133, 151, 171–72, 190, 193, 195–97, 201–2; condom and lubricant usage among, 170, 172–78, 192–94, debates concerning, 171, 192, 201; economic marginalization, 170, 196; educating, 192, 194, 195, 199, 201; exclusion of, 6, 133, 168; and foreign funders' mandates, 10, 171; HIV associated with, 169, 190; and marriage, 182, 194–95; prevention carried out by, 172; prevention media and, 16–17, 119, 169–202; redemption of, 170, 195; renunciation of sex work, 196–99, 201; and stable partners, 192–93, 198; stigmatization of, 178, 193, 195, 198; trafficking and sexual slavery, 171–73; women's access to income, 179, 196–97

SFPS (Sante Famille et Prevention du SIDA), 147

Singer, Linda, 111, 114

Smith, Chris, 171

soap operas, 140, 142–44, 168

social marketing, 16, 139, 141, 146–50; HIV/AIDS prevention as commodity, 148; and melodrama, 139, 141. *See also* Prudence condoms

Sow, Alioune, 52

spectatorship: 9, 140

Spivak, Gayatri Chakravorty, 87

state sovereignty, 26, 56

Stepan, Jan, 108

sterility: abortion leading to, 129; fears of, 129, 166; grounds for divorce, 98n7; and

STDs, 155; sterilization prohibited, 106–8; vs. reproductivity, 129, 160, 166
Stillwaggon, Eileen, 145
"The Story of the Fiancés," 139–41, 157–59, 161, 166–67, 188; acceptance of HIV status, 139; against abortion, 158–59; class, ethnic, and generational conflict, 157, 159, 160, 162, 166; HIV-discordant couple, 157, 159, 161–63, 167; living with HIV in heteronormative family, 161–63, 166; melodrama, 16, 159, 162; telenovela happy endings, 165–66
structural adjustment and austerity, 60n50, 150; affecting prevention campaigns, 21–22, 136, 150–51, 177, 179; civil service cuts, 73, 101; ; cuts in health-care spending, 101, 106n27, 151, 175, 205; failures of, 151; foreign funders' mandates, 4, 20, 111, 133, 150–51; impact children, women, and the poor, 27, 60n50, 111nn40–41, 150, 179; and neoliberal ideology, 14, 19–20, 199and the World Bank, 19–20, 151
subalternity, 26, 97
Super Girl (Super Go), 1, 3, 203–4, 205n6; empowering girls with HIV education, 205–6; foreign funders, 204
Sweetheart, 178
SYNARES (Syndicat national de l'enseignement supérieur), 60
SYNESCI (Syndicat national des enseignants de secondaire de Côte d'Ivoire), and PETV, 60–62

Tchelley, Hanny Brigitte, 128, 138, 147
telenovela, 16, 96, 120–21, 140–45, 157, 165, 167–68, 189; *AIDS and the City 3* as, 143–45; and HIV prevention, 145, 154, 168, 189; and public education, 142–44
Thomas, Lynn M., 179n19
Tiacoh, Gabriel, 46–47
Tiébé, Alain Djédjé (also known as Mousso Dousso and Pierre Wintin Wintin), 51, 85n113
Tomkins, Silvan, 80
Toungara, Jeanne, 19n3, 60n48, 62, 98–99, 190
Touré, Kitia, 15, 117, 119; and *Gestures or Life,* 96, 101, 119
traditional culture: leadership, 37, 190, 192; marabouts (fetishers), 170, 182–83, 188; traditional medicine, 44, 129, 131, 135–36, 170, 187–88, witchcraft, 188, 191. *See also* polygamy
transvestites, 21, 37–38
Treichler, Paula, 2
TRIPS (Trade-Related Aspects of International Property Rights), 112n45; blocks purchase or making patented antiretrovirals, 151

UNAIDS (Joint United Nations Programme on HIV/AIDS), 12, 30, 147, 159, 193; Drug Access Initiative, 112n44; and international property rights (TRIPS), 112n45; and PETV, 55; pressuring abortion for HIV-positive women violates human rights, 128
Uncle Otsama. *See* Ndo, Daniel
UNDP (United Nations Development Program), 57n29, 112n45
UNESCO, 55, 57, 85n114, 150n44
UNICEF, 55, 111n40, 124, 193
United Nations, 2, 111n41, 122, 128
U.S. (United States), 45, 112, 140n25, 172, 204; Bush, George W., 121–22, 171, 204; CDC (Centers for Disease Control), 29, 103, 147, 172, 198; Helms Amendment, 121; Mexico City policy (Global Gag Rule), 122, 204; Obama, Barack, 204; Reagan, Ronald, 18n1, 122; Trump, Donald, 204
Université nationale de Côte d'Ivoire, 12
USAID (United States Agency for International Development), 16, 45, 48n95, 145; funds PSI, 16, 445, 121n52, 150; and PETV, 55, 57n29

Vaughan, Megan, 29n40, 97
Vidal, Claudine, 30
Vidal, Laurent, 39, 140n5
Videau, André, 176

Waby Spider, 67
Wardlow, Holly, 159
Watney, Simon, 97
West Germany, 57n29
WHO, 18, 45, 78, 101, 112, 122, 129, 135n70, 174–75
Who's doing that?, 143
Williams, Linda, 140–41, 165

Wintin Wintin and Old Headscarf, 51, 84–85, 91; "500 CFA If You Don't Come" skit, 15, 51, 85–92; comic male protagonists defy HIV warnings, 51, 85–87, 91; and confusion about HIV prevention, 9–12; monkey figuring mischief and trickery, 86, 88; Wintin Wintin misunderstands "socks," 86–89

Wintin Wintin, Pierre. *See* Tiébé, Alain Djédjé

witchcraft: in *Amoin Séry*, 184, 187–88; as attempt to understand suffering, 188; HIV not transmitted by, 155, 188; practices harmful to women, 170; and female sexuality, 188

women, 3, 12, 44, 51, 75–76, 94, 96, 113, 140, 170; and abortion, 95–96, 109–11; and condom usage, 68–69, 76, 89, 96, 114, 124; control heterosexual exchanges, 77, 85, 86–90, 92, 124; feminization of poverty, 150; HIV-positive, 12, 15–16, 114, 116, 199; HIV-positive and pregnant, 15, 95–96, 100–5, 110, 112, 116, 122; management of women's reproduction, 95–96, 118; menstruation, 119, 155; and patriarchal authority, 76, 96, 105, 137, 149; promiscuity of, 81, 84, 131–33, 185, 188; redemption by romance, 114–16; regulation of reproductive capacity, 97, 113, 137; same-sex relations, 31, 87; "second office," 68, 74; support networks, 199–200; targets of satire, 51–52, 75; unable to convince men of need for prevention, 51, 86–89

Woods, Dwayne, 61

World AIDS day, 175, 193

World Bank, 144–45, 151, 155; mandated cuts in public spending, 74, 150; neoliberal economic restructuring, 19–20, 35, 74, 151; and PETV, 55, 56n24, 57n29, 63. *See also* neoliberalism; structural adjustment and austerity

WTO, 112n45, 151

Yéo, Souleymane Ouattara, 75n96

Zaouru, Zadi, 52
zidovudine. *See* AZT
Zigré, Alexis Don, 147, 166n59

www.ingramcontent.com/pod-product-compliance
Lightning Source LLC
Chambersburg PA
CBHW030134240426
43672CB00005B/125